AF755034

STEM CELLS - LABORATORY AND CLINICAL RESEARCH

STEM CELLS IN DISEASE

STEM CELLS - LABORATORY AND CLINICAL RESEARCH

Additional books in this series can be found on Nova's website under the Series tab.

Additional e-books in this series can be found on Nova's website under the e-books tab.

STEM CELLS - LABORATORY AND CLINICAL RESEARCH

STEM CELLS IN DISEASE

PRASAD S. KOKA
EDITOR

New York

Copyright © 2012 by Nova Science Publishers, Inc.

All rights reserved. No part of this book may be reproduced, stored in a retrieval system or transmitted in any form or by any means: electronic, electrostatic, magnetic, tape, mechanical photocopying, recording or otherwise without the written permission of the Publisher.

For permission to use material from this book please contact us:
Telephone 631-231-7269; Fax 631-231-8175
Web Site: http://www.novapublishers.com

NOTICE TO THE READER

The Publisher has taken reasonable care in the preparation of this book, but makes no expressed or implied warranty of any kind and assumes no responsibility for any errors or omissions. No liability is assumed for incidental or consequential damages in connection with or arising out of information contained in this book. The Publisher shall not be liable for any special, consequential, or exemplary damages resulting, in whole or in part, from the readers' use of, or reliance upon, this material. Any parts of this book based on government reports are so indicated and copyright is claimed for those parts to the extent applicable to compilations of such works.

Independent verification should be sought for any data, advice or recommendations contained in this book. In addition, no responsibility is assumed by the publisher for any injury and/or damage to persons or property arising from any methods, products, instructions, ideas or otherwise contained in this publication.

This publication is designed to provide accurate and authoritative information with regard to the subject matter covered herein. It is sold with the clear understanding that the Publisher is not engaged in rendering legal or any other professional services. If legal or any other expert assistance is required, the services of a competent person should be sought. FROM A DECLARATION OF PARTICIPANTS JOINTLY ADOPTED BY A COMMITTEE OF THE AMERICAN BAR ASSOCIATION AND A COMMITTEE OF PUBLISHERS.

Additional color graphics may be available in the e-book version of this book.

Library of Congress Cataloging-in-Publication Data

ISBN: 978-1-62257-169-7

Published by Nova Science Publishers, Inc. † New York

Contents

Preface

Totipotent embryonic stem cells (ESC) differentiate into different pluripotent stem cells such as of the hematopoietic lineage that home to bone marrow, liver, and fetal adnexa (placenta: mesenchymal stem cells, trophoblasts, mesenchymal amnionic and chorionic membrane, and amniotic fluid-umbilical cord); mesenchymal lineage that are directed to bone marrow and placenta. It has been reported in this book that even the brain glial lineage contain mesenchymal stem cell (MSC) like features which generates evidence for the presence or differentiation into MSC of the ESC in brain and potentially implicate the neural stem cells in the admixture or involvement of MSC.

It is for the first time that experimentally induced generation and isolation of cancer stem cells (CSC) but with the fusion of hematopoietic stem cells (HSC) in vivo, is contained as content in this book. This methodology can be extended to the use of stem cells of totipotent, pluripotent and even multipotent lineages.That the CSC have been induced in the absence of various cellular components makes this a unique method of generation of CSC that can also apply besides HSC, to CSCs of other ESC derived cells such as the ESCs themselves, or the neural stem cells (NSC), cardiomyocytes, etc. Such CSCs can be used to study the mechanisms of malignancies (eg. myelodysplasticity in the case of CSC generated with HSC) and the efficacy of potential therapies for various cancers, since the "stemness" in the CSCs is expected to be lacking in the at least "pure" cancer cells and thus the susceptibility to various cancer antigen marker therapies may prove to be differential. If a cancer drug is not discriminative between a CSC and its cancer origin cell then such a drug may either be specific to the stem cell marker antigen, or eliminate cancer cells in totality.

The reported formation of intracranial tumors by human brain derived stem-like cells in immunocompetent rats may be suggestive of the inability of the immune cells of the species to cross the blood brain barrier. However the mesenchymal stem cell features of the glioblastoma cells may potentially make these glial cells more plastic and attribute these cells with aggressive proliferative capability.

Hematopoietic stem cells and their visualization using the dorsal skinfold chamber model is another important feature content of this book. Whereas the any other stem cells are no less important in the species biology, the HSC are involved in immunity and constantly fight infections. A point of significance that is to be noted herein is that the induced lineage directed differentiation of ESCs is extremely useful to study their mechanisms of further differentiation and experimental evaluations. For example, the hepatocytes induced to be derived from ESCs have significant applications to toxicological assessments in vitro and even the culturing of hepatitis c virus for its virology and development of therapies. Similarly, the HSCs that can be made to be differentiated using hyaluronan as reported herein in this book are extremely useful in basic and clinical experimental science such as the studies on their differentiation mechanisms, reconstitution, and autologous and allogeneic genetically engineered bone marrow transplantation.

In summary, this is a book that consists of some important and novel reports that the stem cell scientific community should further undertake without any bias that this *Journal of Stem Cells* is one of lower impact factor. In fact, it is the responsibility of this scientific community to note that only those of high profile institutionally projected journals to generate high impact factors which feed in a biased commercially oriented advantageous cycle of directed publications and citation indices are a retardation of scientific development even as we have advanced into the 21st century.

In: Stem Cells in Disease
Editor: Prasad S. Koka
ISBN: 978-1-62257-169-7
© 2012 Nova Science Publishers, Inc.

Chapter I

Induction Characterization and Targeting of Human Hematopoietic Cancer Stem Cells

***Menghua Zhang*[1], *Peter Dias*[1], *Boris Minev*[2*] and *Prasad S. Koka*[1,#]**
[1] Laboratory of Stem Cell Biology,
Torrey Pines Institute for Molecular Studies, San Diego, California, US
[2] Moores UCSD Cancer Center, UCSD Division of Neurosurgery,
University of California, San Diego, La Jolla, California, US

Abstract

Tumors contain a minority population of cancer stem cells (CSC) that maintain the tumor. In marked contrast to the CSC, the tumor cells have either no capacity or a markedly diminished capacity, to form new tumors. Therefore, to treat cancer effectively, the CSC must be eliminated. The tumor will rapidly recur if the therapy eliminates cancer cells but spares a significant population of the cancer stem cells.

We report here for the first time the utilization of the SCID-hu Thy/Liv chimeric small animal model system for induction of human cancer stem cells and their early detection. This model system allows long-term systemic human T-cell reconstitution in vivo, and also provides both human antigen-presenting cells (APCs) and effector cells for induction of anti-tumor immune responses. We were able to generate human hematopoietic cancer stem cells (HCSC) using the SCID-hu Thy/Liv system, and confirmed the expression of both the CD34 marker and two human tumor antigens in these cells. Importantly, we observed an enhanced expression of several embryonic stem cell markers in the HCSC, as well as morphological appearance typical for

[*] Corresponding Author: Boris Minev, MD; Email bminev@ucsd.edu, Moores UCSD Cancer Center, UCSD Division of Neurosurgery, University of California, San Diego, 3855 Health Sciences Drive, La Jolla, California 92093, US

[#] Corresponding Author: Prasad S Koka, PhD. Email pkoka@tpims.org, Laboratory of Stem Cell Biology, Torrey Pines Institute for Molecular Studies, 3550 General Atomics Court, San Diego, California 92121, US; Current address to which correspondence should be addressed: Poornaprajna Institute of Scientific Research, Bidalur Post, Devanahalli, Bangalore, India. Email: prasad.koka@poornaprajna.org.

undifferentiated cells, suggesting the acquisition of highly malignant aggressive properties. Therefore, these findings are an important step in our understanding of the mechanisms involved in the early formation of the cancer stem cells, and in demonstrating the stem cell origin of cancer.

Keywords: SCID-hu, human hematopoietic organ, cancer stem cells

In many tissues, a cellular hierarchy exists in which a small population of stem cells is responsible for the production of the mature cells of the organ. The stem cells maintain themselves through a process known as self-renewal. Similarly, tumors contain a minority population of cancer stem cells (CSC) that maintain the tumor [1]. The CSC can give rise to both more CSC as well as cancer cells without the “stemness”. In marked contrast to the CSC, these latter cells have either no capacity or a markedly diminished capacity, to form new tumors. Therefore, to treat cancer effectively, the CSC must be eliminated. The tumor will rapidly recur if the therapy eliminates cancer cells but spares a significant population of the cancer stem cells.

Self-renewal of embryonic or the further differentiated pluripotent stem cells consists of two events: (a) Formation of a new stem cell and (b) formation of a progenitor cell that can undergo proliferation and differentiation but not further self-renewal [1]. Abnormal regulation of normal self-renewal leads to leukemia (blood cancer) or other types of cancer [2]. In malignancies, unregulated self-renewal is the cause of uncontrolled proliferation of cells. It is hypothesized that there exist in vivo a few cancer stem cells that cause de novo proliferation even in the presence of therapies that target and kill most of the existing cancer cells [1].

In order to demonstrate a stem cell origin of cancer, we will need to understand the early formation of CSCs. Mutations in the genes that cause self-renewal like STAT5A, and those involved in multilineage CD34+ progenitor stem cell differentiation such as c-mpl [3], may be inducers of CSC. Mutations in JAK2 and c-mpl induce myeloproliferative disorders [4]. A metastasis model of human prostate cancer in NOD/SCID-hu mice has been established [5]. Constitutive activation of STAT5 is associated with several leukemias, chromosomal aberrations, and the transformation of hematopoietic cells to cytokine independent growth [6].

The SCID-hu Thy/Liv chimeric small animal model system [7] appears to be ideally suited for induction of human cancer stem cells and their early detection. This model system consists of functional human hematopoietic organ that maintains hematopoiesis and allows the reconstitution of human CD34+ progenitor hematopoietic stem cells (HSC) in a fresh stromal microenvironment, or in the host circulatory system [7, 8]. A NOD/SCID-hu Thy/Liv system has been used to generate humanized immune responses *in vivo* utilizing the host vascular and cytokine physiology [8]. Importantly, this model system allows long-term systemic human T-cell reconstitution *in vivo*. The HLA-restricted immune responses utilize the human T-cells (CD8 and CD4), B cells, dendritic cells, monocytes and macrophages. Thus, this model provides both human antigen-presenting cells (APCs) and effector cells for induction of anti-tumor immune responses [8]. We have engrafted the human CD34 positive hematopoietic cancer stem cells (HCSC) and the CD34 negative cancer cells into the SCID-hu Thy/Liv [7] to determine if there is a greater degree of metastasis in mice injected with the HCSC compared to those injected with the original cancer cells lacking the CD34 hematopoietic stem cell phenotype.

Results

We have induced the human hematopoietic cancer stem cells (HCSC) by utilizing the small animal SCID-hu Thy/Liv model system in vivo.

SCID-hu Thy/Liv Model System. The HCSC were generated as shown in the schematic below.

A cell-cell fusion or endocytosis in the SCID-hu Thy/Liv implants between the injected mel-624 cancer cells and the human CD34+ cells of the implants may occur in the generation of HCSC. This may also include exchange of genetic material and/or metabolic cooperation due to the mel-624 and CD34+ cell to cell contact and interactions.

Engraftment of Mel-624 tumor cells in vivo. The Melanoma-624 cells [9, 10] were transferred by injection ($5x10^4$ cells in 100μl) into the Thy/Liv implants of SCID-hu mice. Ten days later, cells from the tumors that formed in the SCID-hu Thy/Liv implants were isolated and the human CD34+ cancer stem cells were purified by AutoMacs, according to manufacturer's protocol.

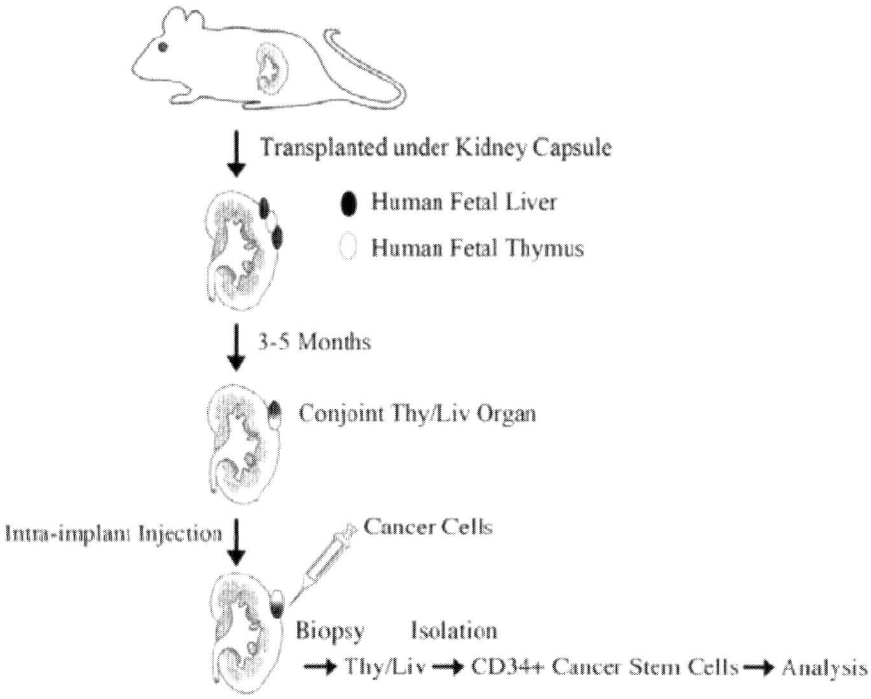

Figure 1. Schematic illustration of the construction and use of the SCID-hu Thy/Liv small animal model system. SCID mice received simultaneous transplants of 1-3 mm pieces of human fetal thymus and liver of 18-24 weeks gestation (Advanced Bioscience Resources, Alameda, CA) under the renal capsule and the resulting conjoint organ was allowed to grow for 3-5 months to generate a SCID-hu animal [7]. The tumor or cancer cells were injected into the Thy/Liv implants. CD34+ cells were isolated from these implants 3-5 weeks post-injection and the HCSC were derived as described below. These HCSC were initially cultured for 3-4 weeks in the presence of hematopoietic growth factors: IL-3, IL-6, GM-CSF and SCF. Thereafter the cells were maintained in culture in RPMI 1640 with 10% FBS.

Morphology of the induced hematopoietic cancer stem cells (HCSC) and its comparison with that of original melanoma-624 cancer cells. During the initial 7-10 days of culture of the mel-624 and HCSC following trypsinization and reseeding, the cells grow as monolayers (Figure 2).

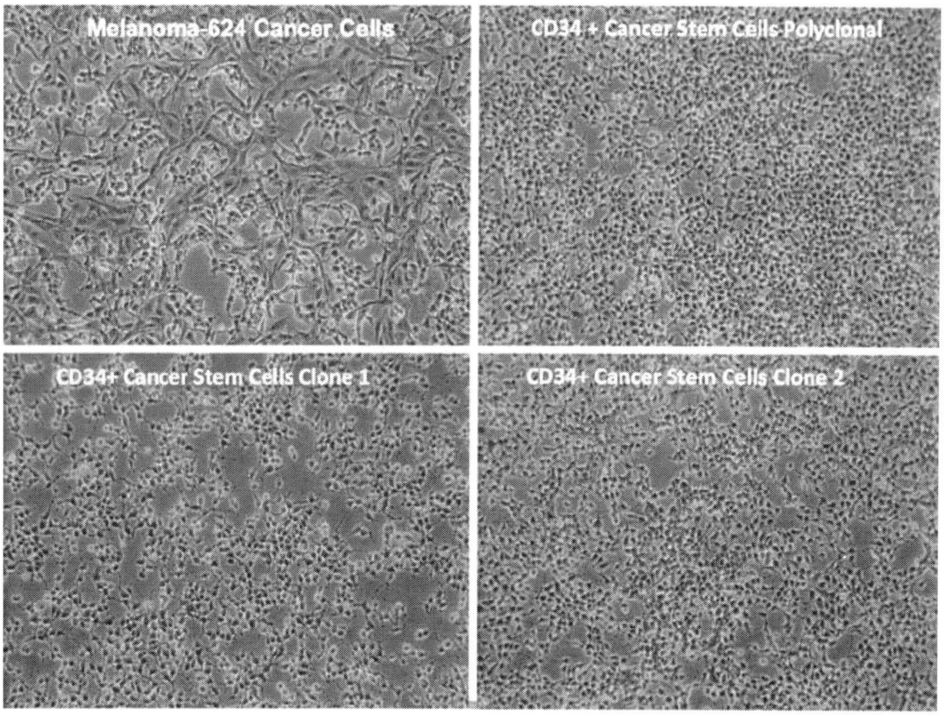

Figure 2. Morphology of the melanoma-624 cancer cells and the mel-624 induced and derived HCSC. The HCSC induced in vivo in the SCID-hu Thy/Liv implants are cultured in parallel (upper right and lower panels) with the original mel-624 cells (upper left panel). The upper right panel shows a polyclonal culture of the HCSC. This culture was cloned in 96-well plates by limiting dilution and HCSC clones 1 and 2 were derived in culture. Clones 1 and 2 are shown in the lower left and right panels, respectively.

The mel-624 cells maintain their fibroblast / strap cell-like morphology in which a large population of cells has a larger cytoplasm to nuclear ratio. In contrast, the HCSC showed smaller cytoplasm to nuclear ratio, with the cells exhibiting an undifferentiated appearance. This type of morphological change is frequently described in various carcinomas during epithelial to mesenchymal transition (EMT) that is associated with the acquisition of highly malignant aggressive properties of the tumors.

Formation of foci by human melanoma-624 cancer cells induced human CD34+ hematopoietic cancer stem cells. Similar to the normal benign primary CD34+ hematopoietic progenitor cells that form colonies in the semi-solid media of methylcellulose (myeloid, CFU-GM; and erythroid, BFU-E) and megacult-C (megakaryocytoid, CFU-MK) , the HCSC form colony-like foci after 7-10 days in culture in the liquid medium (Figure 3).

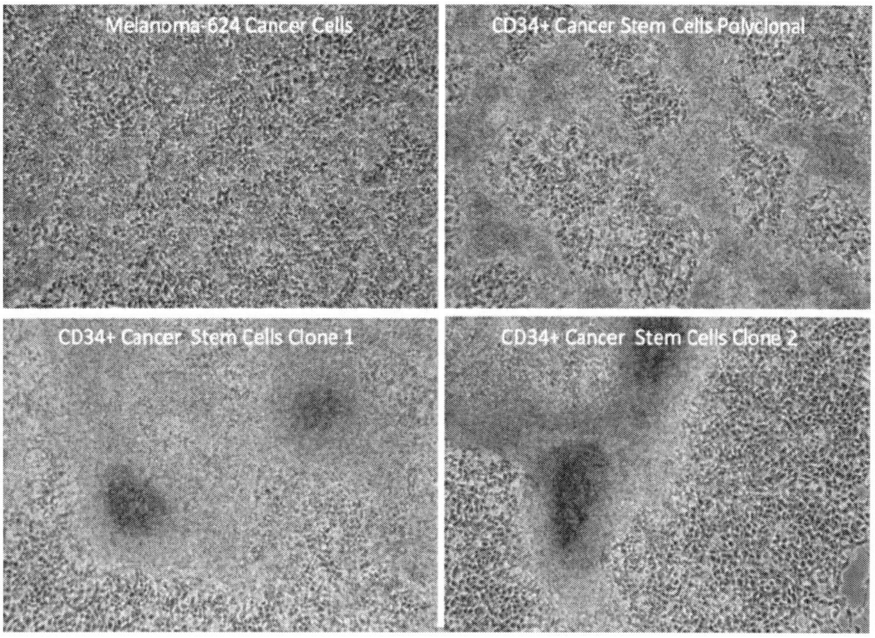

Figure 3. Formation of foci or multi-layered cellular aggregates by the CD34+ cancer stem cells in late cultures in anchorage independent liquid medium. The polyclonal culture was derived from tumors that formed in SCID-hu Thy/Liv implants after isolation by magnetic bead separation for CD34+ cells. This polyclonal culture developed numerous foci in culture. Two of these foci/colonies were carefully picked and each was cloned by limiting dilution in 96-well plate. A representative subclone from each cloning was expanded and used for further characterization (clones 1 and 2). The polyclonal culture and two clones derived from it exhibited similar morphological characteristics and growth properties.

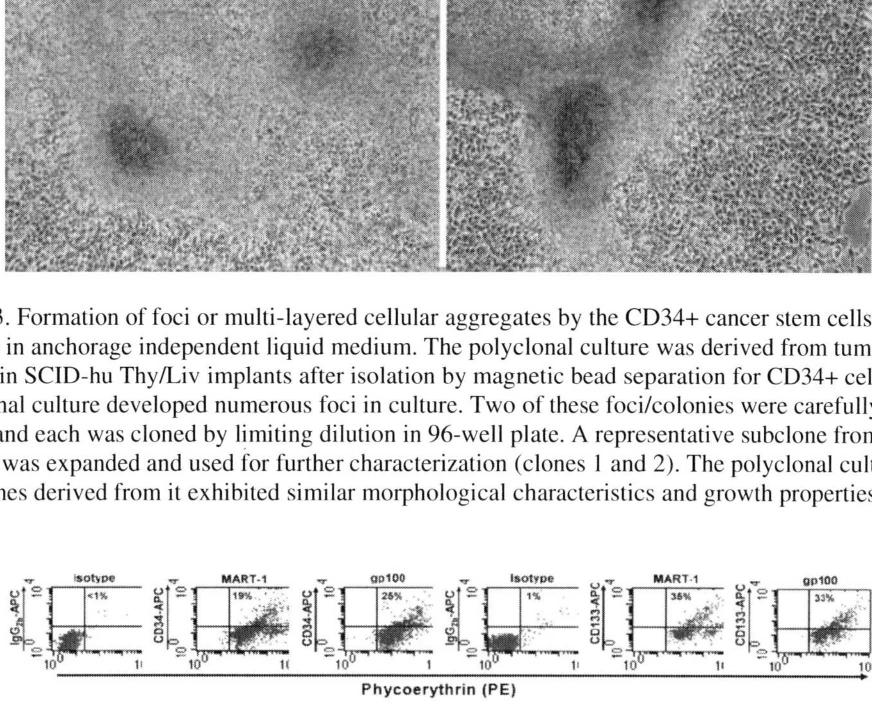

Figure 4. Induction of Melanoma-624 cancer stem cells in SCID-hu implants. Expression of the MART-1 and gp100 tumor antigens is induced in CD34+ hematopoietic progenitor stem cells, in vivo. The cells that were positive for expression of both tumor antigens and CD34 are shown in the upper right quadrants of the histograms. The percentages of expression of these tumor antigens by these cells are indicated within the FACS histograms. Staining with CD34 and CD133 was carried out by surface binding of the anti-CD34-FITC antibodies and MART-1 and gp100 antibodies conjugated with PE were used for staining of the tumor antigens. Isotype control staining is also shown. All the antibodies consist of the IgG2b isotype which is used to set the quadrants.

This is further support that the HCSC are in fact, generated as a result of direct contact, interactions, and/or fusion, of mel-624 cancer cells and primary CD34+ hematopoietic progenitor stem cells in the SCID-hu Thy/Liv implants in vivo. Normal primary CD34+ cells require semi-solid media, methylcellulose or megacult-C, for differentiation. They have a finite lifespan (generally 2 weeks) and do not form colonies in liquid media when grown in the presence of cytokines. The fact that our generated HCSC grow in liquid medium with colony-like foci formation is further evidence that these HCSC cells are of the CD34+ stem cell origin. The indefinite growth of these HCSC in anchorage independent liquid media also supports both the cancer and stem cell characteristics of these cells through expression of the melanoma tumor and the CD34+ antigens, respectively. Induction of melanoma tumor antigen expression in human CD34+ hematopoietic stem cells through cell-cell interaction in vivo. We have induced HCSCs using Mel-624 cancer cells (CD34-) in the benign human CD34+ cells of the SCID-hu implants through cell-cell contact in vivo. The putative fetal liver derived CD34+ hematopoitic stem cells of the SCID-hu implants expressed MART-1 and gp100 melanoma tumor antigens (Figure 4). The data suggest that we can use these melanoma tumor antigens to target the induced HCSC.

Immunohistochemistry of the HCSC compared to the original cancer cells was performed as follows. The cells were first grown in tissue culture flasks coated with collagen and then seeded in chamber slides. The HCSC in the beginning have a tendency to form monolayers like the original cells but they later form clusters on top of the monolayers. The CD34+ HCSC shown in Figure 5 are in fact, clusters of cells. Immunohistochemistry supports the staining patterns of the HCSC determined by FACS as well in Figure 3 thus indicating that these induced hematopoietic cancer stem cells express both melanoma tumor antigens and the CD34 marker of the progenitor stem cells. SOX17 is an important gene that is expressed in the early stages of embryonal development but loses its expression postnatally [11]. However, and our unpublished data show that upon injection of recombinant SOX17, high level of cellular proliferation is induced in certain hematopoietic tissues such as liver. Enhancement of SOX17 expression may be occurring in the HCSC clones due to cellular micro-environmental factors in the implants, or it may also be inherent in the primary CD34+ cells which will be evaluated.

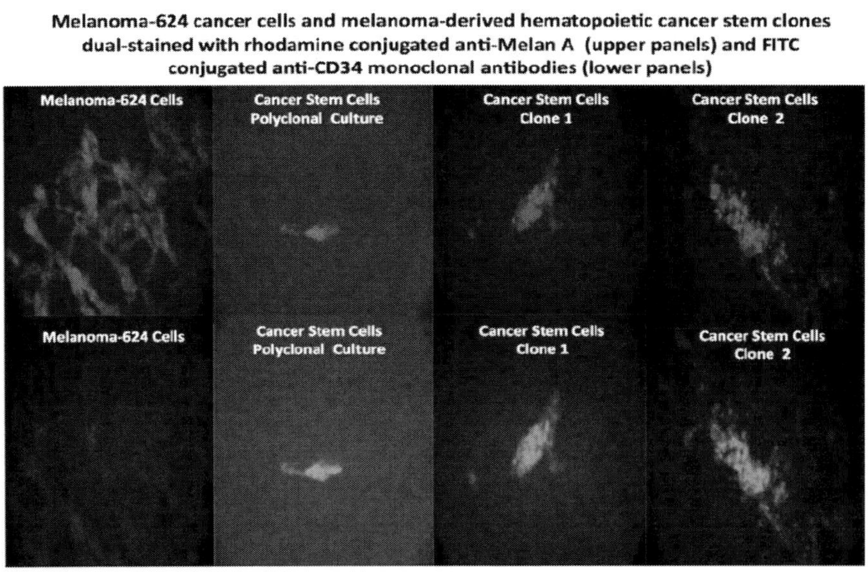

Figure 5. Immunohistochemistry of Mel-624 cells and the hematopoietic cancer stem cells (HCSC). The cells were seeded on chamber slides coated with collagen and allowed to attach for 2 days. The cells in the three right upper and lower panels are clusters of HCSC with similar morphology as the normal human CD34+ cells when they grow in methyl cellulose. As expected, the lower left most panel does not show staining for the CD34 antigen but is positive for anti-Melan-A tumor antigen (upper left most panel). The HCSCs loosely attach to these chamber slides and most fell off during the staining procedure leaving small aggregates for imaging.

Systemic humanized NOD/SCID-hu (Thy/Liv) model and circulation of human cells involved in immune responses: We have used the systemic NOD/SCID-hu model [8] for our studies directed at formation of human hematopoietic cancer stem cells (Figure 6). Purified blood derived CD34+ cancer stem cells were analysed by FACS for purity (data not shown). Since human antigen presenting cells and cytotoxic T lymphocytes are in the blood circulation of these animals, this NOD/SCID-hu model system enables testing of the effects of the human CTL-directed killing of the HCSC versus original cancer cells in vivo.

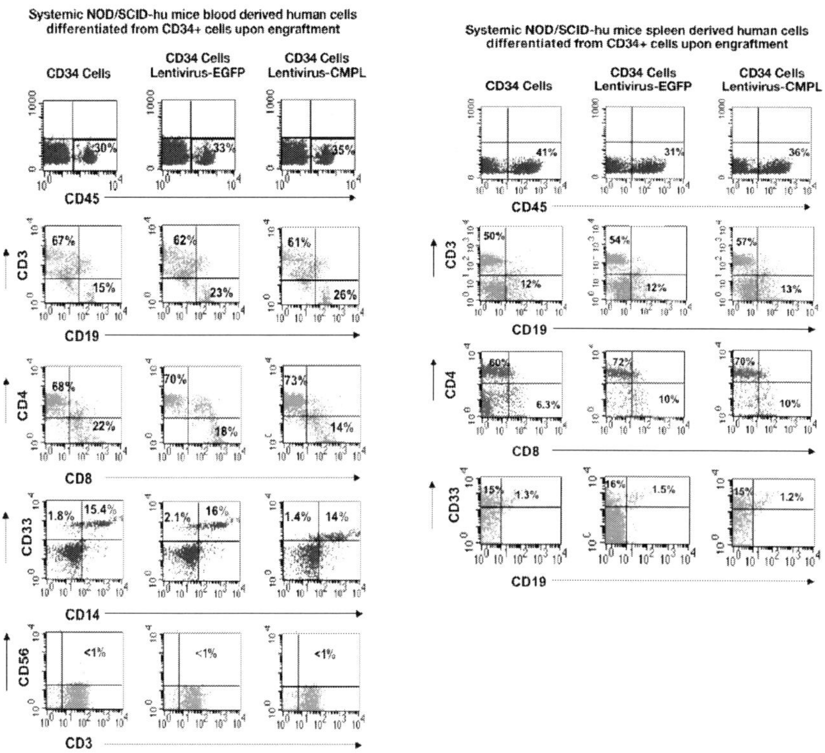

Figure 6. Reconstitution of autologous human CD34+ cells in the development of the systemic NOD/SCID-hu and differentiation of these CD34+ cells in vivo, into multiple lineages, that play a role in immune responses. The untransduced or lentivirus-transduced CD34+ cells were injected intravenously into the SCID-hu Thy/Liv animals. The human CD34+ cells were derived from the blood (left histogram panels) and spleen (right histogram panels) of these animals 6 months post-engraftment and analyzed by flow cytometry. We have detected the following human cell types upon differentiation of the human CD34+ cells: CD45, leukocytes; CD19, B cells; CD3, thymocytes; CD4 and CD8, T cell subsets; CD33, myeloid cells; CD14, macrophages; CD56, NK cells. The human cells were first detected by their human specific CD45 antigen expression and then gated on this population to detect the other human cell antigens or phenotypic markers.

Discussion

In this study we demonstrated for the first time a successful induction of CD34+ hematopoietic cancer stem cells (HCSC) are in the SCID-hu Thy/Liv implants following injection of tumor cells (Mel-624). A cell-cell fusion or endocytosis in the SCID-hu Thy/Liv implants between the injected Mel-624 cancer cells and the human CD34+ cells of the implants may occur in the generation of HCSC. This may also include exchange of genetic material and/or metabolic cooperation due to these mel-624 cell and CD34+ cell contact and interactions.

Expression of certain genes discussed herein is altered by the transformation of the normal primary CD34+ progenitor stem cells into tumor antigen bearing cells with anchorage independent growth in the absence of hematopoietic growth factors (IL-3, IL-6, GM-CSF, SCF) and in liquid media for indefinite periods of time. We suggest that engraftments of these HCSC into secondary SCID/NOD/SCID-hu recipients or into nude nu/nu mice cause growth of tumors or leukemias. Introduction of these HCSC into the SCID-hu and NOD/SCID-hu animals are expected to induce malignancies in the human host cells of the animals. Such malignancies may have different characteristics between those caused by the HCSC compared to the original cancer cells possibly due to acquisition of growth properties of anchorage independence by the CD34+ cells.

The induction and characterization of HCSC using cancer cells and CD34+ cells will undoubtedly contribute to the development of new therapeutic strategies aimed at eradicating the tumorigenic stem cell subpopulation within cancer. The ability to prospectively identify, isolate and study cancer stem cells will significantly alter the way we think about, prevent, and treat cancer. The use of the NOD/SCID-hu model system for studying the CSCs is a novel approach that has not been previously used. Therefore, the findings of this study may be translated to clinical applications, which can benefit many patients with cancer to help reduce the human suffering and the impact of this disease.

Acknowledgments

This work was supported by NIH grant R01HL079846 to PSK and R21CA104047 to BM.

References

[1] Zou G-M. Cancer stem cells in leukemia, recent advances. *J. Cell Physiol.* 213:440-447, 2007.

[2] Jamieson CHM, Weissman IL, Passegue. Chronic versus acute myelogenous leukemia: A question of self-renewal. *Cancer Cell* 6:531-533, 2004.

[3] Hitchcock IS, Chen MM, King JR, Kaushansky K. YRRL motifs in the cytoplasmic domain of the thrombopoietin receptor regulate receptor internalization and degradation. *Blood* 112:2222-2231, 2008.

[4] Gibson SE, Schade AE, Szpurka H, Bak B, Maciejewski JP, His ED. Phospho-STAT5 expression pattern with the MPL W515L mutation is similar to that seen in chronic myeloproliferative disorders with JAK2 V617F. *Human Pathol* 39: 1111-1114, 2008.

[5] Yonou H, Yokose T, Kamijo T, et al. Establishment of a novel species- and tissue-specific metastasis model of human prostate cancer in humanized non-obese diabetic/severe combined immunodeficient mice engrafted with human adult lung and bone. *Cancer Research*, 61:2177-2182, 2001.

[6] Wierenga ATJ, Vellenga E, Schuringa JJ. Maximal STAT5-induced proliferation and self-renewal at intermediate STAT5 activity levels. *Molec Cell Biol.* 28:6668-6680, 2008.

[7] Sundell IB, Koka PS. Chimeric SCID-hu Model as a Human Hematopoietic Stem Cell Host that Recapitulates the Effects of HIV-1 on Bone Marrow Progenitors in Infected Patients. *J. Stem Cells* 1: 283-300, 2006.

[8] Melkus MW, Estes JD, Padgett-Thomas A, Gatlin J, Denton PW, Othieno FA, Wege AK, Haase AT, Garcia JV. Humanized mice mount specific adaptive and innate immune responses to EBV and TSST-1. *Nature Med,* 12:1316-1322, 2006.

[9] Cormier JN, Hijazi YM, Abati A, Fetsch P, Bettinotti M, Steinberg SM, Rosenberg SA, Marincola FM. Heterogenous expression of melanoma-associated antigens and HLA-A2 in metastatic melanoma in vivo. *Int J. Cancer,* 75:517-524, 1998.

[10] Marincola FM, Hijazi YM, Fetsch P, Salgaller ML, Rivoltini L, Cormier J, Simonis TB, Duray PH, Herlyn M, Kawakami Y, Rosenberg SA. Analysis of expression of the melanoma-associated antigens MART-1 and gp100 in metastatic melanoma cell lines and in in situ lesions. *J. Immunother Emphasis Tumor Immunol* 19:192-205, 1996.

[11] Jang Y-Y, Sharkis SJ. Fetal to adult stem cell transition: knocking sox17 off. *Cell* 130, 2007.

In: Stem Cells in Disease
Editor: Prasad S. Koka
ISBN: 978-1-62257-169-7
© 2012 Nova Science Publishers, Inc.

Chapter II

The Bone Marrow Stem Stromal Imbalance –A Key Feature of Disease Progression in Case of Myelodysplastic Mouse Model

Madhurima Das, Sumanta Chatterjee, Pratima Basak, Prosun Das, Jacintha Archana Pereira, Ranjan Kumar Dutta, Malay Chaklader, Samaresh Chaudhuri and Sujata Law*
Stem Cell Research and Application Unit, Department of Biochemistry and Medical Biotechnology, School of Tropical Medicine, Kolkata, India

Abstract

Myelodysplastic syndromes (MDSs) represent a spectrum of disorders that are generally thought to arise from a defective hematopoietic stem cell leading to clonal, dysregulated hematopoiesis. Although it is generally agreed that the marrow microenvironment plays a role in the biology of MDS, it is unclear whether this represents an intrinsically abnormal stromal compartment derived from the MDS clone. Hematopoiesis requires cooperation between progenitors and a variety of functionally and phenotypically different cell types that form the bone marrow stroma. Stromal abnormalities suspected to contribute to the pathology of bone marrow disorder with impaired hematopoiesis. Several studies on human MDS bone marrow microenvironment revealed functional alteration and increased cellular apoptosis thus contribute to the pathology of the disease progression.

In this present study, we have investigsated alterations in the hematopoietic microenvironment and underlying mechanisms involved in the disease progression of MDS animal model. We presented the results of bone marrow single cell culture study,

* Corresponding Author: Dr. Sujata Law, Assistant Professor (Stem Cell Biology), Stem Cell Research and Application Unit, Department of Biochemistry and Medical Biotechnology, Calcutta School of Tropical Medicine, 108, C R Avenue, Kolkata-700073, India. E-mail:- msuj2002@yahoo.co.in Cell Phone: 9051259521.

Long term bone marrow adherent culture study (LTBMC) and their functional efficacy, flowcytometric characterization of stem (Sca1+c-kit+) and stromal (Sca1+CD44+) progenitor cell population and expression level of extracellular apoptosis marker (Annexin v) in the bone marrow cells of MDS animal model. Bone marrow single cell culture study of MDS animal showed impairment in the normal cellular generation, proliferation and presence of apoptic cells. Long term liquid Bone marrow stromal cell colony formation assay from MDS bone marrow cells showed significant difference in the colony formation and their maintenance than the control groups of animals. Immune functional capacity of the bone marrow stromal cells through cell mediated immune (CMI) parameter study denoted defects in the stromal microenvironment. Decreased expression of bone marrow long-term primitive hematopoietic population and stromal progenitor population depicted bone marrow abnormality in case of MDS animal model, which bears significant correlation with high expression level of apoptosis marker in the bone marrow cells.

From the above experimental study we tried to highlight the abnormal bone marrow microenvironment and alteration in the bone marrow cell surface marker expression, which could be the probable mechanism of evolution and disease progression in case of MDS animal model.

Keywords: Myelodysplastic syndrome (MDS), Long term primitive population. Stromal progenitor, Apoptosis

Introduction

Hematopoietic microenvironment plays a key role in the physiology of the hematopoietic system [1, 2, 3, and 4]. Bone marrow microenvironment or stroma is made up of several cell types and extra cellular matrix molecules which in contrast, form an adjustable microenvironment that can modulate quiescent state of stem cells, their self renewal, proliferation, maturation and apoptosis [5, 6]. Stromal cells represent a heterogeneous population of cells including fibroblasts endothelial cells and tissue macrophages [7, 8]. Stromal cells can exert their effect on hematopoietic stem cells via direct cell-cell interaction as well as by releasing suitable factors [9]. This matrix is the supportive structure that can be assumed as the nursery of the progenitors and growing cells in the bone marrow [10, 11, 12, and 13]. The growth and differentiation of hematopoietic stem and progenitor cells in the bone marrow depend on the signals from the stromal matrix. Healthy stromal matrix provides a legitimate stem cell generation. The balance between stem cells and stromal cells helps in the maturation of stem and progenitor cells [14, 15, 16, and 17].

Myelodysplastic syndrome (MDS) is characterized as intravascular bone marrow disease [18]. The hypercellular bone marrow and cellular dysplastic morphology, dysfunction, and impaired differentiation of the hematopoietic stem cells are different facets of the same abnormal MDS clone [19, 20, and 21]. In MDS, aberration occurs in stem cell population of bone marrow that gives rise to multiple abnormal lineages [22].

The most primitive pluripotent HSCs population in mice is characterized by the expression of bone marrow Stem Cell antigen-1(Sca-1), c-kit tyrosine kinase receptor (The receptor for Stem Cell factor, SCF) [23,24].This primitive HSC population have the maximum self-renewal potential, proliferative capacity and bone marrow repopulating ability and at the same time they maintain all the cells of lymphoid and myeloid lineages over long term [25,26]. Maintenance of primitive HSC population within the bone marrow (BM) depends on the interaction with the hematopoietic microenvironment, which supports proliferation, differentiation and survival of the stem cells. In several hematological malignancies, the primitive HSC population gets affected and homeostatic balance between stem cell and stromal microenviroment gets disrupted and ultimately gives rise to hypoplastic or hyperplastic marrow failure condition [27, 28, 29, and 30].

The functional integrity of the hematopoietic microenvironment in MDS is yet an unexplored area. Initial studies on human bone marrow cells revealed that composition and function of adherent cell layers in long-term cultures were similar to those of their normal counterparts, suggesting that the MDS-derived hematopoietic microenvironment (HM) is normal [31,32]. On other hand, subsequent studies by different groups showed a deficient and defective hematopoietic-supportive capacity and abnormal cytokine production by MDS stromal cells [33, 34, 35 and 36].

CD44 marker was expressed by leukocyte, erythrocyte and nonhematopoietic cells and mediates cell attachment to extracellular matrix [37]. Adhesion molecule like, CD44 is widely expressed, multifunctional cell surface glycoprotein that has been implicated in the regulation of normal hemopoiesis [38]. It can mediate adhesion of bone marrow progenitors to adherent stromal layer and plays an important role in angiogenesis, cell proliferation and apoptosis. In case of many bone marrow disorders, the expression of CD44 is altered [39]. Up-regulation of CD44 signaling may also enhance apoptosis in fibroblasts; neutrophils etc. and enhance proinflammatory signals [40]. McKenna and Cotter suggested that increased rate of apoptosis in case of early stage MDS is due to abnormal expression of CD44 [41].

The normal hematopoiesis requires a complex interplay between the hematopoietic cells and the marrow microenvironment which is necessary for switching on several proliferation and differentiation signaling cascade [42, 43]. Multipotent stromal cells (MSC), derived from bone marrow stromal progenitor (Sca-1+, CD44+) populatioon, [44, 45] is essential for physiological activities of normal cells. Maintenance of proper interaction between progenitor cells with the marrow endothelial and stromal cell elements are important for the regulation of hematopoiesis [46].

The ineffective hematopoiesis in case of MDS (despite the increase in bone marrow cellularity) may be due to high rate of intramedullary apoptosis of the bone marrow myeloid precursor cells. In MDS, apoptosis may be the mechanism of the premature cell death, accounts for impaired clonogenic growth [47]. It has been stated that changes in MDS bone marrow microenvironment leads to the secretion of high levels of negative signals (TNF-α, interferon γ etc.), which could be the explanation of the high apoptosis in human MDS [48]. There is still controversy between abnormal stem cell generation, maturation and differentiation procedure and generation of multipotentiality of MDS stem cells within bone marrow. Abnormal functional and structural rearrangement of MDS initiating cells can be demonstrated by the expression of several surface markers [49].

Recently, we have developed a mouse model of MDS that represents all of the critical features of the human disease by administering N-ethyl N-nitrosourea (ENU) through intraperitoneal route in murine model. Subsequent studies of complete peripheral hemogram, Bone marrow cellular architecture, bone marrow cytochemistry and early stem cell marker expression have confirmed the MDS development [50]. Here we attempted to decipher the story of anomalous co-existence of the bone marrow stem and stromal population and the abnormality of bone marrow microenvironment by means of bone marrow short term single cell culture, long term liquid bone marrow stromal cell culture assay, primitive stem and stromal progenitor marker expression along with extra cellular apoptotic marker investigation.

Materials and Methods

Mice and Disease Induction

Inbred Swiss albino mice of mixed sexes for both the normal control (n=24) and experimental (n=24) groups (maintained in our own animal house) formed the animal of choice. They were maintained with standard diet and pure water ad libitum. MDS animal groups were prepared by single dose intraperitoneal injection of N-ethyl N-nitrosourea (ENU) at a dose rate of 80 mg/kg body weight in adult mice (above five months) [50-51]. Control group of animals also received an equal volume of saline.

Isolation of Bone Marrow Cells

Animals were sacrificed after thirty days of exposure with N-ethyl N-nitrosourea (ENU), by cervical dislocation. Long bones (femur, tibia and fibula) were isolated for the preparation of bone marrow materials. Using a syringe with 26-gauge needle the flushing of the bone was done with RPMI 1640 (Sigma, USA) media without fetal bovine serum (FBS). Isolated bone marrow cells were taken from both the treated animals and normal sham control groups for further studies.

Bone Marrow Short-Term Single Cell Culture Study

For the short-term single cell culture, bone marrow cells (2-2.5 X 10^6 cells /ml) were suspended in 35mm culture plates (Corning, New York) containing 3 ml RPMI-1640 (Sigma, USA) media supplemented with 20% FBS (Lonza, USA) and maintained at 37ºC. The cultures were thoroughly observed in 24, 48 and 72 hours using an inverted microscope at 40x magnification [52].

Viability Study of Bone Marrow Single Cell Culture

Cell viability study was done by trypan blue dye exclusion assay. After incubation of 24, 48 and 72 hours an equal volume of bone marrow single cell suspension from each culture plate was mixed with 0.2% trypan blue dye solution and the cell viability was determined by counting alive and dead cells by hemocytometer chamber.

Establishment of Long Term Liquid Bone Marrow -Stromal Cell (LTLBM-SC) Culture

In the long-term adherent cell culture, the bone marrow derived cells were suspended in RPMI-1640 (Sigma,USA) at a concentration of 5×10^6 cells/ml of media, supplemented with

20% (FBS), 100 U/ml penicillin, 100 U/ml streptomycin and 0.01% (V/V) β mercaptoethanol.

Four 65 x15 mm petridishes each for the experimental and control groups were plated with 4 ml of media containing $5x10^6$ cells/ ml and placed in a CO_2 incubator at 37°C. At every 72 hours interval the media was drained off and fresh media supplemented with 20% FBS and 0.01% (v/v) 2β mercaptoethanol, added for the maintenance of the culture. Stromal cells were confluent by 4-6 wk and colonies were scored using an inverted microscope [52].

Studies on Cell Mediated Immune (CMI) Parameters of Adherent Cells Derived from Long Term Culture

The functional efficacy of the bone marrow adherent cells from long term liquid bone marrow culture has been carried out in each group. After 18 days of culture from each normal and experimental group, non-adherent cells were decanted and adherent cells were obtained by 0.25% trypsin and 0.01% EDTA treatment. After collection, adherent cells were thoroughly washed for 2-3 times in PBS and finally suspended in RPMI-1640 media for further study as follows:

a. Nitroblue Tetrazolium (NBT) Reduction Assay

As described earlier [28, 53, 54] effector: target ratio was maintained at 10:1 in the presence of NBT, which is reduced to blue formazan as phagocytosis proceeds. The preparation was incubated for 18 hours at 37°C and finally the reaction was stopped by adding 0.1N chilled HCl and the pellet was extracted by boiling with pyridine for the reduced blue formazan to appear in the supernatant.

The intensity of colour assayed by spectrophotometer at 540 nm provided a direct measure of the extent of phagocytosis. Results were expressed as percentage (%) of phagocytosis.

b. Cytotoxicity Assay

The Effector: Target ratio has been maintained at 10:1. Approximately 1×10^6 bone marrow cells/ml were incubated with 1×10^5 /ml tumour cells (Sarcoma- 180) for 18 hours at 37°C and finally an equal volume of cell suspension was mixed with equal volume of 0.4% trypan blue dye solution and the tumour cell viability was determined by counting through hemocytometer chamber[28, 53, 54].

Flowcytometric Analysis of sca-1+c-kit+Receptor of Hematopoietic Stem Cells (HSCs)

Monoclonal antibodies against Sca-1, c-kit was obtained from BD-Biosciences, USA. Approximately $1x10^6$ bone marrow cells/ ml were incubated for 30 minutes at 37°C in the dark with 2μl of phycoerythrin (PE) labeled anti mouse Sca-1 mAb and 2μl of fluorescence isothyocyanate (FITC) conjugated c-kit mAb and then washed twice in PBS to wash off the excess fluorescence. Stained cells were analyzed with BD-FACS Calibur (Becton Dickenson, USA) using cell quest pro software.

Flowcytometric Expression Profiling of BM Stromal Progenitor (Sca1+ CD44+) cells

Flowcytometry was used to detect the expression of combination of markers that are associated with Stromal progenitor cells (Sca1+ CD44+) under normal and diseased condition. Bone marrow cells were washed and fixed with 3% paraformaldehyde (PFA). $1x10^6$ PFA fixed cells/ml was treated with 2µl each of mouse anti Sca-1 PE and anti CD44 FITC (BD-Biosciences, USA) conjugated mAbs. All the tubes were incubated in dark at 37ºC for 30 minutes. Finally the cells were washed in PBS and analyzed by BD FACS calibur (Becton-Dickenson, USA), using cell quest pro software.

Flowcytometric AnnexinV Expression of Bone Marrow Cells for Early Apoptosis Detection

Bone marrow cellular apoptosis profile was monitored by extracellular apoptosis marker like Annexin v on bone marrow cells from the normal control as well as the experimental MDS mice model.

To analyze early stage apoptosis, $1x\ 10^6$ bone marrow cells/ml were fixed with PFA and incubated with 2µl of mouse FITC-conjugated anti mouse annexin V (e-bioscience, Sandiego, USA) .The cells were incubated for 30 min at 37˚C, washed and analyzed on a FACS Caliber flow cytometer (Becton Dickinson, USA).

Statistical Analysis

Statistical analysis of results was performed using Students't-test of the standard deviation from the mean of different data. A probability of $p<0.01$ was considered statistically significant.

Results

Bone Marrow Single Cell Culture Study

The short-term culture of bone marrow cells from both the MDS [Figure (1b, d and f)] and normal groups of animals [Figure 1(a,c and e)] were maintained for a short term i.e for 72 hours. The photographic images taken by a Olympus inverted microscope equipped with a 10×0.25 NA Plan Achromat objective lens, the BM cell culture of ENU induced MDS mice showed striking difference as early as 24 hrs where number of cells were lower in the MDS group in contrast to the normal healthy cellular proliferation pattern[Figure 1a, b]. Apoptosis begins after 48hrs in the bone marrow single cell culture of the treated animal group and cells become more granular, fragile and apoptic bodies containing remnants of cell organelles appeared in the culture medium which was absent in the normal counterpart [Figure 1c, d]. After 72 hrs, cell number decreased in treated animal group and piknotic bodies appeared in the cells which denoted high rate of apoptosis [Figure 1e, f].

Bone Marrow Single Cell Culture Viability Study

From 10 random fields, total number of cells and number of cells stained with trypan blue were counted by Olympus light microscope with a 40x objective lens. As evident from the data (Figure. 2) the viability of the bone marrow derived cells were found to be highly reduced in MDS mice group compared to that of normal mice and data of viable cell percentage of different time period was presented.

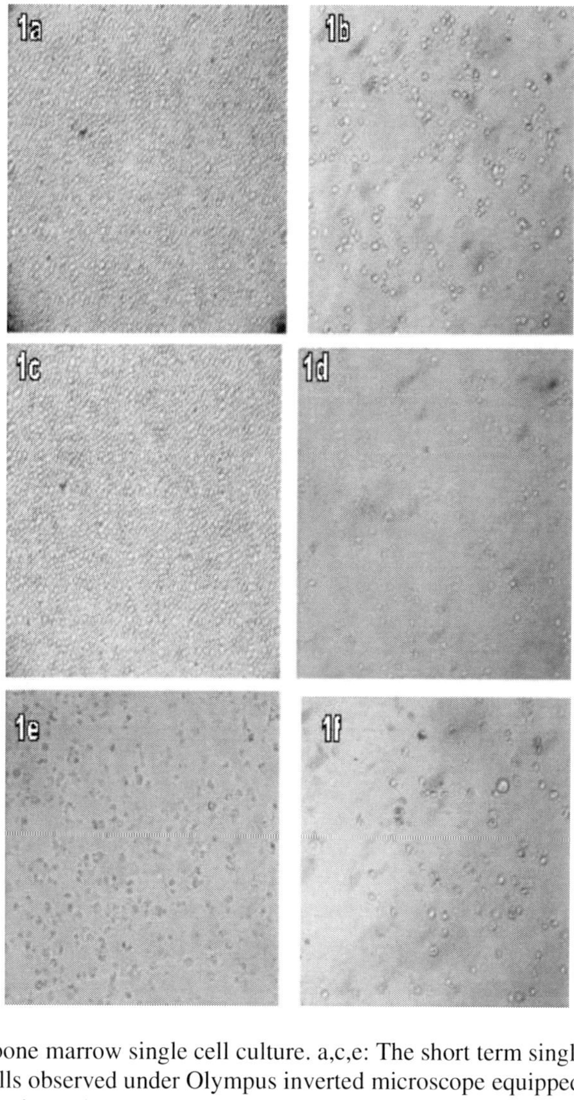

Figures 1(a-f). Mouse bone marrow single cell culture. a,c,e: The short term single culture of normal mouse bone marrow cells observed under Olympus inverted microscope equipped with a 10×0.25 NA Plan Achromat objective lens, showed normal growth pattern at 24, 48 hours and 72 hours. b,d,f: The single cell culture of ENU induced MDS mice, showed lower number of cell generation after 24hrs under inverted microscope at 10×0.25 NA Plan Achromat objective lens. MDS BM showed stunted cell generation after 48 hrs and cells became more granular, apoptic bodies containing remnants of cell organelles appeared in the culture medium which was absent in normal counter part. After 72 hrs there was significant decrease in the cell number with appearance of piknotic bodies in MDS animal bone marrow culture.

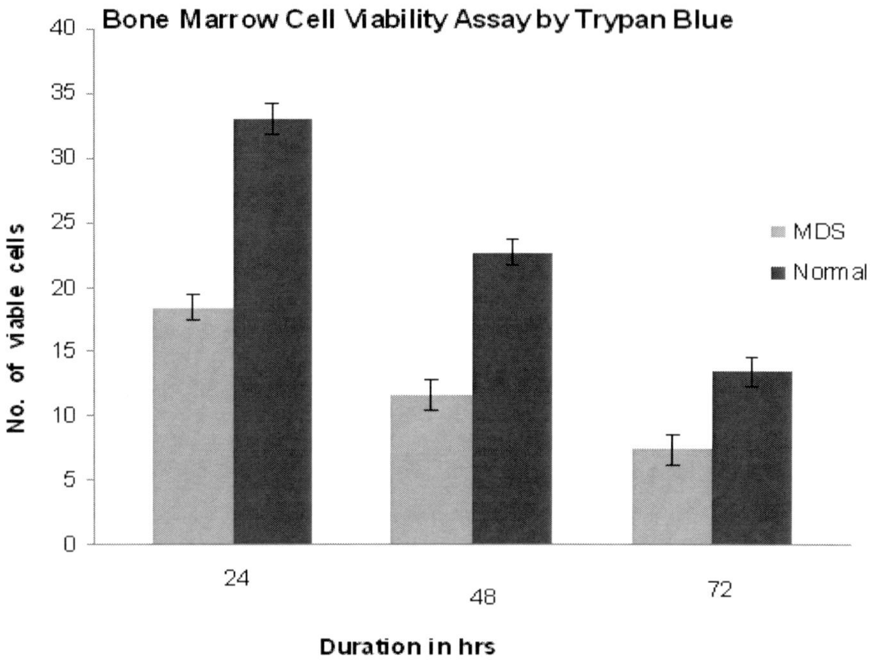

Figure2. Percentage of viable cells were shown at 24, 48, 72hrs in short term single cell culture by Trypan blue dye exclusion method. As the duration of the bone marrow single cell culture increased the percentage of viable cells was decreased in case of MDS bone marrow compare to the normal.

Establishment of Long Term Liquid Bone Marrow -Stromal Cell (LTLBM-SC) culture

To study adherent stromal cell culture, the treated and normal bone marrow cell cultures were observed up to 6 weeks. Initiation of adherent cell layer formation was observed after 7-8 days in normal and MDS animal groups. Adherent cell colonies derived from MDS bone marrow showed increased generation of fibroblast like cells with cluster of cell colonies [Figure 3a, b] after 14 days.

Particularly in case of MDS culture, colony confluence was reached after 21 days, which was one week earlier than the normal adherent colonies. Large number stromal fibroblastic colonies with macrophagic and endothelial precursors were generated, which formed the stromal feeder layer [Figure 3c, d].

After achieving the stromal colony confluence, stromal cell generation was retarded and number of fibroblastic colonies rapidly decreased in MDS adherent culture. In contrast normal stromal cell colonies were healthy in nature even after 4 weeks (28 days) of culture and maintained for 6 weeks. The decreased adherent colony number in MDS compared to the normal essentially pointed towards the defects in functional maturation / terminal differentiation of the MDS stromal progenitor cells.

A graphical representation of the quantitative data of stromal colony formation significantly showed the difference between MDS and normal counterpart in respect of stromal colony maintenance [Figure 4].

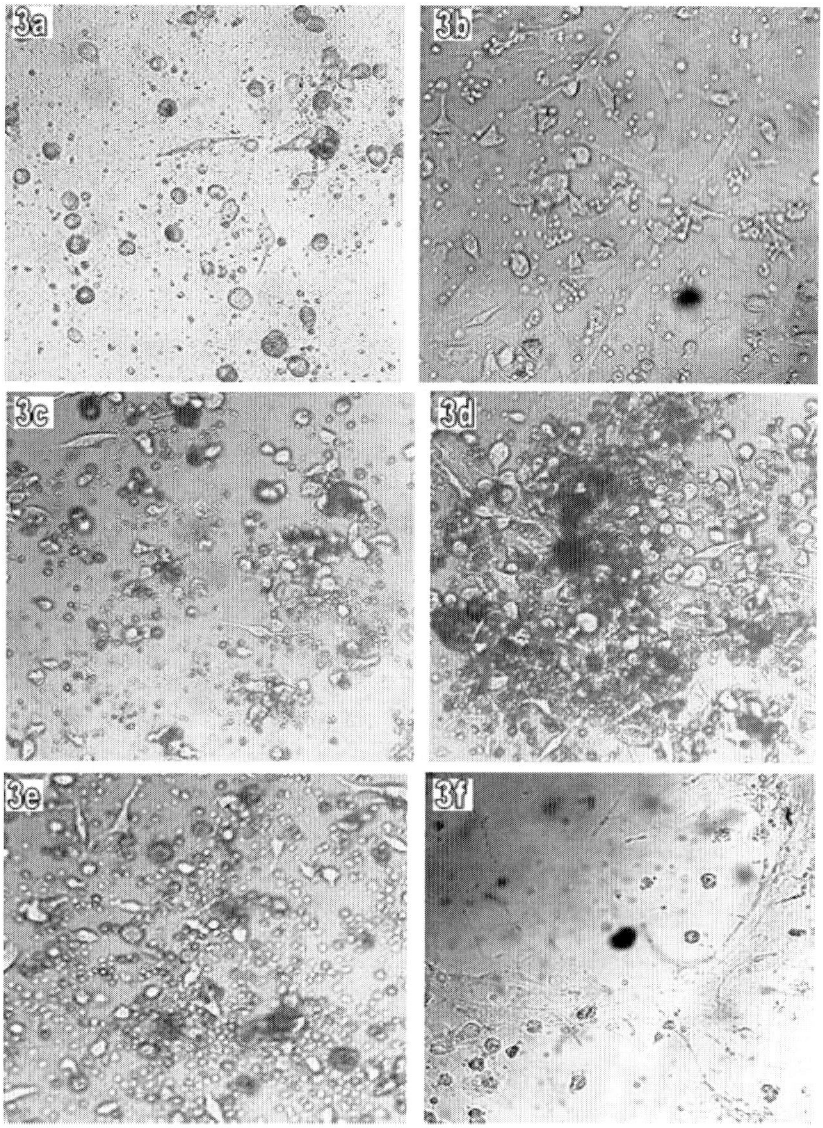

Figure3 (a-f): Mouse Long term liquid bone marrow–stromal cell (LTLBM-SC) culture. a, b: After 14 days, in contrast to normal, fibroblastic colonies were predominant in MDS stromal culture and a bed of adherent cell layer was formed. The score of MDS stromal colony formation was significantly high. c, d: In MDS, stromal adherent colony confluence was reached after 21 days which was one week earlier than the normal counterpart. e, f: After 28 days, adherent colonies dissoluted rapidly and generation of healthy stromal progenitor cell was hampered and the number of stromal precursors declined faster in MDS culture. But, in case of normal counter part, cells were proliferating in a regular fashion with the generation of healthy precursor cell.

After 16 days adherent culture, the photographic images of stromal culture plates (leishman staining) by Olympus light microscope at 100X objective lens showed abnormal stromal precursor formation in case of MDS [Figure 5a], which also denoted the defective maturation aspects of MDS bone marrow in respect to normal [Figure 5b].

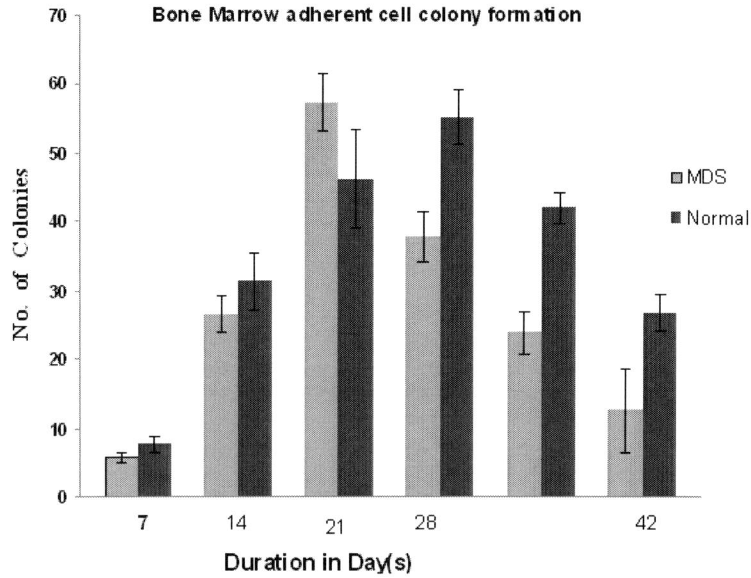

Figures 4. Bone marrow adherent colony forming assay, the number of adherent colony formation is shown at different time periods. Growth rate of adherent colonies in MDS group was higher than the normal and colony confluence reached one week earlier in comparison to normal. After 21 days, the numbers of colonies in case of MDS, decreased rapidly and at 42 days (6 weeks) very few colonies remained in the culture in contrast to normal.

5a) MDS stromal culture (By leishman staining) 5b) NBM stromal culture (By leishman staining)

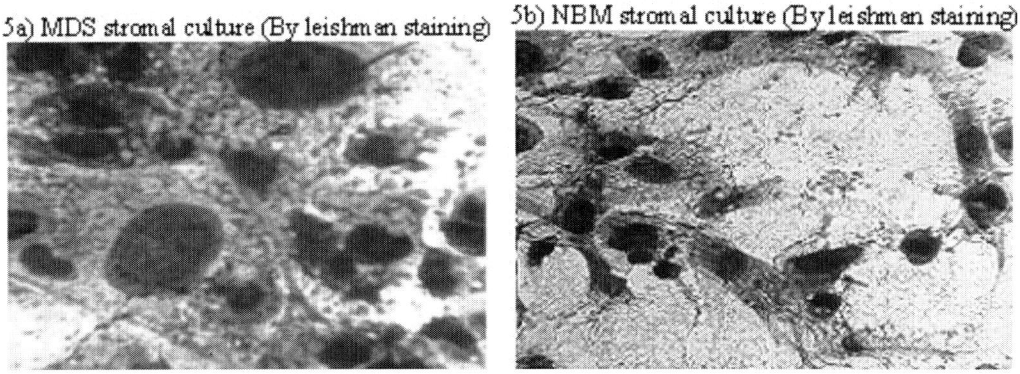

Figures 5 (a,b) Leishman staining of Bone marrow stromal culture. After 16 days culture, Leishman staining of bone marrow stromal cells of the normal (Figure 5b) and ENU treated MDS (Figure 5a) animals showed presence of immature and abnormal stromal precursor cells in the treated group. Appearance of giant cells in the treated group represented dysplastic nature and abnormal differentiation of bone marrow adherent cells.

Immune Functional Efficacy of Bone Marrow Stromal Adherent Cells

Functional alteration of the bone marrow stromal cell was assayed by cell mediated immune parameters (CMI) through a) Nitroblue Tetrazolium (NBT) Reduction Assay (phagocytic capacity) and b) cytotoxicity assay of experimental and control groups of animals.

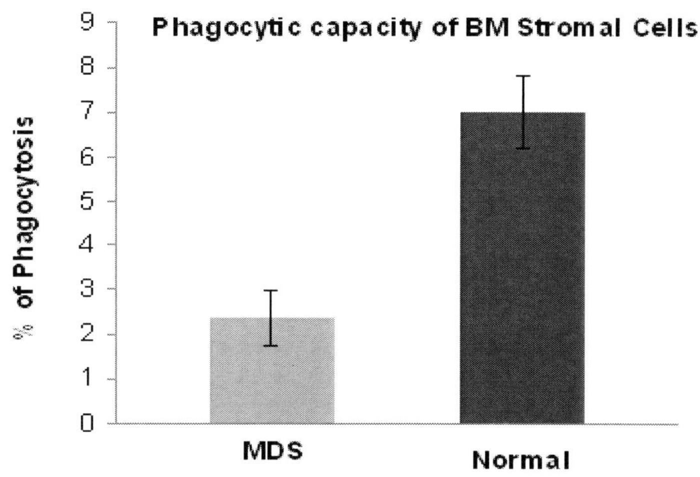

Figures 6a.The phagocytic capacity of the bone marrow stromal cells from ENU exposed MDS group of animals was compared to the normal. The MDS group showed a significant reduction in the phagocytic capacity compared to the normal control group.

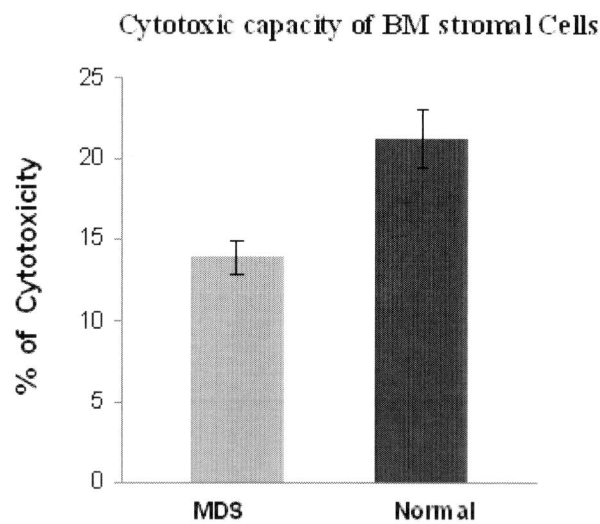

Figures 6b. Cytotoxic efficacy of the bone marrow stromal cells from ENU exposed MDS group of animals was compared with the normal group. The MDS group showed a significant reduction in the cytotoxic efficacy compared to the normal healthy group of animals.

a) NBT Reduction Assay (phagocytic capacity)
   Phagocytic capacity as observed by NBT reduction test revealed a decreased efficacy in experimental group of mice compared to the normal counterpart. The percentage of phagocytosis was 7±0.81 in normal and 2.35 ±0.62 in (Mean±SD) ENU induced MDS mice ($p < 0.001$) [Figure 6a].
b) *Cytotoxic efficacy.* As evident from the data the cytotoxic efficacy of the bone marrow adherent cells were highly reduced in ENU exposed MDS mice compared to that of normal group. The percentage of cytotoxic capacity was 21.23±1.80 in normal and 13.91±1.03 (Mean±SD) in ENU induced MDS mice ($p < 0.005$) [Figure 6b].

Flowcytometric Analysis of sca-1+c-kit+Receptor of Hematopoietic Stem Cells (HSCs)

Phenotypic characterization of Sca1 and c-kit receptor expression by bone marrow primitive stem cells indicated presence of a highly down regulated Sca1+c-kit+ cell population in the MDS animal group (3.44%) [Figure 7b] as compared with normal (9.38%) [Figure 7a].

(7a)

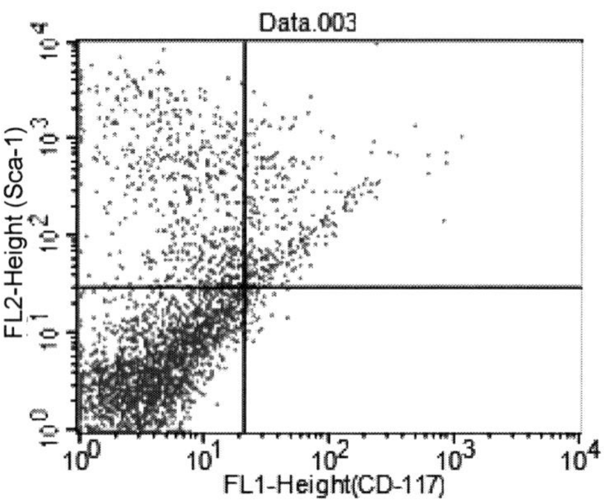

Quadrant Statistics

Gated Events: 3208 Total Events: 10000

Quad	Events	% Gated
UL	606	18.89
UR	301	9.38
LL	2267	70.67
LR	34	1.06

(7b)

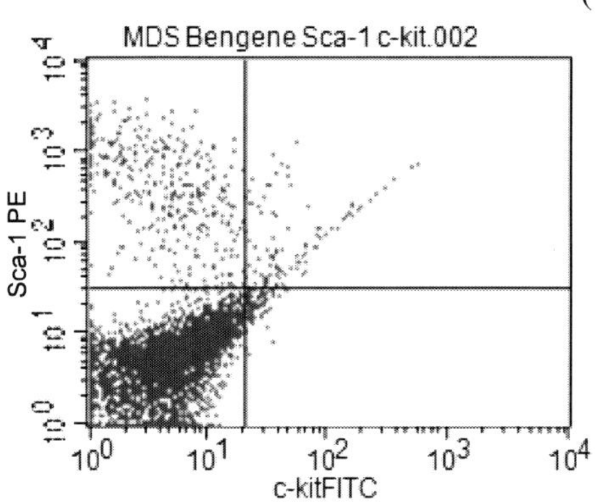

Quadrant Statistics

File: MDS Bengene Sca-1 c-kit.002 Gated Events: 5231

Total Events: 10000

Quad	% Gated
UL	7.09
UR	2.14
LL	89.08
LR	1.68

Figure 7(a,b). a)Phenotypic characterization of Sca-1+ and c-kit+ receptor expression in normal BM cells (Figure 7a) indicated 9.38% dual positivity and in ENU treated MDS. b) Animal the population decreased to 3.44%.

Flowcytometric Expression Profiling of BM Stromal Progenitor (Sca1+ CD44+) Population

Phenotypic characterization of the bone marrow derived stromal progenitor (Sca1+CD44+) cells demonstrated decreased stromal progenitor population in the MDS group as (19.09%) [Figure 8b] compared to the normal (34.64%) [Figure 8a]. The results documented a significant abnormality in stromal progenitor population in MDS bone marrow which demonstrated alteration in phenotypic expression of bone marrow derived progenitors.

Annexinv Expression Study to Detect Early Apoptosis Pattern

Apoptosis or programmed cell death has an important role in maintaining cellular homeostasis in differentiated hematopoietic cells. High Annexin v positivity of the bone marrow cells were exhibited by ENU induced MDS animals (10.96%) [Figure 9b] as compared to the normal (1.29%) counter part [Figure 9a], which denoted an enhanced bone marrow cellular apoptosis level in MDS animals.

(8a)

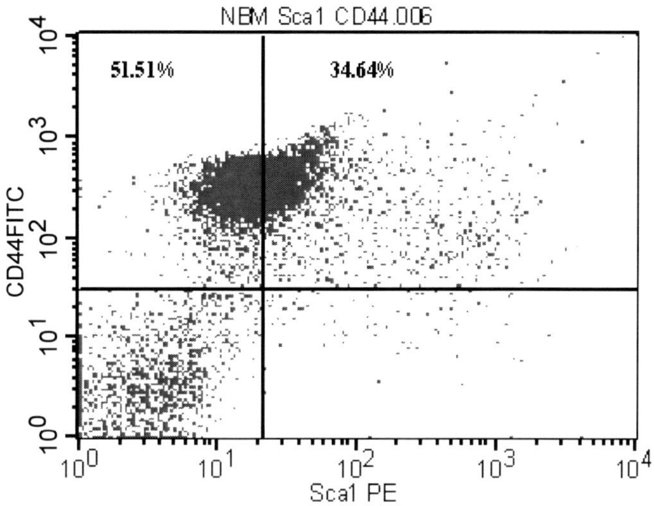

(8b)

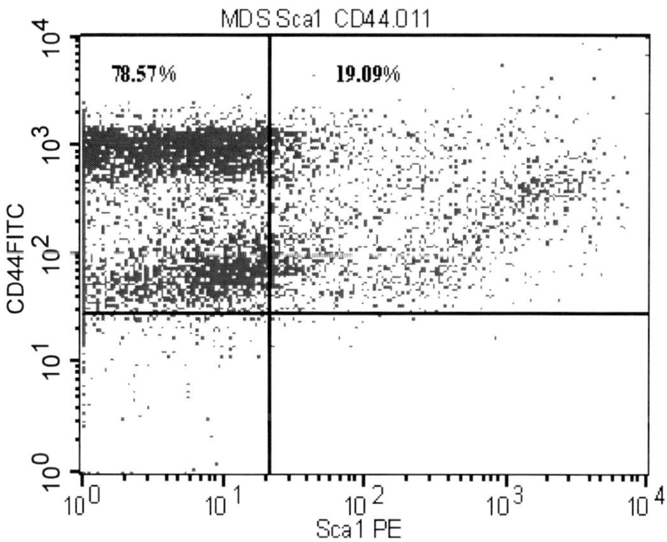

Figures 8a and 8b. Phenotypic characterization of stromal progenitor cell marker (Sca1+ and CD44+) expression by the normal (34.64%) and MDS (19.09%) bone marrow cells depicted depletion in the stromal progenitor cell population in MDS animal group.

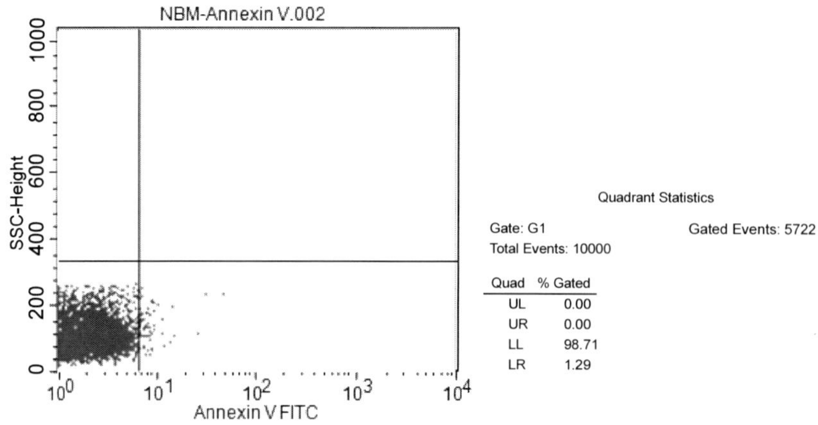

Figures 9a. Phenotypic characterization of Annexin v receptor expression from the Normal bone marrow cells showed 1.29% Annexin v positivity.

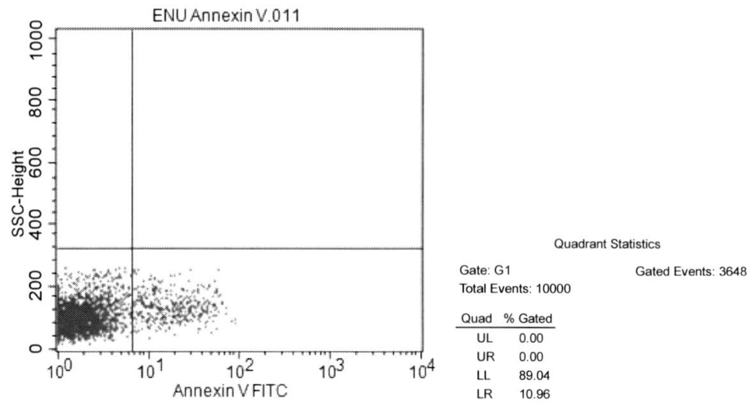

Figure 9b. Phenotypic characterization of Annexin v receptor expression from ENU induced MDS bone marrow cells showed 10.96% Annexin v positivity, which denoted high rate of apoptosis signaling.

Discussion

Interactions between stem cells and their microenvironment regulate their maintenance, proliferation, differentiation and migration into the blood circulation. At all stages of development there is a continuous need to renew senescent blood cells that are ultimately lost from the peripheral blood by days, weeks or months after undergoing terminal differentiation. To prevent depletion, the haemopoietic cells requires a system that not only maintains a self-renewing stem cell pool, but also has the potential to differentiate into all types of highly specialized mature blood cells through a process referred to lineage specification. The association between hematopoietic progenitor and their microenvironment is responsible for cellular steady state growth kinetics. In certain hematological disorders abnormal bone marrow microenvironment seems to contribute to the pathobiology of the bone marrow disorder mainly by hampering the normal hematopoiesis [55]. MDS is a heterogeneous group of disorders characterized by impaired peripheral blood cell production (cytopenias) and most commonly a hypercellular, dysplastic-appearing bone marrow. This incredibly complex spectrum of hematopoietic stem cell disorders thought to arise from abnormalities in stem cell-bone marrow microenvironment interactions or in immune function, although the stem/progenitor cell defects may also arise due to an abnormal environment in which they reside.

In our present study we have used N-ethyl N-nitrosourea (ENU), a potent carcinogen to induce Myelodysplastic syndrome (MDS) in adult 5-6 months old Swiss Albino mice that resembled human MDS [50].

Retarded growth rate of the bone marrow cells and decrease in viable cell percentage [Figure 2] in the short-term single cell culture of the bone marrow cells from the MDS mice [Figure 1.(a-f)] explained the incapability in maintenance of bone marrow derived cells for short period of time, which in other hand denoted defective differentiation cascade of the bone marrow cells. The high rate of apoptosis in MDS actually conveyed that the bone marrow cells were already crippled either by function or by morphology.

Long term liquid BM stromal cell culture was done for the structural and functional characterization of the stromal hematopoietic microenvironment. BM stromal micro-nvironment in terms of both structure and function help to enlighten the disease progression in case of MDS [Figure 3(a-f)]. In contrast to the normal scenario, the adherent culture of MDS bone marrow cells revealed the accelerated generation of stromal fibroblastic colonies. With the high proliferation rate of fibroblastic cells, stromal adherent colony confluence reached one week earlier in case of MDS than the control group [Figure 4]. After the formation of stromal bed, the bone marrow microenvironment from MDS failed to continue the generation and maintenance of the stromal adherent colonies. The enhanced proliferation rate of stromal fibroblast may be to combat the high apoptic nature of MDS BM cells. Leishman staining of bone marrow adherent layer showed presence of abnormally large size stromal progenitor cells which was absent in normal counterpart [Figure 5a,5b]. This also describes the abnormal maturation and differentiation process of stromal progenitor cell in MDS marrow. The functional efficacy of the stromal adherent layer showed abnormality of the bone marrow microenvironment. The immune efficacy of adherent layer from MDS group in terms of phagocytic capacity and cytotoxic efficacy compared to the normal depicted by deficient phagocytic [Figure 6a] and reduced cytotoxic efficacy [Figure 6b]. This result could be explained by quantitative and qualitative deterioration of the bone marrow microenvironment in MDS. From the above mentioned results we can hypothesize that there must be deregulation in the proliferative and functional expression, which could be the reason for microenvironmental abnormality in case of MDS.

The flowcytometric analysis of bone marrow stem (Sca-1+c-kit+) cell compartment represented a quantitative loss in long term primitive hematopoietic progenitor cells. Our data typically showed a significantly decreased (Sca1+c-kit+) HSC population in MDS (3.44%) compared to the normal (9.38%)[Figure 7a,7b].This could be explained by impairment in normal hematopoietic differentiation in case of MDS bone marrow which failed to support healthy generation of stem cells. The quantitative depression in the primitive (sca1+c-kit+) HSC population is also associated with bone marrow stromal cell abnormality, which we are discussing later plays a critical role during hematopoiesis.

CD44 is one of the most widely expressed, multifunctional cell surface glycoprotein that has important role in the hematopoiesis. It helps in the interaction between bone marrow stromal layer and hematopoietic progenitor population [39]. It has also been described as a leukocyte homing receptor and serves an important role in myelopoiesis. Abnormal expression of CD44 in many hematological diseases is associated with disease progression [56]. In our study, increased CD44 (78.57%) [Figure 8a,b] expression reflects the leukocyte retention enhancement within MDS bone marrow, resulting in impairment of differentiation and maturation of the bone marrow cells. Stromal progenitor population i.e. (Sca-1+CD44+) represented by depressed expression profile in MDS bone marrow (19.09%) than the normal counterpart (34.64%) [Figure 8a, b]. The over expression of CD44 marker denoted the altered phenotypic expression by MDS bone marrow cells and the depressed stromal progenitor population denoted abnormal differentiation and maturation of bone marrow stem and stromal population, which focused on the defects of bone marrow microenvironmental components in MDS [57].

Apoptosis or programmed cell death has an important role in maintaining the cellular homeostasis in differentiated hematopoietic cells [58, 59]. Apoptosis may be triggered in cells by intrinsic DNA damage or in cells that have an abnormal growth factor milieu; both mechanisms could contribute to the accelerated apoptosis observed in MDS. AnnexinV expression in MDS bone marrow (10.96%) (Figure 9b) denoted higher expression pattern compared to normal (1.29%) (Figure 9a) This high rate of apoptosis affected not only the hematopoietic cells, but stromal cells too, as MDS is a clonal disease and the abnormal cells may be producing noxious factors that poison the BM microenvironment. Simultaneously, the lesion in MDS may be in pluripotential stem cells, which affect stromal cells because of strong interrelationship [20, 47].

In conclusion, we can say that the abnormalities in the MDS BM microenvironment were generated via interactions with bone marrow stem and stromal cells. It is also evidenced that bone marrow microenvironment in case of MDS facilitates the survival, differentiation, and proliferation of stromal progenitor cells, and serves as a nourishing bed not only for normal but also abnormal hematopoietic cells and thus helps in disease progression. High apoptosis of bone marrow cells is another vital point that needs to be reconsidered for the defective clonogenicity of MDS bone marrow progenitors. So we can conclude that our investigations into the stromal microenvironment and the interaction between stem and stromal components in MDS will be helpful for understanding the mechanism and disease progression and will leave ample scope for future stem-stroma based therapeutic purposes.

Acknowledgments

We are thankful to the Department of Science and Technology (Government of India) and Department of Science and Technology (Government of West Bengal) for their sponsorship. We are grateful to the Director, Calcutta School of Tropical Medicine (Kolkata) for his encouragement and support for the successful completion of the work.

References

[1] Friedenstein AJ, Latzinik NV, GroshevaAG, Gorskaya UF (1982) Marrow microenvironment transfer by heterotopic transplantation of freshly isolated and cultured marrow cells in porous sponges. *Exp. Hematol.* 10: 217 – 227.

[2] Tavassoli M, Friedenstein A (1983) Hemopoietic stromal microenvironment. *Am J Hematol* 15: 195-203.

[3] Lemischka IR. (1997) Microenvironmental regulation of hematopoietic stem cells. *Stem Cells* 15(suppl 1): 63-68.

[4] Taichman RS (2005) Blood and bone: two tissues whose fates are intertwined to create the hematopoietic stem-cell niche. *Blood* 105(7): 2631-2639.

[5] Till, J. E., McCulloch, E. A. (1964) A stochastic model of stem cell proliferation based on the growth of spleen colony-forming cells. *Proc. Natl Acad. Sci.(USA)* 51:29—36.

[6] McCulloch, C.A, Strugurescu, M.,Hughes, F., Melcher, A.H. and Aubin JE (1991) Osteogenic progenitor cells in rat bone marrow stromal populations exhibit self-renewal in culture. *Blood* 77(9): 1906-1911.

[7] Hasthorpe, S., Bogdanovski, M., Rogerson, J., and Radley, J.M. (1992). Characterization of endothelial cells in murine long-term marrow culture. Implication for hemopoietic regulation. *Exp. Hematol.* 20:476–481.

[8] Chazaud, B., Sonnet, C., Lafuste, P., Bassez, G., Rimaniol, A.C., Poron, F., Authier, F.J., Dreyfus, P.A., and Gherardi, R.K. (2003). Satellite cells attract monocytes and use macrophages as a support to escape apoptosis and enhance muscle growth. *J. Cell Biol.*163, 1133–1143.

[9] Bentley, S. A. (1981) A close range cell-cell interaction required for stem cell maintenance in continuous culture. *Exp. Hematol* 9(3): 308-312.

[10] Weiss, L (1976) The hematopoietic microenvironment of bone marrow: An ultrastructural study of the stroma in rats. *Anat. Rec.*186: 161-184.

[11] Mayani, H., Guilbert, L.J., Janowska-Wieczorek, A.(1992) Biology of the hemopoietic microenvironment. *Eur. J. Haematol* 49:225–33.

[12] Honczarenko M, LE Y, Swierkowski M,Ghiran I, Glodek AM, Silberstein LE. (2006) Human Bone Marrow Stromal Cells Express a Distinct Set of Biologically Functional Chemokine Receptors. *Stem cells* 24:1030–1041.

[13] Scadden, D.T. (2006) The stem cell niche as an entity of action. *Nature* 441:1075–9.

[14] Dennis JE, Charbord P. (2002)Origin and Differentiation of Human and Murine Stroma. *Stem cells* 20:205-214.

[15] Hubin F, Humblet C,Belaid Z,Lambert C,Boniver J,Thiry A and Defresne MP(2005) Murine Bone Marrow Stromal Cells Sustain In Vivo the Survival of Hematopoietic Stem Cells and the Granulopoietic Differentiation of More Mature Progenitors. *Stem Cells* 23:1626–1633.

[16] Law S and Chaudhuri S. (2008) Stem Cell Niche, the Microenvironment and Immunological Crosstalk. *Cellular and Molecular Immunology* 5(2):107-112.

[17] Law S and Chaudhuri S. (2007). Niche Theory, Stem-Stromal Imbalance and Aplastic Anaemia. *Journal of Stem Cells*, 2 (4).

[18] Cazzoala M and Malcovati L. (2005) Myelodysplastic syndromes – coping with ineffective haematopoiesis. *N. Eng. J. Med* 352(6):536 – 539.

[19] Janssen J WG, Buschle, M., Layton, M., Drexler, H.G. ,Lyons J, Berghe HV(1989) Clonal Analysis of Myelodysplastic Syndromes: Evidence of Multipotent Stem Cell Origin. *Blood* 73(1): 248-254.
[20] Vardiman JW (2006) Hematopathological Concepts and Controversies in the Diagnosis and Classification of Myelodysplastic Syndromes. *American Society of Hematology* 199-204.
[21] Nimer SD (2008) MDS: A Stem Cell Disorder—But What Exactly Is Wrong with the Primitive Hematopoietic Cells in This Disease? *American Society of Hematology*. 43-51.
[22] Liesveld JL, Jordan CT, Gordon L, Phillips II (2004) The hematopoietic stem cell in myelodysplasia. *Stem Cell* 22:590-599.
[23] Zhao Y, Lin Y, Zhan Y, Yang G, Louie J, Harrison DE, Anderson WF. (2000) Murine Hematopoietic stem cell characterization and its regulation in BM transplantation. *Blood* 96(9): 3016-3022.
[24] Shizuru JA, Negrin RS, Weissman IL (2005) Hematopoietic stem and progenitor cells: clinical and preclinical regeneration of the hematolymphoid system. *Annu. Rev. Med.* 56: 509-538.
[25] Harrison DE, Stone M, Astle CM. (1990)Effects of transplantation on the primitive immunohematopoietic stem cell. *J. Exp. Med.* 172: 431-437.
[26] Harrison DE, Jordan CT, Zhong RK, Astle CM.(1993) Primitive hematopoietic stem cells: direct assay of most productive populations by competitive repopulation with simple binomial, correlation and covariance calculations. *Exp. Haematol.*; 21: 206-219.
[27] Chatterjee S, Basak P, Das P, Das M, Pereira JA, Dutta R K,Chaklader M, Chaudhuri S, Law S (2010) Primitive Sca-1 Positive bonemarrow HSC in mouse model of Aplastic Anemia: a comparative study through flowcytometric analysis and scanning electron microscopy. *Stem Cells International*: 1-7 .
[28] Chatterjee S, Chaklader M Basak P, Das P, Das M, Pereira JA, Dutta R K, , Chaudhuri S, Law S (2010) An Animal Model of Chronic Aplastic Bone Marrow Failure Following Pesticide Exposure in Mice. *International Journal of Stem Cells* 3:54-62.
[29] Okada S, H. Nakauchi, K. Nagayoshi, S. I. Nishikawa, Y.Miura, and T. Suda,(1992) In vivo and in vitro stem cell function of C-kit- and Sca-1-positive murine hematopoietic cells. *Blood* 80 (12). 3044–3050.
[30] Haylock, D. N. Williams, B. Johnston, H. M (2007) Hemopoietic stem cells with higher hemopoietic potential reside at the bone marrow endosteum. *Stem Cells* 25 (4): 1062–1069.
[31] Coutinho, L.H., Geary, C.G, Chang J., Harrison, C., Testa, N.G (1970) Functional studies of bone marrow hematopoietic and stromal cells in the myelodysplastic syndrome (MDS). *Br. J. Haematol* 75:16-25.
[32] Tauro S, Hepburn MD, Peddie CM, Bowen DT , Pippard MJ.(2002)Functional disturbance of marrow stromal microenvironment in the myelodysplastic syndromes. *Leukemia* 16:785–790.
[33] Aizawa S, Hiramoto M, Hoshi H, Toyama K, Shima D, Handa H(2000). Establishment of stromal cell line from an MDS RA patient which induced an apoptotic change in hematopoietic and leukemic cell in vitro. *Exp. Hematol.* 28:148–155.

[34] Flores-Figueroa E,Gutiérrez-Esp´ındola G ,Montesinos JJ, Mar´ıa Arana-Trejo R, Mayani H (2002) In vitro characterization of hematopoietic microenvironment cells from patients with myelodysplastic syndrome. *Leuk Res.* 26 :677–686.

[35] Michalopoulou S, Micheva I, Kouraklis-Symeonidis A, Kakagianni T, Symeonidis A, Zoumbos NC(2004) Impaired clonogenic growth of myelodysplastic bone marrow progenitors in vitro is irrelevant to their apoptotic state. *Leuk Res* 28:805–812.

[36] Mayani H. (2007) Abnormal stromal cells in Myelodysplastic Syndromes: Genomics presents further evidence.(Guest editorial). *Leuk Res* 31 :577–578.

[37] Trowbridge, I. S., Lesley, J., Schulte, R., Hyman, R. and Trotter, J.(1982). Biochemical characterization and cellular distribution of a polymorphic, murine cell-surface glycoprotein expressed on lymphoid tissues. *Immunogenetics* 15, 299-312.

[38] Khaldoyanidi, S., Schnabel, D., Fohr, N. and Zoller, M. (1997) Functional activity of CD44 isoforms in haemopoiesis of the rat. *Br. J. of Haematol* 96:31-45.

[39] Liu J, Jiang G. (2006) CD44 and Hematologic Malignancies. *Cellular and Molecular Immunology.* 3(5):359-365.

[40] Seoh J-Y, Woo S-Y, Im A, Yj K, Park HY, Lee S, Lee MA, Yoo E-S , Huh J-W, Ryu K-H , Lee S-N, C W-S, Seong C-M. (1999) Distinct patterns of apoptosis in association with modulation of CD44 induced by thrombopoietin and granulocyte-colony stimulating factor during ex vivo expansion of human cord blood CD34+cells. *Br. J. of Haematol.* 107: 176-185.

[41] McKenna SL, Cotter TG.(1997) Functional aspects of apoptosis in hematopoiesis and consequences of failure. *Adv. Cancer Res.*71:121–164.

[42] Okubo, T.,Matsui, N., Yanai, N., Obinata, M., (2000). Stroma dependent maintenance of cytokine responsive hematopoietic progenitor cells derived from long -term bone marrow culture. *Cell Struct Funct.* 25(2), 133-9.

[43] Yamada , M., Suzu, S., Tanaka-Douzono, M., Wakimoto, N., Hatake, K., Hayasawa ,H., Motoyoshi, K., (2000). Effects of cytokines on the Proliferation/differentiation of stroma-initiating cells. *J. Cell. Physiol.* 184, 351-5.

[44] Badoo, M., Hill, K., Wilkinson, R., Gaupp, D., Hughes, C., Kopen, G.C., and Phinney, D.G. (2003). Characterization of Mesenchymal stem cells isolated from murine bone marrow by negative selection. *J. Cell Biochem.* 89:1235-1249.

[45] Peister, A., Mellad, J.A., Lason, B.L., Hall, B.M., Gibson, L.F. and Procop D.J. (2004). Adult stem cells from bone marrow (MSCs) isolated from different strains of inbred mice vary in surface epitopes, rates of proliferation, and differentiation potential. *Blood* 103:1662-1668.

[46] Nadri S, Soleimani M, Hossein H.R, Massumi M, Atashi A and Izapanah R (2007) An efficient method for isolation of murine bone marrow mesenchymal stem cells. *Int. J. Dev. Biol.* 51: 723-729.

[47] Raza A. et.al.(1995) Apoptosis in Bone Marrow Biopsy Samples Involving Stromal and Hematopoietic Cells in 50 Patients With Myelodysplastic Syndromes. *Blood,* 86 (1) 268-276.

[48] Kitagawa M, Saito I, Kuwata T, Yoshida S, Yamaguchi S, Takahashi M (1997) Over expression of tumor necrosis factor (TNF)- and interferon (IFN)-by bone marrow cells from patients with myelodysplastic syndromes. *Leukemia* 11:2049–2054.

[49] Elghetany, MT.(1998) Surface marker abnormalities in myelodysplastic syndromes. *Haematologica* 83:1104-1115.

[50] Das M ,Chatterjee S, Basak P, Das P,Pereira JA, Dutta RK,Chaklader M, Chaudhuri S, Law S(2009) Sca-1 / c-Kit Receptor Expression and Apoptosis Pattern in ENU Induced MDS Mice. *JOSC 4(4)* (in press) ISSN: 1556-8539.

[51] Koestner, A; Swenberg, JA; Wechsler, W. Transplacental (1971) Production with Ethyinitrosourea of Neoplasms of the Nervous System in Sprague-Dawley Rats. *Am. J. Physiol* 63(8):39-59.

[52] Soleimani M, Nadri S (2009) A protocol for isolation and culture of mesenchymal stem cells from mouse bone marrow. *Nat. Protoc* 4(1):102-106.

[53] Law Sujata, Maiti D, Palit A, Mazumdar D, Basu K, Chaudhuri Swapna and Chaudhuri S (2001a): Facilitation of Functional compartmentalization of bone marrow cells in Leukaemic mice by biological response modifiers : an immunotherapeutic approach. *Immul. Letters,* 76, 145-152.

[54] Law S, Basu K, Banerjee S, Begum B, Das SP and Chaudhuri S (2001b): Isolation and ex-vivo expansion of Stem cells : physiological manipulation for cytotherapy . *Indian J. Physiol. and Allied Sci.*, 55(3), 114-122.

[55] Bissell MJ, LaBarge MA (2005) Context, tissue plasticity, and cancer: Are tumor stem cells also regulated by the microenvironment? *Cancer Cell* 7 :17-23.

[56] Seoh J-Y, Woo S-Y, Im A, Yj K, Park HY, Lee S, Lee MA, Yoo E-S , Huh J-W, Ryu K-H , Lee S-N, C W-S, Seong C-M. (1999) Distinct patterns of apoptosis in association with modulation of CD44 induced by thrombopoietin and granulocyte-colony stimulating factor during ex vivo expansion of human cord blood CD34+cells. *Br. J. of Haematol.* 107: 176-185.

[57] Schmits R, Filmus J, Gerwin N, Senaldi G, Kiefer F, Kundig T, Wakeham A, Shahinian A,Catzavelos C, Rak J, Furlonger C, Zakarian A, Simard JJL, Ohashi PS,Paige C J, Gutierrez-Ramos JC, and Mak TW(1997) CD44 Regulates Hematopoietic Progenitor Distribution, Granuloma Formation, and Tumorigenicity . *Blood* 90 (6) :2217-2233.

[58] Fadok, V.A., Voelker, D.R, Campbell PA, Cohen JJ, Bratton DI, Henson PM (1992) Exposure of phosphatidylserine on the surface of apoptotic lymphocytes triggers specific recognition and removal by macrophages. *J. Immunol.*148: 2207-2216.

[59] Parker, JE; Mufti, GJ; Rasool, F; Mijovic, A; Devereux, S; Pagliuca, A. The role of apoptosis, proliferation, and the Bcl-2- related proteins in the myelodysplastic syndromes and acute myeloid leukemia secondary to MDS. *Blood*, 2000, 96, 3932-3938.

In: Stem Cells in Disease
Editor: Prasad S. Koka

ISBN: 978-1-62257-169-7
© 2012 Nova Science Publishers, Inc.

Chapter III

Isolation, Characterization and Mobilization of Prostate Cancer Tissue Derived CD133$^+$ MDR1$^+$ Cells

***Satyanarayana Rentala*[*,1] *and Lakshmi Narasu Mangamoori*[2]**
[1]Department of Biotechnology (Engg), GITAM Institute of Technology, GITAM University, Rushikonda, Visakhapatnam, India
[2]Centre for Biotechnology, Institute of Science and Technology, Jawaharlal Nehru Technological University, Hyderabad, India

Abstract

Cancer stem cells undoubtedly exist in many tumor types, including the prostate. CD133 has recently been considered an important marker that represents the subset population of cancer stem cells. The purpose of the present study is to isolate CD133$^+$ and CD133$^-$ cells from normal healthy volunteers and prostate cancer patients to check the prostate stem cells markers and chemokine receptors like CXCR4 for their mobilization. In this study we isolated CD133$^+$ and CD133$^-$ cells using magnetic beads from prostate tissues and peripheral blood samples of normal healthy volunteers and prostate cancer patients (NV-CD133$^+$, NV-CD133$^-$, PC-CD133$^+$and PC-CD133$^-$). The isolated cells were analyzed using flow cytometry and western blot analysis of MDR1, $\alpha_2\beta_1$, CD44, Oct-4 and CXCR4. PC-CD133$^+$ cells displayed higher expressions of CD44, MDR1, Oct-4 and $\alpha_2\beta_1$ expressions with the ability to differentiate into prostate cancer cells. Furthermore, PC-CD133$^+$, highly expressed the chemokine receptor CXCR4 and its ligand SDF1-α. Here we conclude that, PC-CD133$^+$ displayed a higher expression of prostate stem cell markers like CD44, MDR1 and Oct-4 and chemokine receptor CXCR4 and its ligand SDF1-α in peripheral blood and prostate cancer tissue derived CD133+ cells The CXCR4 and SDF1-α expressions will have impact on the mobilization of prostate cancer stem cells (PC-CD133$^+$ cells).

Keywords: Prostate cancer stem cells, CD133, CD44, Multi Drug Resistance1 (MDR1) and CXCR4

[*] Correspondence to: Satyanarayana Rentala, Department of Biotechnology (Engg), GITAM Institute of Technology, GITAM University, Rushikonda, Visakhapatnam-530045, India. E-mail: s.rentala@yahoo.com.

Introduction

Prostate cancer is the most frequently diagnosed cancer in men and is excelled only by lung cancer as the leading cause of cancer-related mortality among men. Despite recent advances in the detection of early prostate cancer, there remains little effective therapy for patients with locally advanced and/or metastatic disease [1-3]. The majority of patients with advanced disease respond initially to androgen ablation therapy, due to the androgen-dependent nature of the vast majority of prostate cancer cells. However, with very high frequency, androgen-independent cancers emerge and subsequently wide spread metastasis occur [4-7]. Autopsy studies show that many older men (and even younger men) who died of other diseases also had prostate cancer that never caused a problem during their lives. These studies showed that 7 or 8 out of 10 men had prostate cancer by age 80. A transmembrane glycoprotein, CD133 (prominin-1) was first recognized in $CD34^+$ progenitor populations from adult blood, bone marrow, and fetal liver cells [8-11]. To improve the patient survival rate, investigation to elucidate the mechanism of tumorigenesis of prostate cancer is needed. Recent data have demonstrated that tumors contain a small subpopulation of cells, i.e., cancer stem-like cells (CSCs) or cancer-initiating cells (CICs), which exhibit a self-renewing capacity and are responsible for tumor maintenance and metastasis[12-14]. Recently, CD133 has been considered an important marker to represent the subset population of CSCs in leukemia, brain tumors, retinoblastoma, renal tumors, pancreatic tumors, colon carcinoma, prostate carcinoma, and hepatocellular carcinoma. Stem cells have been isolated by their ability to efflux Hoechst 33342 dye [2] and are referred to as the ‘‘side population (SP)’’. Our previous publication [16] showed MDR1 in stem cells, enhanced the migration and homing of cultured bone marrow stem cells. However, the gene regulation mechanisms in maintaining the self-renewal and drug resistant properties in putative cancer stem-like cells of prostate tumors are still unclear. Oct-4, which is expressed in pluripotent embryonic stem (ES) and germ cells and has been found, to be a master switch during differentiation by regulating the pluripotent potentials of the stem cell, and Oct-4 [8-10] plays a pivotal role in mammalian development. In this study, the CD133-positive cells ($CD133^+$) and CD133-negative cells ($CD133^-$) were isolated from normal volunteers' (NV) and prostate cancer patients' tissue samples (PC). Our data further demonstrated that only in PC-$CD133^+$, MDR1 and CXCR4 expression in prostate cancer stem cells. These results suggested that the expression of CXCR4 and SDF1-α may play a crucial role in maintaining cancer stem-like and migration of prostate cancer derived $CD133^+$ cells during metastasis.

Materials and Methods

All normal and prostate cancer tissues were procured from Sri Krishna hospital, Krishna (Dist), Andhra Pradesh, India.

Isolation of $CD133^+$ Population from Prostate Cancer Biopsies

The study was approved by the Institutional Ethics Committee/Institutional Review Board. Biopsy samples from both normal (n=6) and prostate cancer patients (n=10) were digested with Trypsin-collagenase mixture (Sigma) to dissociate cells from tissues. Normal prostate tissues were collected from multiple organ donors who had accidental deaths. Organ donor samples from accidental death victims were removed after obtaining consent from next of kin. In all cases, the normal tissues were free from prostate intraepithelial neoplasia and cancer on histological examination. $CD133^+$ cells were isolated from prostate tissues of normal (prostate specific antigen levels < 4ng/ml) and cancer patients (prostate specific antigen levels > 4ng/ml) belonging to age group 60-70 years. Biopsy samples were digested with Trypsin-collagenase mixture (Sigma-Aldrich) to dissociate the cells. $CD133^+$ cells were selected using magnetic beads and analyzed for the presence of CD133 (AC133, Miltenyi Biotech). The purity of $CD133^+$ in the sorted samples was routinely higher than 96%.Cells were selected for CD133 expression (Miltenyi Biotech) from this fraction, using magnetic beads as described by the manufacturer and were analyzed for the presence of CD133 (AC133, Miltenyi Biotech) and MDR1 (Sigma-Aldrich). The purity of $CD133^+$ in the sorted samples was routinely greater than 92% and nearly all these cells also expressed MDR1. The sorted cells were investigated for the expression of Oct-4, CD24, CD44, CXCR-4 and $\alpha_2\beta_1$.

Isolation of $CD133^+$ Population from Peripheral Blood Samples

Mononuclear cells were obtained from normal and prostate cancer patients' buffy coats, on a Ficoll gradient (Biocoll 1077, Sigma). From this fraction, cells were selected for CD133 expression (Miltenyi Biotech) using magnetic beads as described by the manufacturer and were analyzed for the presence of CD133 (AC133, Miltenyi Biotech) and MDR1. The purity of $CD133^+$ in the sorted samples was routinely greater than 94% and nearly all these cells also expressed MDR1. The sorted cells were investigated for the expression of Oct-4, CD24, CD44, CXCR4 and $\alpha_2\beta_1$.

Western Blot Analysis for p53 and SDF1- α

$CD133^+$ cells from peripheral blood and prostate tissue of normal and prostate cancer patients. Samples were lysed by adding SDS sample buffer containing 1 mM orthovanadate, and the samples were processed for Western Blotting. The expression patterns of p53 and SDF1- α (both from Sigma-Aldrich) were detected in normal and prostate cancer patients' biopsies.

Flow cytometry: 5 X 10^5 cells were stained from freshly isolated cells from patient biopsies and peripheral blood samples, by incubating with 50 μl of diluted primary antibodies at $4^{\circ}C$ for 45 min. The cells were washed and stained with secondary antibody and then again washed and fixed with 0.2% paraformaldehyde.

The antibodies used in this study were Biotinylated CD133 (Miltenyi Biotech), Mouse Anti-human MDR1 (Clone F4, Sigma Aldrich), Rabbit anti-human Oct-4 (Sigma Aldrich), Rabbit anti-human CD44 (BD Biosciences – Pharmingen; clone NK-1, labeled with FITC), Rabbit anti-human CD24 (BD Biosciences – Pharmingen; clone NK-1, labeled with FITC), Rabbit anti-human $\alpha_2\beta_1$ (BD Biosciences – Pharmingen; clone NK-1, labeled with FITC), anti-Biotin-PE (Miltenyi Biotec), streptavidin-FITC (Pharmingen), and isotype control antibodies, were procured from Pharmingen. Cells were analyzed on a customized BD FACS Caliber (BD Biosciences, San Jose, CA) using filters of 530/28 BP for FITC and 575/26 BP for PE with a 488-nm argon laser to excite both PE and FITC.

Results

Isolation and Characterization of Prostate Cancer-Derived CD133-Positive Cells

Using the magnetic bead method, we isolated $CD133^+$ cells from tissue samples of six normal healthy volunteers and ten prostate cancer patients. $CD133^+$ cells from normal volunteer (NV-$CD133^+$) and $CD133^+$ cells from prostate cancer patient (PC-$CD133^+$) were characterized by using flow cytometric analysis to investigate the expression profile of various prostate cancer stem cell markers.

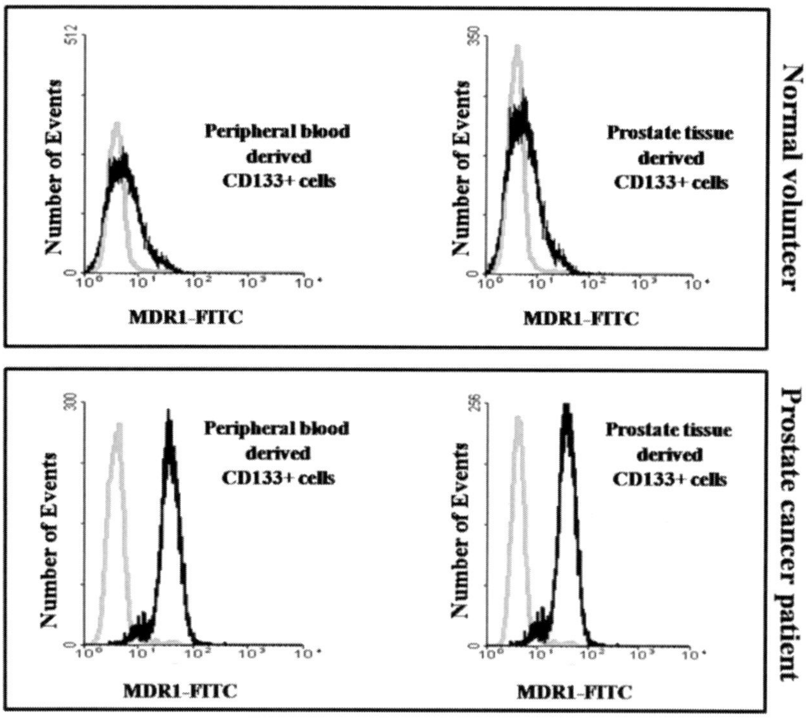

Figure 1. Cellular characterization of MDR1 in $CD133^+$ cells derived from peripheral blood and prostate tissues of normal volunteers and prostate cancer patients: MDR1 was represented as dark line and IgG-isotype control was represented as gray line the in the histogram. The expression of MDR1 in $CD133^+$ cells derived from peripheral blood and prostate tissues of in normal volunteers (n = 6) was represented as the upper panel of the histograms The expression of MDR1 in $CD133^+$ cells derived from peripheral blood and prostate tissues of in prostate cancer patients (n = 10) was represented as the lower panel of the histograms.

More than 97% of CD133$^+$ cells were isolated from prostate tissues, out of which prostate cancer tissue derived CD133$^+$ cells showed more than 92 % cells expressed MDR1 (Figure 1).

Peripheral blood derived CD133$^+$ cells were isolated from normal healthy volunteers and prostate cancer patients. More than 97% of CD133$^+$ cells were isolated from prostate tissues, out of which prostate cancer tissue derived CD133$^+$ cells showed more than 92 % cells expressed MDR1 (Figure 1).

Here we found that CD133$^+$ and MDR1$^+$ cells were significantly less in tissues of normal volunteers than prostate cancer patients.

Characterization of Other Cancer Stem Cell Markers and Mobilization Molecules

CD133$^+$ and CD133$^-$ cells from peripheral blood and prostate tissues of normal volunteers and prostate cancer patient showed a differential expression of Oct-4, CD24, CD44, and $\alpha_2\beta_1$ (Table 1). Oct-4, CD24, CD44, and $\alpha_2\beta_1$ were significantly less expressed in CD133$^+$ cells from normal volunteers than prostate cancer patients (Table 1 – Panel A).

Table 1. Expression of various markers in CD133$^+$ and CD133$^-$ cells: Differential expression of CD44, CD24, Oct-4 and $\alpha\beta_1$ in CD133$^+$ (Panel-A) and CD133$^-$ (Panel-B) cells derived from peripheral blood and prostate tissues of from prostate cancer patients in normal volunteers (n=6) and prostate cancer patients (n=10) was shown in the table.

A

Name of the marker studied in CD133$^+$ cells	Normal volunteer		Prostate cancer patient	
	Peripheral blood derived CD133$^+$ cells	Prostate tissue derived CD133$^+$ cells	Peripheral blood derived CD133$^+$ cells	Prostate tissue derived CD133$^+$ cells
CD44	5 ± 2.1 %	4 ± 2.1 %	87 ± 6.7 %	91 ± 2.3 %
$\alpha_2\beta_1$	4.6 ± 1.3 %	3.2 ± 2.1 %	88 ± 2.6 %	90 ± 3.1 %
CD24	16.5 ± 4.4 %	20 ± 2.1 %	1.5 ± 0.1 %	1.8 ± 0.3 %
Oct-4	1.5 ± 1.2 %	1.7 ± 1 %	67 ± 3.5 %	78 ± 5.1 %

B

Name of the marker studied in CD133$^-$ cells	Normal volunteer		Prostate cancer patient	
	Peripheral blood derived CD133$^-$ cells	Prostate tissue derived CD133$^-$ cells	Peripheral blood derived CD133$^-$ cells	Prostate tissue derived CD133$^-$ cells
MDR1	3.1 ± 1.1 %	4.5 ± 2.1 %	3.3 ± 1.5 %	4.5 ± 2.6 %
CXCR4	2.5 ± 0.5 %	2.2 ± 1.4 %	4.5 ± 2.2 %	5.6 ± 2.2 %
CD44	4.3 ± 1.0 %	5.6 ± 1.5 %	4.7 ± 2.1 %	3.1 ± 0.7 %
$\alpha_2\beta_1$	2.1 ±0.4 %	1.6 ± 0.6 %	1.5 ± 1.1 %	3.1 ± 1.4 %
CD24	25.6 ± 3.4 %	22.4 ± 2.1 %	30.5 ± 3.1 %	28.5 ± 2.5 %
Oct-4	1.5 ± 0.2 %	2.1 ± 0.5 %	1.8 ± 0.4 %	2.3 ± 0.5 %

There was very less expression of MDR1, CXCR4, Oct-4, CD44, and $\alpha_2\beta_1$ in CD133$^-$ cells (Table 1 – Panel B). The expression of chemokine receptor CXCR4 was shown to be high in peripheral blood and prostate cancer tissues of prostate cancer tissues derived CD133$^+$ cells (Figure 2).

Western Blot Analysis for p53 and SDF1- α

Chemokine receptor CXCR4 was expressed in peripheral blood and prostate cancer tissues of prostate cancer tissues derived CD133$^+$ cells as shown in Figure 2. *SDF1-* α, which is a lignad for CXCR4, was expressed in peripheral blood and prostate cancer tissues of prostate cancer tissues derived CD133$^+$ cells as shown in Figure 3. There was low expression of p53 in prostate cancer tissues and β-actin was used as control for all samples.

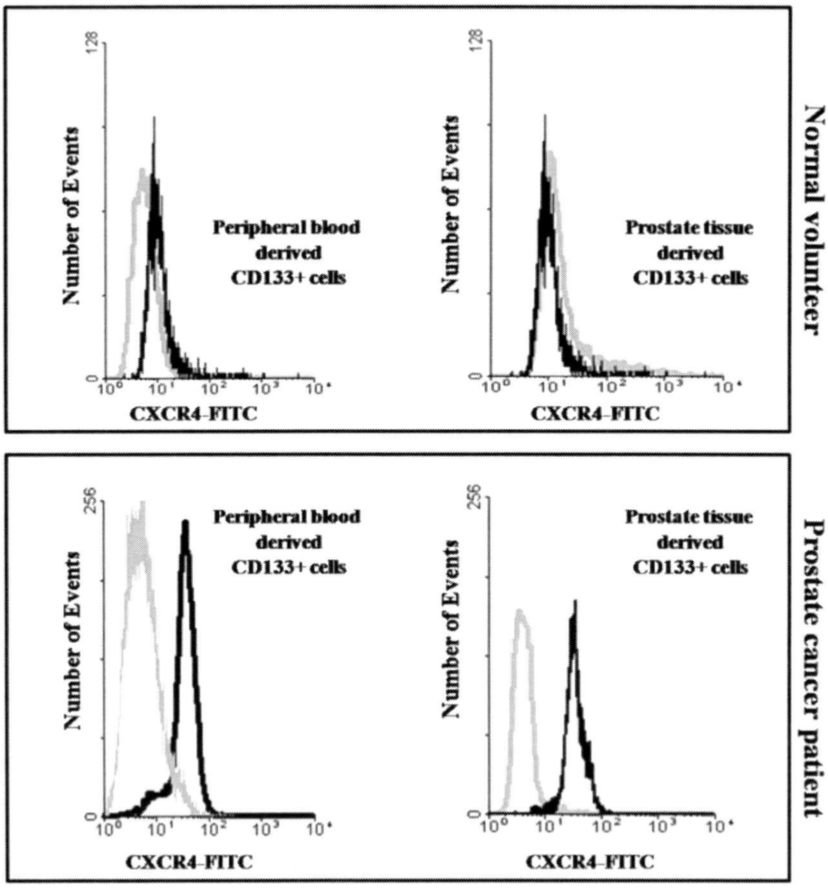

Figure 2. Study of chemokine receptors in CD133$^+$ cells: CXCR4 was represented as dark line and IgG-isotype control was represented as gray line the in the histogram. The expression of CXCR4 in CD133$^+$ cells derived from peripheral blood and prostate tissues of in normal volunteers (n = 6) was represented as the upper panel of the histograms The expression of CXCR4 in CD133$^+$ cells derived from peripheral blood and prostate tissues of in prostate cancer patients (n = 10) was represented as the lower panel of the histograms.

Statistical analysis: Data were analyzed by one–way ANOVA followed by Dunnett's t-test using computerized Graph Pad Instat version 3.05 (Graph Pad software, U.S.A.).

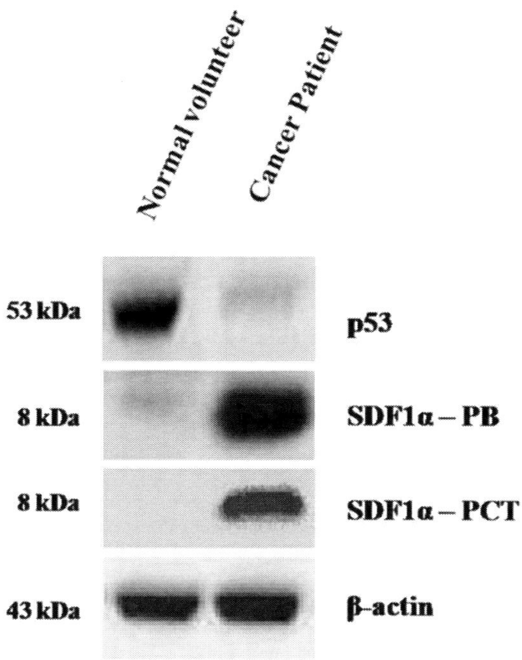

Figure 3. Detection of chemokine SDF1-α in CD133$^+$ cells: Expression of SDF1-α in CD133$^+$ cells derived from peripheral blood and prostate tissues of in normal volunteers and prostate cancer patients was shown using western blot technique. Expression of p53 was also shown to distinguish normal volunteer and prostate cancer **patient**. β- actin was used as positive control.

Discussion

CD133 is known to be a cancer stem cell marker in various adeno-carcinomas. In this manuscript, we reported the isolation of CD133-positive cells (PC-CD133$^+$) and CD133-negative cells (PC-CD133$^-$) from clinical tissue samples and peripheral blood samples. The property of resistance to chemotherapy (MDR1) and irradiation treatment is the major clinical criterion to characterize ''cancer stem-like cells (CSCs)''. The existence of cancer stem-like cells may explain why conventional anti-cancer therapies [1,12,13] are able only to suppress or shrink a tumor but often cannot completely eradicate it, resulting in eventual recurrence. MDR1 expression has been shown to be enhanced in cancer stem cells derived from glioblastoma [2,17,18]. Herein we also checked the expression of MDR1 in CD133$^+$ cells. Peripheral blood and prostate cancer tissues derived CD133$^+$ cells showed a higher expression of MDR1 (Figure 1). CXCR4 is known to regulate migration and development of human acute myelogenous leukemia stem cells in transplanted NOD/SCID Mice. In our manuscript, CD133$^+$ also displayed significant expression profiles of CXCR4 in peripheral blood and prostate tissues of prostate cancer patients (Figure 2). Oct-4 has been suggested as one of four major factors that render the reprogramming capability [3-5] of adult cells into germline-competent-induced pluripotent stem cells. Recently, Oct-4 transcript can be consistently detected in human embryonal carcinomas, testicular germ cell tumors [6-9,16], seminomas, and bladder carcinomas. The expression of Oct-4 has further been shown in human breast cancer stem-like cells [10], suggesting that its expression may be implicated in self-renewal and tumorigenesis via activating its downstream target genes. PC-CD133^{+} also showed higher expression of Oct-4, CD44 and $\alpha_2\beta_1$ (Table 1 – Panel A), but the expression of CD24 was considerably less. CD133^{-} cells did not express MDR1 and CXCR4. The other markers, Oct-4, CD44 and $\alpha_2\beta_1$ were also not shown in CD133^{-} cells (Table 1 – Panel B). *in vitro* studies need to be done to find differentiation capabilities of CD133^{+} and CD133^{-} cells. SDF1-α, which is a ligand for CXCR4 is known migratory factor for cancer stem cells during metastasis. Herein we demonstrated the expression of SDF1-α in peripheral blood and prostate tissues derived CD133^{+} cells from prostate cancer patients. To our knowledge, this is the first study to show that CXCR4 expression in CD133^{+} cells derived from peripheral blood and prostatic tissues of prostate cancer patients. Thus, more investigations are needed to find the role of MDR1, CXCR4, SDF1-α, $\alpha_2\beta_1$ and other integrins in adhesion, migration and differentiation of prostate cancer stem cells during metastasis of prostate cancer.

Conclusion

We demonstrated that PC-CD133^{+} display a higher expression of MDR1, CD44, $\alpha_2\beta_1$ and Oct-4. In addition, our data support the expressions of the CXCR4 which play an important role in the migration of prostate cancer stem cells using CXCR4-SDF1-α mediated signaling.

References

[1] Nakai E, Park K, Yawata T, Chihara T, Kumazawa A et al., Enhanced MDR1 expression and chemoresistance of cancer stem cells derived from glioblastoma, *Cancer Invest.* 2009 Nov;27(9):901-8.

[2] Sigal Tavor, Isabelle Petit, Svetlana Porozov, Abraham Avigdor, Ayelet Dar et al., CXCR4 Regulates Migration and Development of Human Acute Myelogenous Leukemia Stem Cells in Transplanted NOD/SCID Mice, C*ancer research, 2004,* 64, 2817–2824.

[3] SH Lang, FM Frame and AT Collins, Prostate cancer stem cells, *J Pathol* 2009; 217: 299–306.

[4] Jordan CT, Guzman ML, Noble M. Cancer stem cells. *N Engl. J. Med.* 2006; 355: 1253–1261.

[5] Monk M, Holding C. Human embryonic genes re-expressed in cancer cells. *Oncogene* 2001; 20: 8085–8091.

[6] Gidekel S, Pizov G, Bergman Y, Pikarsky E. Oct-3/4 is a dose-dependent oncogenic fate determinant. *Cancer Cell* 2003; 4: 361–370.

[7] Ponti D, Costa A, Zaffaroni N, Pratesi G, Petrangolini G, et al., Isolation and *in vitro* propagation of tumorigenic breast cancer cells with stem/progenitor cell properties. *Cancer Res.* 2005; 65: 5506–5511.

[8] Goodell MA, Brose K, Paradis G, Conner AS, Mulligan RC. Isolation and functional properties of murine hematopoietic stem cells that are replicating *in vivo*. *J Exp. Med.* 1996; 183: 1797–1806.
[9] Jin T, Branch DR, Zhang X, Qi S, Youngson B, Goss PE. Examination of POU homeobox gene expression in human breast cancer cells. *Int. J. Cancer* 1999; 81: 104–112.
[10] Wang P, Branch DR, Bali M, Schultz GA, Goss PE, Jin T. The POU homeodomain protein OCT3 as a potential transcriptional activator for fibroblast growth factor-4 (FGF-4) in human breast cancer cells. *Biochem. J.* 2003; 375: 199–205.
[11] Okita K, Ichisaka T, Yamanaka S. Generation of germline-competent induced pluripotent stem cells. *Nature* 2007; 448: 313–317.
[12] Park I.H, Zhao R, West JA, Yabuuchi A, Huo H, et al., Reprogramming of human somatic cells to pluripotency with defined factors. *Nature* 2008; 451: 141-146.
[13] Kawabata S, Oka M, Soda H, Shiozawa K, Nakatomi K, et al., Expression and functional analyses of breast cancer resistance protein in lung cancer. *Clin. Cancer Res.* 2003; 9: 3052–3057.
[14] Elena Monzani, Floriana Facchetti, Enrico Galmozzi; Elena Corsini, Anna Benetti, et al., Melanoma contains CD133 and ABCG2 positive cells with enhanced tumorigenic potential *Eur. J. Cancer* 2007; 43: 935-946.
[15] Yu J, Vodyanik, MA Smuga-Otto K, Antosiewicz-Bourget J, Frane JL, et al., Induced pluripotent stem cell lines derived from human somatic cells. *Science* 2007; 318: 1917-1920.
[16] Satyanarayana Rentala, Murali Mohan Sagar Balla, Satish Khurana and Asok Mukhopadhaya. MDR1 gene expression enhances long-term engraftibility of cultured bone marrow cells *Biochemical and Biophysical Research Communications*. 2005; 335: 957-964.
[17] Clarke MF, Dick JE, Dirks PB, Eaves CJ, Jamieson CH, et al., Cancer stem cells: perspectives on current status and future directions: AACR Workshop on Cancer Stem Cells. *Cancer Res.*, 2006; 66:9339-9344.
[18] Elkind NB, Szentpe´tery Z, Apa´ti A, Ozvegy-Laczka C, Va´rady G, Olga Ujhelly, et al., Multidrug transporter ABCG2 prevents tumor cell death induced by the epidermal growth factor receptor inhibitor Iressa (ZD1839, Gefitinib). *Cancer Res.* 2005; 65: 1770–1777.

In: Stem Cells in Disease
Editor: Prasad S. Koka

ISBN: 978-1-62257-169-7
© 2012 Nova Science Publishers, Inc.

Chapter IV

Placental Membrane as a Source of Mesenchymal Stem Cells

I. Birgitta Sundell*[*1] and Prasad Koka[1, 2]
[1]Laboratory of Stem Cell Biology, Torrey Pines Institute for Molecular Studies, San Diego, California, US
[2]SVYASA University, 19, Eknath Bhavan, Kempegowdanagar, Bangalore, India

Abstract

Non-embryonic stem cells have the potential for being used in therapeutic attempts to develop treatments for human diseases and injuries. There is an increasing demand for non invasive treatments for a number of diseases and disorders that strike and disable relatively young people that would otherwise have many active years ahead. As longevity increases and we face new challenges in treating patients who suffers from disorders that reduces their quality of life already at middle age. Simple, secure methods to isolate non-embryonic stem cells from different tissues is one step towards making those treatments available to people suffering from Parkinson's disease, spinal cord injury, stroke, burns, heart disease, diabetes, osteoarthritis, and rheumatoid arthritis.

Background

Stem cells have very unique features in that that they can multiply without changing, self-renew, or can differentiate to produce specialized cell types. Stem cells can be derived from both embryonic and non-embryonic tissues, and these stem cells have different characteristics. However, both embryonic and non-embryonic stem cells show potential for developing treatments for human diseases and injuries. Further research is needed to

* Correspondence: I. Birgitta Sundell, Laboratory of Stem Cell Biology, Torrey Pines Institute for Molecular Studies, 3550 General Atomics Court, San Diego, California 92121, USA. Email; bsundell@med.wayne.edu

overcome the technical hurdles between the potential of stem cells and clinical applications that will benefit patients in need. Stem cells, directed to differentiate into specific cell types like neurons, hepatocytes and osteoblasts, offer the possibility of a renewable source of replacement cells and tissues to treat a number of common disabling diseases and disorders, including Parkinson's disease, spinal cord injury, stroke, burns, heart disease, diabetes, osteoarthritis, and rheumatoid arthritis.

Placenta and fetus are both formed at the time of gestation and it is not fully understood how this process is initiated or how it progresses during pregnancy. By the time the fertilized embryo (blastocyst) implants in the uterine wall three differentiated cell types exist: the trophoblast, the epiblast (embryonic or primitive ectoderm), and the primitive endoderm. In the next step the gastrula with the three embryonic germ layers, endoderm, mesoderm, and ectoderm, forms. Thus, the embryonic ectoderm has succeeded the epiblast as the tissue that will generate the body of the embryo. The yolk sac functions only in early embryogenesis when it initiates hematopoiesis and help in the formation of the primary germ cells. Throughout the nine months of pregnancy signal transductions lead to intracellular events by triggering a signal at the surface membrane of the cell. Signals to the cell interior cause change in the activity of a particular gene, and/or other important events. Some stem cells remain undifferentiated and self renew, micro-RNA (miRNA)s may have a role in the self-renewal process. miRNA are post-transcriptional regulators that bind to complementary sequences in the three prime untranslated regions (3' UTRs) of target messenger RNA transcripts (mRNAs), usually resulting in gene silencing. miRNAs are short molecules only 20 to 22 nucleotides long, usually derived from longer RNA molecules [1]. In the micro environment surrounding the stem cells contain elevated levels of let-7 mRNA both in the intracellular and extra cellular compartments suggesting a possible intercellular signaling mechanism through micro-vesicle transfer [2, 3]. Indeed the genetic exchange of miRNA between cells may be essential for cell-cell communication, tissue-specificity and developmental processes leading to differentiation. It has also been reported that expression of miRNA-145 has low expression in self-renewing hESCs, this molecule is upregulated during differentiation. miRNA-145 targets OCT4, SOX2, and KLF4 consequently miRNA-145 represses the 3' untranslated regions of OCT4, SOX2, and KLF4 and serves as a determinant of pluripotency [4].

Embryonic stem cells (ESC) are pluripotent and they have the potential of developing into any of the over 200 different cell types that compose the human body (for example blood cells, heart cells, brain cells, muscle cells, bone cells, etc) upon signal transduction. Pluripotent stem cells can be derived from the inner cell mass of the preimplantation embryo. ESC can not be removed from an embryo without terminating the pregnancy, and great controversy has surrounded investigations of these stem cells since they were first discovered in 1988. These cells are currently not an alternative for use in therapeutic applications.

Fetal stem cells (FSCs) on the other hand can be isolated from fetuses as well as from a variety of extraembryonic tissues such as amniotic membranes, amniotic fluid and placenta. Strong evidence shows that these cells differ functionally from EC with regards to growth rate, morphology, immunophenotype, differentiation potential and engraftment capacity *in vivo*. Nevertheless, FSCs appear to have greater multi-potentiality than adult stem cells. Accessibility makes FSCs a useful therapeutic tool for treatments in a wide range of diseases such as skeletal dysplasia, neurological disease and cancers. These cells could be considered to be an intermediate state between adult and embryonic stem cells. Embryo-like stem cells could be obtained from the placenta's amniotic sac, "amniotic epithelial cells". One placenta contains about 300 million amniotic epithelial cells that could potentially be expanded a hundred fold to 30 billion cells and if they have the same growth capacity as fetal FCS, the number of cells is a crucial factor for the use all forms of stem cells in therapeutic applications. An important step for use these cells is the knowledge of how to harvest, and expand stem cells without maturation of the cells. Further studies of these amniotic cells are required to fully investigate their usefulness in therapeutic applications.

A description of the biological characteristics of stem cells from fetal cord blood and extra embryonic tissues has recently been published by Abdulrazzak and coworkers [5]. Mesenchymal stem cells (MSC) from different tissues seems to be a homogeneous population considering their expression of cell surface markers (Table 1). Amniotic membrane is an attractive source of MSCs because fetal tissues of the placenta are usually discarded and MSCs can be recovered without intrusive or ethically unacceptable procedures. Amniotic membrane is avascular and neither does it contain nervous or lymphatic tissues. Amniotic membrane gets oxygen and nutrients from the surrounding chorionic fluid, amniotic fluid and fetal surface blood vessels. The membrane is just a matrix of extra cellular proteins that holds the cells.

Table 1. Surface makers expressed on MSC from bone marrow (BMC, amniotic membrane (AMC), and chorionic membrane (CMC) [17, 18]

BMC	BMC	AMC	CMC		BMC	AMC	CMC
CD1a	-	-	-	CD44	+	+	+
CD3	-	-	-	CD90	+	+	+
CD14	-	-	-	CD105	+	+	+
CD34	-	-	-	CD13	+	+	+
CD133	-	-	-	CD29	+	+	+
CD31	-	-	-	CD54	+	+	+
CD45	-	-	-	CD73	+	+	+
CD36	-	-	-	CD166	+	+	+
HLA class I	-	-	-	CD19	+	+	+
				CD140b	+	+	+
				HLA-ABC	+	+	+

Isolation of MSC from amniotic membrane is fairly easy procedure because the risk of contamination with blood cells, smooth muscle cells, epithelium of endothelial cells are small to none if the membrane is washed in saline or PBS prior to enzyme digestion. Mesenchymal cells from amniotic membrane are usually referred to as Amniotic Membrane-human Mesenchymal Stromal Cells (AM-hMSC) as recommended by the International Society for Cellular Therapy. Amniotic membrane is avascular and neither does it contain nervous or lymphatic tissues.

Only 1% of the cells in cultures of human amniocentesis specimens obtained for prenatal genetic diagnosis express the surface antigen c-Kit (CD117), or stem cell factor receptor [6]. Stem cells derived from amniotic fluid express mesenchymal markers (CD29, CD44, CD73, CD90 and CD105) [7-9] but do not express hematopoietic lineage (CD45) or hematopoietic stem cells (CD34, CD133) markers.

Cells from amniotic fluid are also positive for stage-specific embryonic antigen (SSEA)-4, but negative for surface markers characteristic of ES and embryonic germ (EG) cells [10-12]. Over 90% of the cells expressed the transcription factor Oct4, which has been associated with the maintenance of the undifferentiated state and the pluripotency of ES and EG cells [13]. However the amniocentesis procedure represents a risk for miscarriage, and cells for therapeutic applications needs to be obtained without risk for the cell donor.

Preparation of Mesenchymal Stem Cells for Therapeutic Use

AM-hMSCs have a large capacity for self-renewal while maintaining their multipotency and are therefore a potentially valuable source of stem cells for therapeutic applications. Mesenchyme is considered to be an embryonic connective tissue, it consists of unspecialized cells set in a gelatinous substance. These cells are totipotent and they later form connective tissue, bone, cartilage, and the circulatory and lymphatic systems [14] by moving from their place of origin to other areas/tissues.

On this schematic drawing of the mammalian foetal membranes at term the amnion forms the inner most lining of the sac which directly surrounds and protects the foetus (Figure 1). The amnion MSC is a monolayer that secretes a thick basement membrane which consists of a variety of collagens including types II, IV and V, and proteins such as laminin, nidogen and fibronectin. Different enzymatic digestions methods have been used for the isolation of MSCs, we suggest using 0.2% collagenase IV considering that the matrix contains mainly collagen. A specific enzyme is less likely to digest underlaying layers and allow for a contamination with the underlaying layers of fibroblasts.

Mesenchymal cells from amniotic membrane collected postpartum were cultured for 14 days in either of the two serum free media MethoCult or MesenCult (Stem Cell Technologies, Vancouver, BC, Canada). Amnion was digested in 0.2% collagenase IV for 30 min at 37°C, cells were washed in PBS, spun at 1000x*g* and plated in sterile Petri dishes with collagen coating at a density of 30,000 cells per cm^2.

It is essential to avoid using pretreated tissue culture dishes as they are coated with plasma components which may interfere with the results of this experiment. MesenCult have been shown by the manufacturer to sustain mesenchymal cell cultures of CD19+ /CD105+/CD73+ cells and deplete contaminating hematopoietic cells (CD45+/CD11b+) efficiently, see Table1 for mesenchymal cell surface markers. An equal number of cells from the same donor was simultaneously cultured in MethoCult, a media that is optimized to sustain erythroid progenitors (BFU-E), granulocyte-macrophage progenitors (CFU-GM, CFU-M, CFU-G), and multi-potential granulocyte, erythroid, macrophage and megakaryocyte progenitors (CFU-GEMM).

At 14 days of culture no viable colonies of cells were observed in MethoCult while cultures in MesenCult were healthy and viable (Figure 2), this supports the previous observations that AM-hMSCs are totipotent rather than pluripotent stem cells.

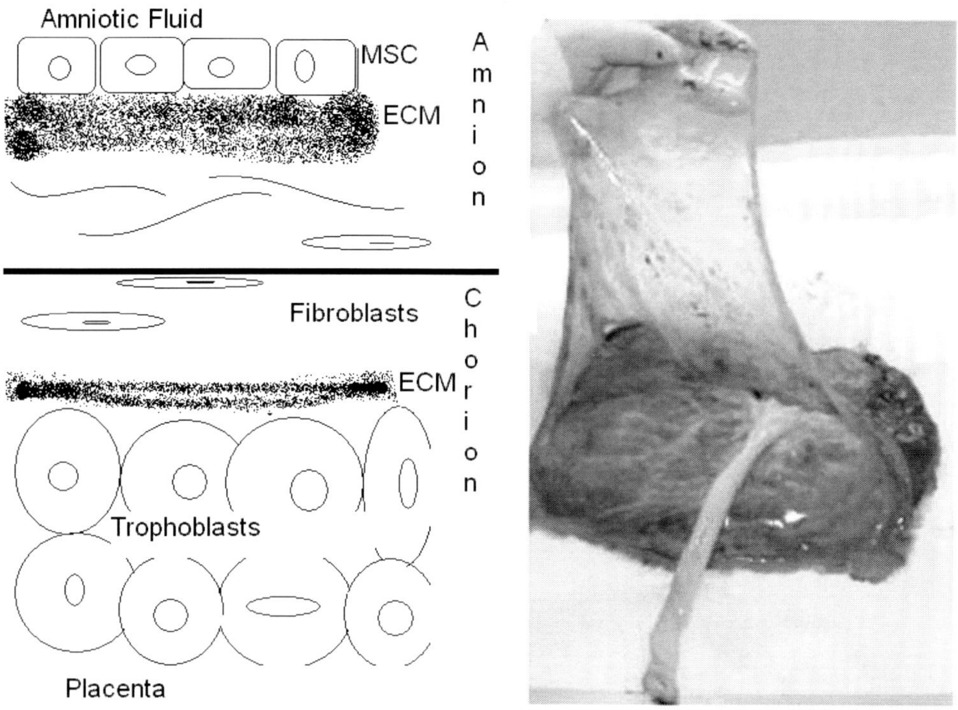

Figure 1. The amniotic membrane is the thin innermost layer of placenta, almost fused with the chorion in a way that the two are one membrane (left panel). Amnion consists of a thin epithelial layer, a thick basement membrane of extra cellular matrix proteins (ECM) and an avascular stroma. In the amniotic membrane there are two cell types present, they are of different embryological origin: mesenchymal cells from mesoderm and epithelial cells from ectoderm. The chorionic membrane contains fibroblasts and trophoblasts. For mesenchymal stem cell isolation the two mebranes should be separated prior to enzymatic digestion.

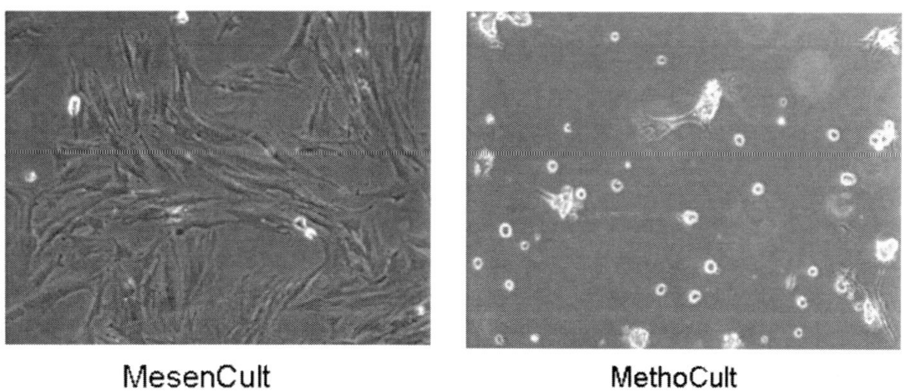

Figure 2. Cells isolated from amniotic membrane were isolated and plated in 35 mm dishes (20,000 cell/plate) coated with collagen. Left panel. Cells were cultured for 10 days in mesenchymal expansion medium (MesenCult, Stem Cell Technologies). The cultures were confluent at day 10. Right panel. Cells were cultured for 10 days in hematopoietic expansion medium (MethoCult, Stem Cell Technologies). There were no colonies of cells on the plates, only a few cells did survive. Culture in serum free expansion media supports the notion that amniotic cells are over 90% pure mesenchymal cells with pluripotent capacity. Cell culture using expansion media is one way to purify the cells isolated from amniotic membrane. Similar results was obtained by Soncini et al 2007 (21).

Therapeutic Use of AM-hMSC in Osteoarthritis

Data from the Center of Disease Control (CDC) shows that osteoarthritis a leading cause of knee problems and replacement surgery affects 27 million American adults. Annually 500,000 total knee replacement surgeries are performed. Given the increased number of obese people in the US this number may increase significantly. As many as 1 in 2 people will get some form of osteoarthritis in their lifetime. If methods can developed to delay or substitute surgeries using stem cell transplants it represents significant benefits and some studies shows that stem cells repair knee cartilage [16-19].

Investigators have found gene expression to be similar but with small differences in MSC derived from different tissues [20]. It is one possibility that gene expression is developed on site and all pluripotent MSC would develop the same gene expression profile if moved to the same site. Further studies remains to fully elucidate the mechanisms that govern maturation and differentiation of MSC. In a case study Centeno et al [16] isolated MSC from the iliac crest of a patient, expanded them ex vivo and infused the cells back in to the patient. In the patients arthritic knee c new cartilage growth was observed and the patient reported improved mobility and decreased discomfort. In theory AM-hMSCs could possibly used in a similar application, this would require extensive studies to ensure that no adverse effects develop by using cells from different donor.

Conclusion

Mesenchymal stem cells from amniotic membranes could become one alternative for treatment of osteoarthritis. Infusion of bone marrow derived mesenchymal stem cells in to knees with osteoarthritis have shown that the cells will produce cartilage and improve the quality of life for the treated patients [18]. Artificial joints is costly and the surgery itself poses risks so replacement surgery should be the last alternative following less invasive yet efficient treatments. Mesenchymal stem cells from amniotic membranes are easy to isolate and placentas is not in short supply.

Acknowledgment

Supported by Ramalingaswami Fellowship (Department of Biotechnology, India).

References

[1] He L, Hannon GJ. MicroRNAs: small RNAs with a big role in gene regulation. *Nat. Rev. Genet.* 5 (2004), pp. 522–531.

[2] Chen TS, Lai RC, Lee MM, Choo AB, Lee CN, Lim SK. Mesenchymal stem cells secretes microparticles enriched in pre-microRNAs. *Nucleic Acids Res.* 2010; 38(1): 215-24.

[3] Koh W, Sheng CT, Tan B, Lee QY, Kuznetsov V, Kiang LS, Tanavde V. Analysis of deep sequencing microRNA expression profile from human embryonic stem cells derived mesenchymal stem cells reveals possible role of let-7 microRNA family in downstream targeting of hepatic nuclear factor 4 alpha. *BMC Genomics*. 2010;11 Suppl 1:S6.

[4] Xu N, Papagiannakopoulos T, Pan G, Thomson JA, Kosik KS. MicroRNA-145 regulates OCT4, SOX2, and KLF4 and represses pluripotency in human embryonic stem cells. *Cell*. 2009;137(4):65.

[5] Abdulrazzak H, Moschidou D, Jones G, Guillot PV. Biological characteristics of stem cells from foetal, cord blood and extraembryonic tissues. *J. R. Soc. Interface*. 2010 Aug 2547-58.

[6] De Coppi P, Bartsch G Jr, Siddiqui MM, Xu T, Santos CC, Perin L, Mostoslavsky G, Serre AC, Snyder EY, Yoo JJ, Furth ME, Soker S, Atala A. Isolation of amniotic stem cell lines with potential for therapy. *Nat Biotechnol*. 2007 Jan;25(1):100-6.

[7] Tsai, M.S., Lee, J.L., Chang, Y.J., Hwang, S.M. Isolation of human multipotent mesenchymal stem cells from second-trimester amniotic fluid using a novel two-stage culture protocol. *Hum. Reprod*. 2004; 19: 1450–1456.

[8] Barry, F.P., Boynton, R.E., Haynesworth, S., Murphy, J.M., Zaia, J. The monoclonal antibody SH-2, raised against human mesenchymal stem cells, recognizes an epitope on endoglin (CD105). *Biochem. Biophys. Res. Commun*. 1999; 265: 134–139.

[9] Barry, F., Boynton, R., Murphy, M., Haynesworth, S., Zaia, J. The SH-3 and SH-4 antibodies recognize distinct epitopes on CD73 from human mesenchymal stem cells. *Biochem. Biophys. Res. Commun*. 2001; 289: 519–524.

[10] Thomson, J.A., Itskovitz-Eldor J., Shapiro SS, Waknitz MA., Swiergiel JJ., Marshall VS., Jones JM. Embryonic stem cell lines derived from human blastocysts. *Science* 1998; 282: 1145–1147.

[11] Carpenter, M.K., Rosler, E., Rao, M.S. Characterization and differentiation of human embryonic stem cells. *Cloning Stem Cells* 2003; 5: 79–88.

[12] Shamblott, M.J., Axelman J., Wang S., Bugg EM., Littlefield JW., Donovan PJ., Blumenthal PD., Huggins GR., Gearhart JD. Derivation of pluripotent stem cells from cultured human primordial germ cells. *Proc. Natl. Acad. Sci. USA* 1998; 95: 13726–13731.

[13] Pan, G.J., Chang, Z.Y., Scholer, H.R., Pei, D. Stem cell pluripotency and transcription factor Oct4. *Cell Res*. 2002; 12: 321–329.

[14] Anna M. Wobus. Stem Cells. *Springer*. 2008, pp.248.

[15] Births, Marriages, Divorces and Deaths. Provisional Data for 2009. *National Vital Statistics report* 2010; 58: 25.

[16] Centeno CJ, Busse D, Kisiday J, Keohan C, Freeman M, Karli D. Increased knee cartilage volume in degenerative joint disease using percutaneously implanted, autologous mesenchymal stem cells. *Pain Physician*. 2008;11(3):343-53.

[17] Horie M, Sekiya I, Muneta T, Ichinose S, Matsumoto K, Saito H, Murakami T, Kobayashi E.Intra-articular Injected synovial stem cells differentiate into meniscal cells directly and promote meniscal regeneration without mobilization to distant organs in rat massive meniscal defect. *Stem Cells*. 2009;27(4):878-87.

[18] Nejadnik H, Hui JH, Feng Choong EP, Tai BC, Lee EH. Autologous bone marrow-derived mesenchymal stem cells versus autologous chondrocyte implantation: an observational cohort study. *Am. J. Sports Med.* 2010;38(6):1110-6.
[19] Pabbruwe MB, Kafienah W, Tarlton JF, Mistry S, Fox DJ, Hollander AP. Repair of meniscal cartilage white zone tears using a stem cell/collagen-scaffold implant. *Biomaterials.* 2010; 31(9): 2583-91.
[20] Segawa Y, Muneta T, Makino H, Nimura A, Mochizuki T, Ju YJ, Ezura Y, Umezawa A, Sekiya I. Mesenchymal stem cells derived from synovium, meniscus, anterior cruciate ligament, and articular chondrocytes share similar gene expression profiles. *J. Orthop. Res.* 2009; 27(4):435-41.
[21] Soncini M, Vertua E, Gibelli L, Zorzi F, Denegri M, Albertini A, Wengler GS, Parolini O. Isolation and characterization of mesenchymal cells from human fetal membranes. *J. Tissue Eng. Regen. Med.* 2007;1(4):296-305.

In: Stem Cells in Disease
Editor: Prasad S. Koka

ISBN: 978-1-62257-169-7
© 2012 Nova Science Publishers, Inc.

Chapter V

Human Glioblastoma Cells Display Mesenchymal Stem Cell Features and Form Intracranial Tumors in Immunocompetent Rats

Adriana M. Nakahata[1,2], *Daniela E. Suzuki*[1,2], *Carolina O. Rodini*[2], *Márcia C. L. Pereira*[1,2], *Luciana Janjoppi*[1,2] *and Oswaldo K. Okamoto*[2*]

[1]Departamento de Neurologia e Neurocirurgia, Disciplina de Neurologia Experimental, Universidade Federal de São Paulo, SP, Brazil

[2]Centro de Estudos do Genoma Humano, Departamento de Genética e Biologia Evolutiva, Instituto de Biociências, Universidade de São Paulo, SP, Brazil

Abstract

Isolation of highly tumorigenic stem-like cells from human glioblastoma specimens and cell lines has been focusing on their neural stem cells properties or capacity to efflux fluorescent dyes. Here, we report that, under standard culture conditions, human glioblastoma cells of the U87MG cell line display a predominant mesenchymal phenotype and share some of the *in vitro* properties of mesenchymal stem cells. Moreover, these cells were capable of forming tumors in immunocompetent rats. Infiltrative intracranial tumors could be detected 15 to 30 days post-stereotaxic cell injection within the motor cortex. Tumors were comprised by pleomorphic and mitotically active cells and displayed necrotic and hemorrhagic foci, which are common features of human glioblastomas. This rather unexpected *in vivo* tumorigenesis in the

* Corresponding author: Oswaldo Keith Okamoto. Present address: Centro de Estudos do Genoma Humano, Departamento de Genética e Biologia Evolutiva, Instituto de Biociências, Universidade de São Paulo. Rua do Matão 277, Cidade Universitária, Caixa Postal 05508-090 São Paulo, SP, Brazil. Phone: (55 11) 3091-7501. e-mail: keith.okamoto@usp.br.

absence of immune suppression more closely mimics the physiological milieu encountered by tumor cells and could be explored as a xenograft orthotopic model of human glioblastomas to address new therapeutic approaches, particularly those involving immune effector mechanisms.

Keywords: glioblastomas, mesenchymal stem cells, immunocompetent rats, xenograft orthotopic model

Introduction

Small subsets of cells displaying stem cell characteristics and tumorigenic capability have been identified in a number of solid tumors including breast, brain, colon, prostate, lung, melanoma, pancreatic, and head and neck tumors [1-8]. These cancer stem cells are thought to be responsible for tumor initiation, tumor recurrence after conventional cytotoxic therapy, and metastasis. Due to their clinical relevance, cancer stem cells are natural targets for therapeutic development in tumors of poor prognosis such as glioblastoma multiforme (GBM), the most common primary malignant tumor of the central nervous system [9]. Mean survival rate of patients with GBM stands below 16 months and no effective treatment is currently available for this highly aggressive brain tumor.

In GBM, cancer stem cells have been identified based on the expression of CD133 antigen, an integral membrane glycoprotein of 97kDa. Initial studies have reported that as few as one hundred CD133+ cells are sufficient to initiate tumors *in vivo,* while injections of thousands of the remaining cells composing the tumor bulk consistently fail or form new tumors at lower yield in immunocompromised mice [1, 2, 5, 7]. Furthermore, GBM stem cells display enhanced ability to efflux conventional anti-cancer drugs such as doxorubicin, etoposide, carboplatin, and BCNU [10-13], and are less sensitive to radiation, most likely due to an exacerbated expression of *MDR1* and DNA repair genes, respectively [14-15].

CD133+ stem cells have also been isolated and characterized in several GBM cell lines [16-19], establishing a useful experimental model to study cancer stem cell biology and to evaluate new therapeutic strategies aiming at selectively targeting this subset of highly tumorigenic cells. Nonetheless, recent studies have reported the characterization of tumorigenic stem-like cells that do not express CD133 in GBM [20-21]. Neural stem cells lacking CD133 expression have also been characterized in humans and mice [22] raising interesting questions regarding CD133 as a bona fide marker of tumorigenic GBM stem cells.

In this study, we report that human GBM cells from the U87MG cell line display a predominant mesenchymal stem cell (MSC) phenotype. These cells express typical MSC markers such as CD44, CD90, and CD105, and are capable of undergoing adipogenic, osteogenic, and chondrogenic differentiation *in vitro*. Furthermore, these MSC-like GBM cells express low levels of HLA-DR and form infiltrative intracranial tumors when injected in immunocompetent rats. Pleomorphism, necrosis, and hemorrhages could be detected in the brains of rats harboring tumors, resembling common features of human GBM. This *in vivo* tumorigenic process in the absence of immune suppression more closely mimics the natural conditions encountered by tumor cells and could be explored as a xenograft orthotopic model of human GBM to address new therapeutic approaches for malignant gliomas.

Materials and Methods

Cell Culture

The human GBM cell line U87MG was kindly provided by Dr. Suely K. N. Marie from the Laboratory of Medical Investigation (LIM15) at the University of São Paulo. Cells were grown in Dulbecco's-modified Eagle's Medium-Low Glucose (DMEM-LG, Invitrogen), supplemented with 2 mM L-glutamine, 10% bovine fetal serum, 100 U/mL penicillin, and 100 μg/mL streptomycin, in a humidified atmosphere at 37°C with 5% CO_2.

Flow Cytometric Immunophenotyping

In order to analyze cell-surface expression of typical MSC markers, cells were incubated at 4°C for 30 minutes with the following monoclonal antibodies to human antigens: CD14-FITC, CD29-PE, CD31-PE, CD133-PE, CD44-PE, CD45-PerCP-Cy5, CD73-PE, CD90-APC, CD166-PE, HLA-DR-PerCP-Cy5 (Becton Dickinson), CD105-PE (Chemicon), with respective isotype controls IgG2a (FITC), IgG1 (PE), IgG1 (PerCP Cy-5.5), and IgG1 (APC) (Becton Dickinson). Cells were rinsed twice with cold PBS and fixed with cold, freshly prepared 1% paraformaldehyde (Sigma-Aldrich). A minimum of 30.000 fluorescent cellular events were acquired on the FACSAria flow cytometer and analyzed with FacsDiva software (Becton Dickinson).

In Vitro Cell Differentiation Assays

GBM cells were subjected to adipogenic, osteogenic, and chondrogenic differentiation *in vitro*, according to standard protocols [23]. Briefly, cells were grown in six-well culture plates as described above. After reaching 80% confluence, cells were transferred to Minimum Essential Medium Alpha Medium (α-MEM, GIBCO Invitrogen) supplemented with either adipogenic medium (10% FBS, 1μM dexamethasone, 100 μg/mL 3-isobutyl-1-methylxanthine, 5 μg/mL insulin, and 60 μM indomethacin), osteogenic medium (10% FBS, 0,1 mM dexamethasone, 10 μM β-glycerophosphate, and 50 μg/mL ascorbic acid), or chondrogenic medium (10% FBS, 50 μg/mL ascorbic acid, 10 ng/mL TGF-β, and 6,25 μg/mL insulin). Cells were cultivated for three weeks and stained with Oil Red O, Alizarin Red, or PAS/Alcian Blue to access intracellular lipid accumulation, extracellular matrix calcification, and chondrogenic proteoglycans, respectively. Human MSCs isolated from cord blood and bone marrow were included in the assays as positive controls.

In Vivo Tumor Xenograft Model

Adult male Wistar rats (200-250g) were anesthetized with ketamine hydrochloride (90 mg/kg, i.p.) and xylazin hydrochloride (10 mg/kg, i.p.). After shaving a small area on their heads, the animals were positioned in a stereotaxic frame (KOPF® Model 1430, Germany).

The scalp was sterilized with iodine and 70% ethanol and a median incision of approximately 1.5 cm was made. The cranial cavity was assessed by a right frontal hole using an electric mini-drill (Micromotor LB100, Beltec). A total of 10^6 GBM cells were resuspended in 5 μL of DMEM-LG medium without serum and inoculated with a high precision microsyringe (model 701RN, Hamilton Co.) into the motor cortex, 2.0 mm anterior to bregma, 2.0 mm lateral to midline, and 2.0 mm ventral to dura [24], at a 0.5 μL/min rate. At the end of cell injection, the needle was kept in the incision for 5 minutes and removed slowly to prevent cell suspension from flowing back. Sham animals received 5 μL of vehicle only. The scalp was closed with 2-0 silk suture and the animals housed under standard controlled conditions (7:00 AM/7:00 P.M. light/dark cycle; 20-22°C; 45-55% humidity) with food and water *ad libitum*. Histological analysis was performed 15 or 30 days post-intracranial implantation of tumor cells. All efforts were made to minimize animal suffering as proposed by the International Ethical Guideline for Biomedical Research (CIOMS/OMS, 1985). The study was approved by the Ethics Committee for animal research of the Federal University of São Paulo, Brazil (CEP 2003/07).

Histological Analysis

Animals were deeply anaesthetized with sodium pentobarbital, 75mg/kg i. p., and decapitated. Brains were removed from the skull, frozen in cold isopentane solution (Sigma-Aldrich Corporation, St. Louis) at -25 °C, and then sectioned at 20 μm on a cryostat. Coronal histological sections of the tumor xenograft and surrounding brain area were mounted on silanized microscope slides (Star Frost ®, Knittel-Gläser, Germany), and stained with hematoxylin-eosin or according to the Nissl method. Microscope images were captured by an ExwaveHAD Color video digital camera (Sony) attached to a Nikon Eclipse E600 microscope, using the WinAVI Video Capture software.

Immunofluorescence

Human cells were detected in rat brains by immunofluorescence using antibodies specific to human DNA. Brain slices were obtained as described above. Histological sections were blocked with 10% FBS, 5% bovine serum albumin (BSA), and 0.1% Triton X-100 in PBS for 1 hour at room temperature and incubated at 4°C overnight with primary antibody (mouse anti-human nuclei CAT# MAB1281, Chemicon International, California, USA) at a 1:20 dilution, followed by incubation with secondary anti-mouse IgG antibody at a 1:100 dilution for 2 hours at room temperature. Tissues were counterstained with 5μg/mL 4',6-Diamidino-2-phenylindol (DAPI) and microscope slides mounted in Vectashield medium (Vector Laboratories). Immunofluorescence analysis was performed in a Zeiss Imager Z1 Apotome microscope with epi-fluorescence, or using an argon ion laser scan microscope LSM 410 (Zeiss – Jena, Germany). Images were captured and digitalized with the Axiovision 4.8 software.

Results

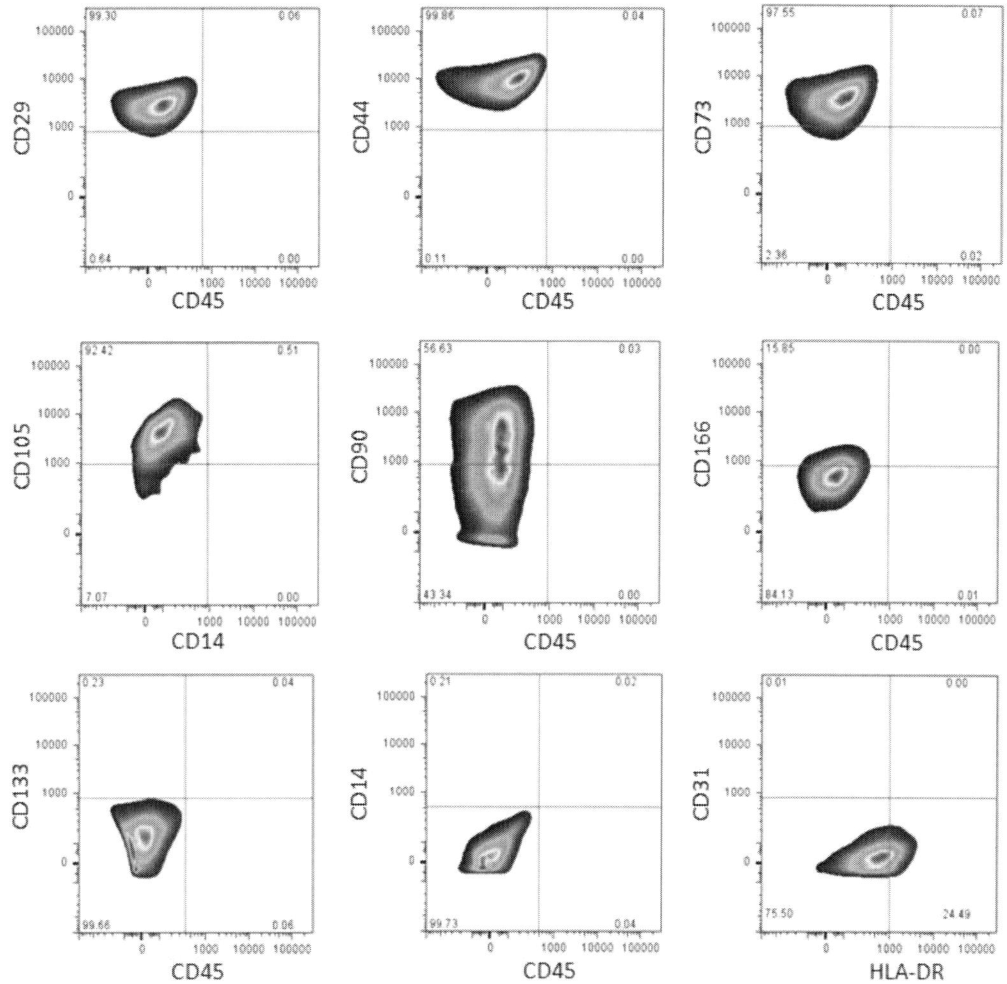

Figure 1. Flow cytometry analysis of cell surface markers in human glioblastoma cells. U87MG cells labeled positively for typical mesenchymal cell markers such as CD29, CD44, CD73, CD105, CD90, and CD166. Similarly to mesenchymal stem cells, U87MG cells lack expression of CD133, CD45, CD14, CD31, and HLA-DR. Heat map code: the highest and the lowest concentration of cells are depicted in the red and dark blue areas of the plots, respectively.

Under standard culture conditions, U87MG glioblastoma cells were found to express cell membrane proteins that are typical mesenchymal markers such as CD29, CD44, CD166, CD90, CD105, and CD73. On the other hand, neither hematopoietic (CD45, CD133, CD14, HLA-DR) nor endothelial (CD31) markers were detected on the surface of U87MG cells by flow cytometry (Figure 1). Such immunophenotype is identical to that of human MSCs. In fact, this flow cytometric immunophenotyping is one useful and widespread criterion to characterize human MSCs from different biological sources including bone marrow, umbilical cord and adipose tissue. Another critical parameter used in the characterization of human MSC is the *in vitro* cell differentiation capability towards adipogenic, osteogenic and chondrogenic cell lineages. Noteworthy, under proper conditions, glioblastoma cells were also found to have multipotent properties similar to those reported by MSC. When cultured in chondrogenic medium, glioblastoma cells displayed a round-shaped morphology with pericellular proteoglycan deposition evidenced by PAS/Alcian Blue staining (Figure 2 A-C). Osteogenic differentiation was also observed for some glioblastoma cells based on Alizarin Red staining of intracellular calcium deposits (Figure 2, D-F). Furthermore, under adipogenic differentiation conditions, glioblastoma cells underwent cell morphology change and displayed multiple intracellular lipid-rich vacuoles, as identified by Oil-red O staining (Figure 2, G-I).

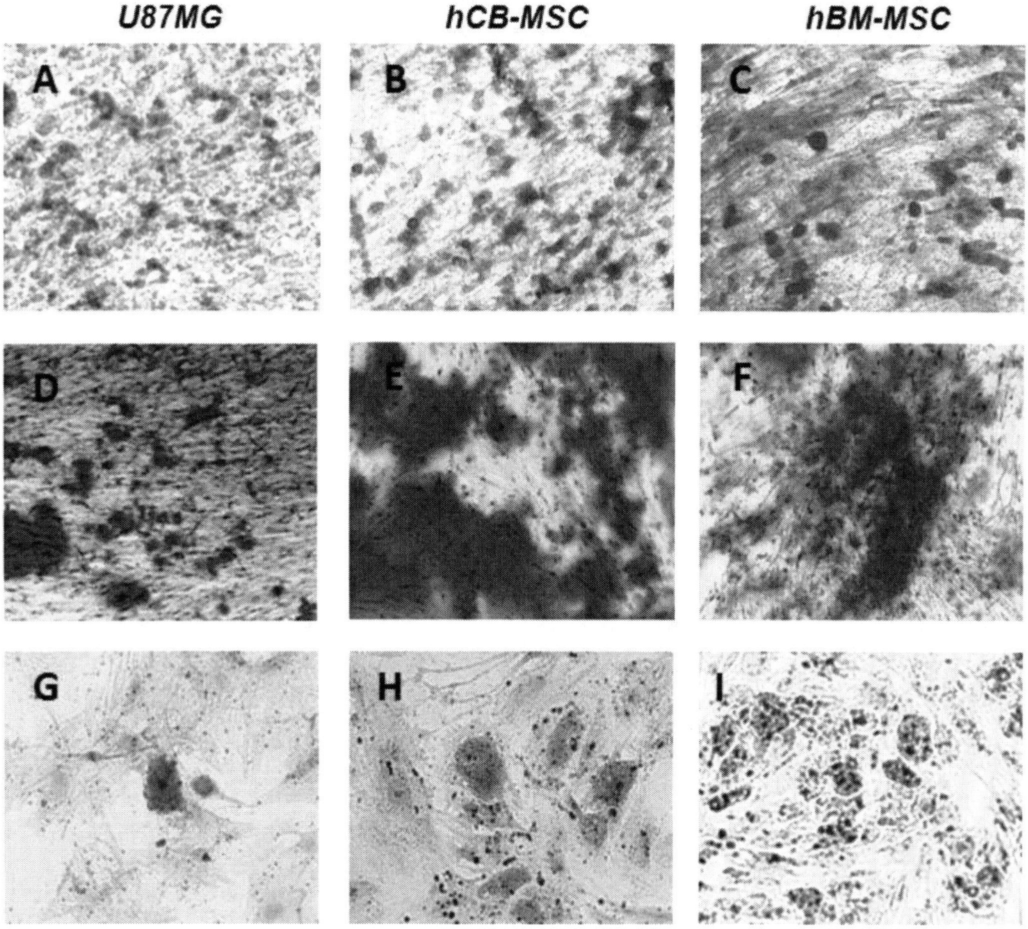

Figure 2. In vitro plasticity of human glioblastoma cells. U87MG cells were capable of differentiating into cells of mesodermal lineage. Monolayer cultures were stained with PAS/Alcian Blue to access chondrogenic differentiation (A-C). Osteogenic differentiation based on calcium deposition was shown by Alizarin Red (D-F). Adipogenesis was detected by the formation of intracytoplasmic lipid droplets stained with Oil red O (G-I). Human mesenchymal stem cells from cord blood (hUC-MSC) and bone marrow (hBM-MSC) were included in the assays as positive controls of cell differentiation.

Upon stereotaxic injection within the motor cortex of immunocompetent rats, U87MG cells formed intensely cellularized tumors. Human tumor xenografts could be visualized 15 days-post injection, characterized by growth of glioblastoma cells in the injection space and local cell spreading into the adjacent brain tissue, including the cortical surface close to the injection site (Figure 3, A). Viable tumor cells were visualized by Nissl staining (Figure 3, B, D). Tumor xenografts were confirmed by immunofluorescence with antibody specific to human DNA (Figure 3, C).

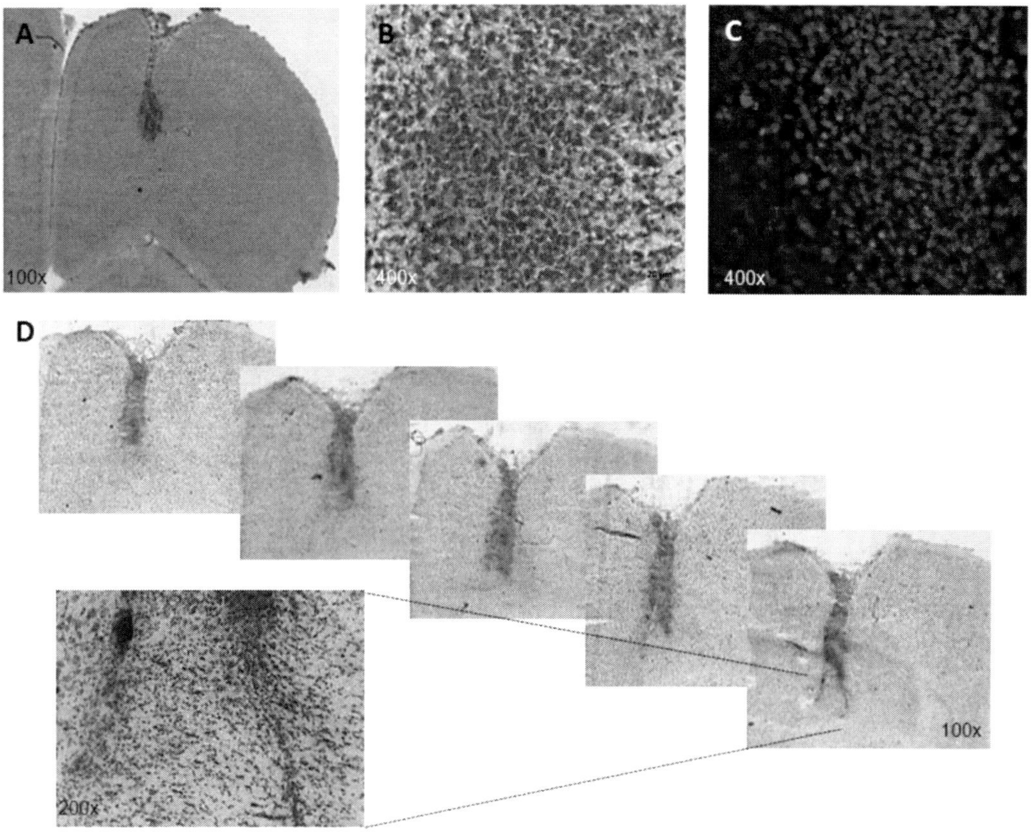

Figure 3. Human glioblastoma xenografts in immunocompetent rats. U87MG cells were able to form intracranial tumors after stereotaxic injection into the motor cortex. (A) Intensely cellularized tumors could visualized 15 days post-injection. (B) Viable pleomorphic cells in the center of the tumor mass. (C) Co-localization of DAPI and anti-human nuclei fluorescence confirming presence of U87MG cells in the same region depicted in B. (D) Serial brain slices displaying tumor cell spreading into the parenchyma and cortical regions. A = HE staining; B and D = Nissl staining; C = immunofluorescence.

After 30 days of cell injection, larger intracranial tumor xenografts were noticed. Mitotically active glioblastoma cells displaying pleomorphic morphology were detected in the center of the tumor mass, where necrotic and/or hemorrhagic foci could also be observed (Figure 4). Infiltrative cell growth was more evident at this later stage, forming a gradient of cell density at the brain-tumor interface. Tumors displayed an irregular board with cells infiltrating into the parenchyma, either isolated or in small clusters (Figure 4, A-C). Invasion of tumor cells toward the corpus callosum, caudate-putamen, and perivascular spaces was also found in some cases (figure 4, D-F). All animals survived the surgical procedure and no signs of motor deficits and body weight loss were observed during the course of tumor development.

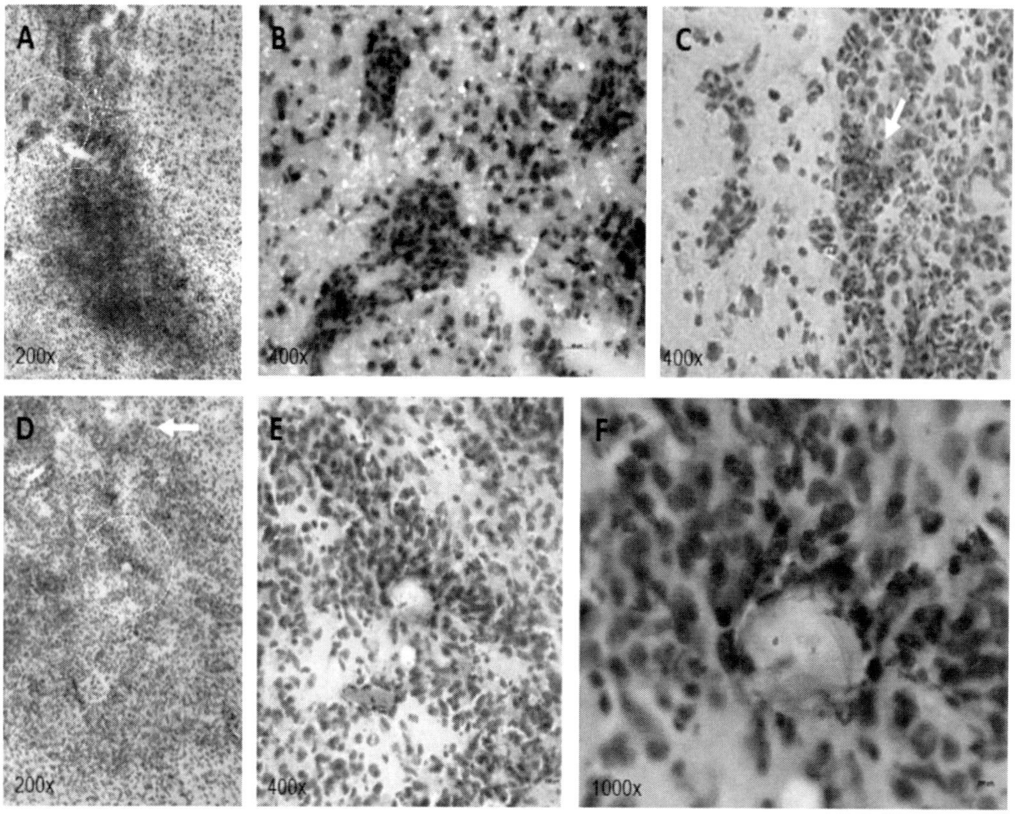

Figure 4. Anatomo-pathological features of human U87MG tumor xenografts. (A) Necrosis and areas of more highly packed tumor cells were evident within intracranial tumors developed 30 days post-injection. The tumor-brain border was often irregular due to local invasion of tumor cells. (B) Magnification of a border region (dashed circle in A), showing tumor cell islets penetrating the surrounding brain tissue. (C-F) Areas of hemorrhage (white arrows in C and D) and perivascular concentration of tumor cells (dashed circle in D; E and F).

Discussion

Human glioblastoma cell lines display variable tumorigenic activity *in vivo*. The different proportion of cancer stem cells in each cell line could partially explain such variability. *In vitro* expansion and intracranial tumor development can be exacerbated by serial passage of stem-like GBM cells *in vivo*. Secondary cell lines established from tumor xenografts developed by orthotopic implantation of GBM stem-like cells are enriched in tumorigenic cells, which preserve the same karyotypic features, molecular signature, and multipotency of their parental cells [25].

Bao and co-workers [26] have shown that the proportion of CD133+ stem cells in short-term cultures of the human GBM cell line A172 and primary GBM cultures is significantly increased after ionizing radiation treatment. Human glioma xenografts derived from irradiated cultures were also enriched in $CD133^+$ cells relative to untreated cultures. Such increment in CD133+ cell fraction correlated with enhanced tumor growth and vascularity in nude mice.

Enrichment of stem-like cells can also be achieved by changing the culture conditions. When using medium suitable for neural stem cell cultivation, Qiang and co-workers [18] where able to increase the proportion of CD133+ cells as well as side population (SP) cells in U87MG, A172 and U251 GBM cell line cultures. The SP cells are named by their disposition in flow cytometry plots and correspond to those cells with increased efficiency in efflux fluorescent dyes. Such SP is comprised by highly tumorigenic cells displaying self-renewal and multi-lineage differentiation capabilities. The proportion of SP cells in common GBM cell lines such as SK-MG-1, U87MG, U373MG, KNS42 and U251 is usually lower than 2%, although larger percentages may be obtained by progressively increasing the concentration of serum-free neural stem cell medium [16].

Recent studies describing the characterization of GBM stem-like cells lacking CD133 expression suggest the existence of distinct subsets of CSC or changes in CSC features depending on the culture conditions [20-21]. Interestingly, in addition to the reported neural stem cell-like properties, our results indicate that U87MG cells also display features of MSC. These findings are in agreement with the recent report of cells with mesenchymal phenotype in whole specimens of human glioblastomas [27]. Furthermore, Ricci-Vitiani and co-worker [28] reported CD133+ stem cells isolated from human glioblastomas to be multipotent and capable of differentiating into cells of mesenchymal type, in addition to neural cells. Here we show that a MSC phenotype can be preserved in an established GBM cell line. Through a detailed *in vitro* characterization, U87MG cells were found to display full MSC antigen markers, including low HLA-DR expression, in addition to multipotent differentiation capability, which had not been previously demonstrated. Interestingly, MSC properties have recently been found for cells undergoing epithelial-to-mesenchymal transition which is a process involved in tumor invasion and metastasis [29].

More unexpectedly was the ability of a human glioblastoma cell line to form intracranial tumors in rats without immunosuppression. Tumor xenografts were found in rat brains for at least 30 days, displaying basic features of human GBM. Gliomas are known to scape tumor-specific immunity by different mechanisms involving both intrinsic properties of glioma cells, as well as microenvironmental factors [30-31]. Intracranial growth of U87MG cells and ensuing tumor formation could have been facilitated by virtue of the immune privileged nature of the central nervous system. Indeed, in a xenograft glioma model, tumors have been generated through implantation of C6 rat glioma cells into the brain of adult and neonatal normal mice, with largest tumors attained between 21 and 28 days post-implantation. Conversely, subcutaneous inoculation of C6 cells in the same mice did not form tumors [32].

Furthermore, it is well established that MSC are poorly immunogenic since they lack constitutive HLA-class II expression and display immunosuppressive activity [33]. Similarly, U87MG cells were also found to express low levels of HLA-class II and should be expected to have low immunogenic potential, although it remains to be investigated whether additional immunomodulatory properties could contribute with its tumorigenic capability in immuno-competent rats.

In conclusion, our findings reveal that human glioblastoma U87MG cells display typical properties of MSC *in vitro*, express low levels of HLA-DR, and are able to form intracranial tumors in immunocompetent animals. To our knowledge, this is the first report of tumor development through implantation of human glioblastoma cells into rats not subjected to either genetically or pharmacologically forms of immunosuppression. Since such conditions more closely mimics the physiological milieu encountered by tumor cells within the brain, the intracranial implantation of U87MG cells in immunocompetent rats could be used as an alternative xenograft orthotopic model of human glioblastoma. Some of the anticipated uses of such model would include the study of gliomagenesis as well as of new molecular therapy approaches for malignant astrocytomas, including monoclonal antibodies with immune effector toxicity, and tumor vaccines.

Acknowledgments

The authors thank Mariane Secco for technical assistance, Dr. S. Marie for providing the U87MG cell line, and Dr. L.R.Travassos for kindly providing access to his cell culture facility. This work was supported by grants from INCT-Células Tronco em Doenças Genéticas Humanas, CNPq, CAPES, and FAPESP. COR, DES, AMN, MCLP, and LJ were recipients of fellowships from CAPES and CNPq.

Conflict of Interest Statement

No authors declared any potential conflicts of interest. The authors alone are responsible for the content and writing of this paper.

References

[1] Al-Hajj, M., Wicha, M.S., Benito-Hernandez, A., Morrison, S.J., Clarke, M.F.. Prospective identification of tumorigenic breast cancer cells. *Proceedings of the National Academy of Sciences of the United States of America,* 2003;100, 3983–3988.

[2] Singh, S.K., Hawkins, C., Clarke, I.D., Squire, J.A., Bayani, J., Hide,T., Henkelman, R.M., Cusimano, M.D., Dirks, P.B. Identification of human brain tumour initiating cells. *Nature,* 2004;432, 396–401.

[3] Collins, A.T., Berry, P.A., Hyde, C., Stower, M.J., Maitland, N.J. Prospective identification of tumorigenic prostate cancer stem cells. *Cancer Research,* 2005; 65,10946–10951.

[4] Patrawala, L., Calhoun, T., Schneider-Broussard, R., Li, H., Bhatia, B., Tang, S., Reilly, J.G., Chandra, D., Zhou, J., Claypool, K., Coghlan, L., Tang, D.G. Highly purified CD44+ prostate cancer cells from xenograft human tumors are enriched in tumorigenic and metastatic progenitor cells. *Oncogene,* 2006;25, 1696–1708.

[5] Li, C., Heidt, D.G, Dalerba, P., Burant, C.F., Zhang, L., Adsay, V., Wicha ,M., Clarke, M.F., Simeone, D.M. Identification of pancreatic cancer stem cells. *Cancer Resarch,* 2007;67,1030–1037.

[6] O'Brien, C.A., Pollett, A., Gallinger, S., Dick, J.E. A human colon cancer cell capable of initiating tumour growth in immunodeficient mice. *Nature,* 2007;445, 106–110.

[7] Prince, M.E., Sivanandan, R., Kaczorowski, A., Wolf, G.T., Kaplan, M.J., Dalerba, P., Weissman, I.L., Clarke, M.F., Ailles, L.E. Identification of a subpopulation of cells with cancer stem cell properties in head and neck squamous cell carcinoma.

Proceedings of the National Academy of Sciences of the United States of America, 2007;104, 973–978.

[8] Ricci-Vitiani, L., Lombardi, D.G., Pilozzi, E., Biffoni, M., Todaro, M., Peschle, C, De Maria, R. Identification and expansion of human colon-cancer-initiating cells. *Nature*, 2007;445, 111–115.

[9] Okamoto, O.K., Perez, J.F. Targeting cancer stem cells with monoclonal antibodies: a new perspective in cancer therapy and diagnosis. *Expert Review Molecular Diagnostics*, 2008;8(4):387-93.

[10] Hirschmann-Jax, C., Foster, A.E., Wulf, G.G., Nuchtern, J.G., Jax, T.W., Gobel, U., Goodell, M.A., Brenner, M.K. A distinct "side population" of cells with high drug efflux capacity in human tumor cells. *Proceedings of the National Academy of Sciences of the United States of America*, 2004;101, 14228-14233.

[11] Hadnagy, A., Gaboury, L., Beaulieu, R., Balicki, D. SP analysis may be used to identify cancer stem cell populations. *Experimental Cell Research*, 2006;312, 3701-3710.

[12] Jørgensen, H.G., Holyoake, T.L. Characterization of cancer stem cells in chronic myeloid leukaemia. *Biochemical Society Transactions*, 2007;35(Pt 5), 1347-1351.

[13] Nakai, E., Park, K., Yawata, T., Chihara, T., Kumazawa, A., Nakabayashi, H., Shimizu, K. Enhanced MDR1 expression and chemoresistance of cancer stem cells derived from glioblastoma. *Cancer Investigation*, 2009;27(9):901-8.

[14] Liu, G., Black, K.L, Yu, JS. Sensitization of malignant glioma to chemotherapy through dendritic cell vaccination. *Expert Review of Vaccines*, 2006;5, 233 – 247.

[15] Phillips, T.M., McBride, W.H., Pajonk, F. The response of CD24($^-$/low)/CD44+ breast cancer – initiating cells to radiation. *Journal of the National Cancer Institute*, 2006;98, 1777–1785.

[16] Yu, S.C., Ping, Y.F., Yi, L., Zhou, Z.H., Chen, J.H., Yao, X.H., Gao, L., Wang, J.M., Bian, X.W. Isolation and characterization of cancer stem cells from a human glioblastoma cell line U87. *Cancer Lett*ers, 2008;28;265(1):124-34.

[17] Wu, A., Oh, S., Wiesner, S.M., Ericson, K., Chen, L., Hall, W.A., Champoux, P.E., Low, W.C., Ohlfest, J.R. Persistence of CD133+ cells in human and mouse glioma cell lines: detailed characterization of GL261 glioma cells with cancer stem cell-like properties. *Stem Cells and Development*, 2008;17(1):173-84.

[18] Qiang, L., Yang, Y., Ma, Y.J., Chen, F.H., Zhang, L.B., Liu, W., Qi, Q., Lu, N., Tao, L., Wang, X.T, You, Q.D., Guo, Q.L. Isolation and characterization of cancer stem like cells in human glioblastoma cell lines. *Cancer Letters*, 2009:279(1):13-21.

[19] Fukaya, R., Ohta, S., Yamaguchi, M., Fujii, H., Kawakami, Y., Kawase, T., Toda, M. Isolation of cancer stem-like cells from a side population of a human glioblastoma cell line, SK-MG-1. *Cancer Letters*, 2010;291(2):150-7.

[20] Beier, D., Hau, P., Proescholdt, M., Lohmeier, A., Wischhusen, J., Oefner, P.J., Aigner, L., Brawanski, A., Bogdahn, U., Beier, C.P. CD133(+) and CD133(-) glioblastoma-derived cancer stem cells show differential growth characteristics and molecular profiles. *Cancer Research*, 2007;67(9):4010-5.

[21] Nishide, K., Nakatani, Y., Kiyonari, H., Kondo, T. Glioblastoma formation from cell population depleted of Prominin1-expressing cells. *PLoS One*, 2009;4(8):e6869.

[22] Sun, Y., Kong, W., Falk, A., Hu, J., Zhou, L., Pollard, S., and Smith, A. CD133 (Prominin) negative human neural stem cells are clonogenic and tripotent. *PLoS One*, 2009;4(5):e5498.

[23] Secco, M., Zucconi, E., Vieira, N.M., Fogaça, L.L., Cerqueira, A., Carvalho, M.D., Jazedje, T., Okamoto, O.K., Muotri, A.R., Zatz, M. Multipotent stem cells from umbilical cord: cord is richer than blood! *Stem Cells,* 2008;26(1):146-50.

[24] Paxinos, G., Watson, C. The rat brain: in stereotaxic coordinates. Academic Press. San Diego, 1995 second edition.

[25] Galli, R., Binda, E., Orfanelli, U., Cipelletti, B., Gritti, A., De Vitis, S., Fiocco, R., Foroni, C., Dimeco, F., Vescovi, A. Isolation and characterization of tumorigenic, stem-like neural precursors from human glioblastoma. *Cancer Research,* 2004;64(19):7011-21.

[26] Bao, S., Wu, Q., McLendon, R.E., Hao, Y., Shi, Q., Hjelmeland, A.B., Dewhirst, M.W., Bigner, D.D., Rich, J.N. Glioma stem cells promote radioresistance by preferential activation of the DNA damage response. *Nature*, 2006;444(7120):756-60.

[27] Rieske, P., Golanska, E., Zakrzewska, M., Piaskowski, S., Hulas-Bigoszewska, K., Wolańczyk, M., Szybka, M., Witusik-Perkowska, M., Jaskolski, D.J., Zakrzewski, K., Biernat, W., Krynska, B., Liberski, P.P. Arrested neural and advanced mesenchymal differentiation of glioblastoma cells-comparative study with neural progenitors. *BMC Cancer*, 2009;9:54.

[28] Ricci-Vitiani, L., Pallini, R., Larocca, L.M., Lombardi, D.G., Signore, M., Pierconti, F., Petrucci, G., Montano, N., Maira, G., De Maria, R. Mesenchymal differentiation of glioblastoma stem cells. *Cell Death Differentiation,* 2008;9:1491-8.

[29] Battula, V.L., Evans, K.W., Hollier, B.G., Shi, Y., Marini, F.C., Ayyanan, A., Wang, R.Y., Brisken, C., Guerra, R., Andreeff, M., Mani, S.A. Epithelial-Mesenchymal Transition-Derived Cells Exhibit Multi-Lineage Differentiation Potential Similar to Mesenchymal Stem Cells. *Stem Cells,* 2010;8:1435-45.

[30] Okada, H., Kohanbash, G., Zhu, X., Kastenhuber, E.R., Hoji, A., Ueda, R., Fujita, M. Immunotherapeutic approaches for glioma. *Critical Reviews Immunology,* 2009:29(1):1-42.

[31] Albesiano, E., Han, J.E., Lim, M. Mechanisms of local immunoresistance in glioma. *Neurosurgery* Clinics of *North America,* 2010;21(1):17-29.

[32] Kaye, A.H., Morstyn, G., Gardner, I., Pyke, K. Development of a xenograft glioma model in mouse brain. *Cancer Research*, 1986;46(3):1367-73.

[33] Morandi, F., Raffaghello, L., Bianchi, G., Meloni, F., Salis, A., Millo, E., Ferrone, S., Barnaba, V., Pistoia, V. Immunogenicity of human mesenchymal stem cells in HLA-class I-restricted T-cell responses against viral or tumor-associated antigens. *Stem Cells,* 2008:5:1275-1287.

In: Stem Cells in Disease
Editor: Prasad S. Koka
ISBN: 978-1-62257-169-7
© 2012 Nova Science Publishers, Inc.

Chapter VI

Visualization of the Hematopoietic Microenvironment: An Alternative Approach Using Intravital Microscopy

***Lyudmila Sikora*[1] *and Sophia Khaldoyanidi*[2,3*#]**
[1] Animal Cell Therapies Inc, San Diego, California, US
[2] Torrey Pines Institute for Molecular Studies, San Diego, California, US
[3]Cascade LifeSciences Inc, San Diego, Callifornia, US

Keywords: Bone marrow, hematopoietic stem cell, stem cell niche, intravital microscopy

The behavior of hematopoietic stem cells (HSCs) is regulated by signals arising from the microenvironment in response to physiological and pathophysiological demands [1]. However, there are significant gaps in our understanding of the biology of this microenvironment that impede progress towards optimizing the therapeutic application of stem cell transplantation. There are many challenges to studying the stem cell microenvironment, including the difficulty in identifying the cellular structure of the bone marrow (BM) hematopoietic niche. Here, we suggest the use of an alternate experimental model to visualize and delineate the anatomical compartments of BM.

Currently, there is no consensus operational definition for the 'HSC niche'. The original observation that "the stem cell is seen in association with other cells which determine its behavior"[2] first suggested the existence of a niche that regulates HSC function. During the mid-1980s it was then postulated that "the fundamental characteristic of a stem cell is self-renewal" [1], suggesting the niche as a microenvironmental structure regulating HSC self-

* Corresponding Author: Sophia K. Khaldoyanidi, MD, PhD, Torrey Pines Institute for Molecular Studies, 3550 General Atomics Court, San Diego CA, 92121. Phone: (858) 597-3879. Fax: (858) 597-3804. E-mail: skhaldoyanidi@tpims.org. www.tpims.org.
# Author contribution summary: Sophia Khaldoyanidi: Conception and design, data analysis and interpretation, financial support, manuscript writing; Lyudmila Sikora: Microsurgery, HSC purification, cell injections and collection of data.

renewal or maintenance. Today, it is increasingly recognized that the niche is responsible not only for HSC maintenance (e.g. self-renewal *versus* differentiation, and survival *versus* apoptosis), but also regulates other vital HSC functions such as proliferation *versus* quiescence and mobilization *versus* retention. Thus, it is clear that the stem cell niche must be multifunctional [3, 4].

This multifunctionality has lead to debate as to whether more than one "niche" exists, which reflects the fact that the anatomical dimensions of the niche have not been delineated. In this regard, another factor that contributes to the complexity of the field is the lack of consensus about the identity of the cell(s) that constitute the HSC niche. While early studies supported a role for stromal fibroblast-like cells in structuring the niche [5], later findings favored the involvement of osteoblasts and BM endothelial cells [6-8], resulting in the nomination of "osteogenic" and "endothelial" BM niches. Suggestions that macrophages are important for HSC function date to the mid-1980s [9 10 11]. However, BM macrophages remained neglected as a structural component of the niche until the recent creation of the macrophage-Fas-induced apoptosis (MAFIA) mouse [12]. It has been demonstrated that ablation of BM macrophages leads to extramedullary hematopoiesis in the MAFIA mice, and subsequent studies have shown that BM macrophages are required to maintain osteoblasts [13], providing strong evidence that macrophages play a critical role in structuring the hematopoietic niche. This phenomenon is likely to involve not only the production of soluble hematopoiesis-regulatory factors and extracellular matrix, but also direct cell-cell interactions between macrophages and other cells in the BM milieu, phagocytosis of cell debris, and differentiation into osteoclasts. Osteoclasts control not only bone resorption, but also osteoblast chemotaxis and thus, formation of the hematopoietic niche [14].

Although there is no doubt that culturing BM cells *in vitro* is a useful experimental model that has provided important information, this approach is not capable of delineating an anatomical structure of the niche, or of identifying the cell-cell interactions that take place during hematopoiesis *in vivo*. The ability to microscopically observe BM in a living animal would be a very useful tool, but marrow cells are surrounded by a thick bone that impedes direct observation and this has presented a major obstacle to delineating BM anatomical compartments, including the stem cells niche(s).

The first attempts to visualize intra-marrow space *in situ* were performed in rabbits [15, 16], and required microsurgical procedures to create a narrow window in the bone, and implant a metallic chamber for long-term observation of the exposed marrow. Undoubtedly, this method is associated with considerable trauma, and chronic pain and distress to the animals.

An alternative *in vivo* methodology allowed direct microscopic observation of the calvaria of the murine skull, which are sufficiently thin to allow visualization of *in situ* cell-cell interactions within the marrow vasculature [17]. This technique was further adapted for visualization of the hematopoietic niche[18]. While extremely informative, this approach also has limitations: 1) Experimental animals cannot be observed for an extended period; 2) The approach cannot be adapted to human tissue; and 3) The marrow cannot be locally manipulated. Thus, there remains a need to develop alternate methods to visualize and manipulate the stem cell niche that circumvents these limitations.

We propose that intravital microscopy using dorsal skinfold chambers is one such approach. Intravital microscopy is widely used in many fields of biology and pathophysiology. In one application, implants of various tissues, such as lung, or tumor spheroids, are inserted into dorsal skinfold chambers of the host animals [19,20]. This approach is non-traumatic and allows observation for at least 2 months. Most importantly, human tissue can be implanted into the chambers, revascularized, and used for experimentation [21, 22].

We have used the dorsal skinfold chamber approach to implant fragments of marrow-containing murine bones for long-term observation of the HSC microenvironment [Figure 1]. To prepare the dorsal skinfold chambers, mice were anesthetized and two identical titanium frames were implanted into a dorsal skin-fold parallel to the dorsum, to sandwich the stretched double layer of skin as described before [20]. One layer of the dorsal skin was completely removed in a circular area, and the remaining underlying skin layer was covered with a coverslip incorporated into one of the frames [Figure 1A]. After recovery from anesthesia, and a 2-3 day convalescence period, fragments of syngeneic marrow-containing femoral bones were placed into the skin chamber over the subcutaneous tissue [Figure 1B]. The transplanted BM isografts were completely revascularized within 7 to 10 days post-transplantation [Figure 1 C, D, and E].

Murine HSCs, which were purified from syngeneic bone marrow using MACS, *ex vivo* labeled with 5-carboxyfluorescein diacetate (CFDA) and injected into the tail vein of chamber-bearing mice, were shown directly by intravital fluorescent microscopy to interact with marrow microvasculature within the skinfold chamber [Figure 1F]. The images were recorded and analyzed *post hoc* to distinguish HSCs within the marrow vasculature from those transmigrating or located outside the vasculature [Figure 1F].

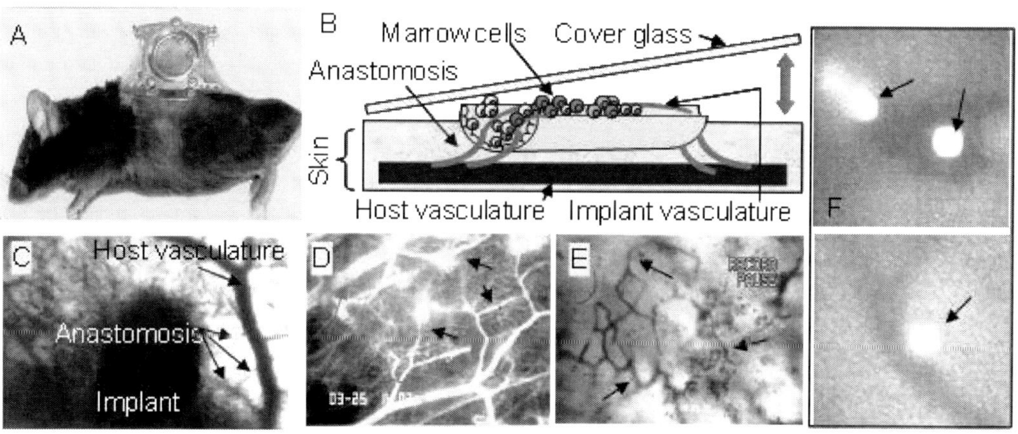

Figure 1. The dorsal skinfold chamber model. A: A C57BL/6 mouse with the implanted titanium dorsal skin chamber. B: Schematic representation of the implanted bone fragment with marrow cells. C: Revascularization of the implant was visualized using light microscopy (x40). D: To confirm the formation of vascular anastomosis between the host vasculature and the implant vasculature, mice were injected with FITC-dextran to visualize the intravascular space (x60). E: The implant vasculature can be visualized by light microscopy. F: Interactions of the CFDA-labeled HSCs with marrow were visualized by stroboscopic epi-illumination using a video-triggered xenon lamp and a Leitz Ploemopak epi-illuminator employing a 12 filter block. The images were recorded through a silicon-intensified tube camera using s X10/0.13 water immersion objective and a SVHS video recorder HC-6600 (x250).

There are several important advantages to this approach: 1) The chamber implants can remain in place for 2 months or longer, allowing the behavior of cells within the implant to be monitored over an extended period; 2) Fragments of marrow-containing bones can be transferred, thus maintaining the anatomical structure of the niche. Minor damage heals naturally during the period of revascularization; 3) The cover glass can be lifted to allow procedures to be performed on the living animal; for example, perfusion of cytokines, small molecules, and antibodies, or staining of implant cells; 4) NOD/SCID mice can be used as the host, allowing implantation of human bone fragments. In conclusion, we believe this novel approach is an important methodological step forward, and will allow visualization of the cellular structure of the hematopoietic niche and study of the molecular mechanisms mediating cell-cell interactions within the niche.

Acknowledgment

This work was supported by National Institutes of Health (grants R41CA126004, R43AI082759 and R21DK067084) and University of California TRDRP (grant 16RT-0134) to SKK.

References

[1] Schofield R. The stem cell system. *Biomed. Pharmacother.* 1983;37(8):375-380.
[2] Schofield R. The relationship between the spleen colony-forming cell and the haemopoietic stem cell. *Blood Cells.* 1978;4(1-2):7-25.
[3] Kiel MJ, Morrison SJ. Uncertainty in the niches that maintain haematopoietic stem cells. *Nat. Rev. Immunol.* Apr 2008;8(4):290-301.
[4] Scadden DT. The stem-cell niche as an entity of action. *Nature.* Jun 29 2006;441 (7097):1075-1079.
[5] Hackney JA, Charbord P, Brunk BP, Stoeckert CJ, Lemischka IR, Moore KA. A molecular profile of a hematopoietic stem cell niche. *Proc. Natl. Acad. Sci. USA.* Oct 1 2002;99(20):13061-13066.
[6] Calvi LM, Adams GB, Weibrecht KW, et al. Osteoblastic cells regulate the haematopoietic stem cell niche. *Nature.* Oct 23 2003;425(6960):841-846.
[7] Kiel MJ, Yilmaz OH, Iwashita T, Yilmaz OH, Terhorst C, Morrison SJ. SLAM family receptors distinguish hematopoietic stem and progenitor cells and reveal endothelial niches for stem cells. *Cell.* Jul 1 2005;121(7):1109-1121.
[8] Taichman RS, Reilly MJ, Emerson SG. The Hematopoietic Microenvironment: Osteoblasts and The Hematopoietic Microenvironment. *Hematol.* 2000;4(5):421-426.
[9] Crocker PR, Gordon S. Isolation and characterization of resident stromal macrophages and hematopoietic cell clusters from mouse bone marrow. *J. Exp. Med.* Sep 1 1985;162(3):993-1014.
[10] Lee SH, Crocker PR, Westaby S, et al. Isolation and immunocytochemical characterization of human bone marrow stromal macrophages in hemopoietic clusters. *J. Exp. Med.* Sep 1 1988;168(3):1193-1198.
[11] Rich IN. A role for the macrophage in normal hemopoiesis. I. Functional capacity of bone-marrow-derived macrophages to release hemopoietic growth factors. *Exp. Hematol.* Sep 1986;14(8):738-745.

[12] Burnett SH, Kershen EJ, Zhang J, et al. Conditional macrophage ablation in transgenic mice expressing a Fas-based suicide gene. *J. Leukoc Biol.* Apr 2004;75(4):612-623.
[13] Chang MK, Raggatt LJ, Alexander KA, et al. Osteal tissue macrophages are intercalated throughout human and mouse bone lining tissues and regulate osteoblast function in vitro and in vivo. *J. Immunol.* Jul 15 2008;181(2):1232-1244.
[14] Sanchez-Fernandez MA, Gallois A, Riedl T, Jurdic P, Hoflack B. Osteoclasts control osteoblast chemotaxis via PDGF-BB/PDGF receptor beta signaling. *PLoS ONE.* 2008;3(10):e3537.
[15] Branemark PI. Vital microscopy of bone marrow in rabbit. *Scand. J. Clin. Lab. Invest.* 1959;11(Supp 38):1-82.
[16] McCuskey RS, McClugage SG, Younker WJ. Microscopy of living bone marrow in situ. *Blood.* Jul 1971;38(1):87-95.
[17] Mazo IB, Gutierrez-Ramos JC, Frenette PS, Hynes RO, Wagner DD, von Andrian UH. Hematopoietic progenitor cell rolling in bone marrow microvessels: parallel contributions by endothelial selectins and vascular cell adhesion molecule 1. *J. Exp. Med.* Aug 3 1998;188(3):465-474.
[18] Celso CL, Fleming HE, Wu JW, et al. Live-animal tracking of individual haematopoietic stem/progenitor cells in their niche. *Nature.* Dec 3 2008.
[19] Makale M. Intravital imaging and cell invasion. *Methods Enzymol.* 2007;426:375-401.
[20] Khaldoyanidi SK, Glinsky VV, Sikora L, et al. MDA-MB-435 human breast carcinoma cell homo- and heterotypic adhesion under flow conditions is mediated in part by Thomsen-Friedenreich antigen-galectin-3 interactions. *J. Biol. Chem.* Feb 7 2003;278(6):4127-4134.
[21] Lehr HA, Leunig M, Menger MD, Nolte D, Messmer K. Dorsal skinfold chamber technique for intravital microscopy in nude mice. *Am. J. Pathol.* Oct 1993;143(4):1055-1062.
[22] Wallerath T, Witte K, Schafer SC, et al. Down-regulation of the expression of endothelial NO synthase is likely to contribute to glucocorticoid-mediated hypertension. *Proc. Natl. Acad. Sci. USA.* Nov 9 1999;96(23):13357-13362.

In: Stem Cells in Disease
Editor: Prasad S. Koka

ISBN: 978-1-62257-169-7
© 2012 Nova Science Publishers, Inc.

Chapter VII

Endogenous Hyaluronan Participates in Generation of Hematopoietic Cells during Differentiation of Human Embryonic Stem Cells

***Ingrid U. Schraufstatter*[1], *Naira Serobyan*[2], *Valentina Goncharova*[1], *Jeanne Loring*[3] *and Sophia K. Khaldoyanidi*[*1]**
[1]Torrey Pines Institute for Molecular Studies, , San Diego, CA, US
[2]La Jolla Institute for Molecular Medicine, San Diego, CA, US
[3]The Scripps Institute for Medical Research, La Jolla, CA, US

Abstract

Hyaluronan (HA) is an important component of the microenvironment in bone marrow, but its role in regulation of the development of hematopoietic cells is not well understood. To address the role of HA in regulation of human embryonic stem cell (hESC) differentiation into the hematopoietic lineage, we screened for genes encoding components of the HA pathway. Using gene arrays, we found that HA synthases and HA receptors are expressed in both undifferentiated and differentiating hESCs. Enzymatic degradation of HA resulted in decreased numbers of hematopoietic progenitors and lower numbers of CD45+ cells generated in HA-deprived embryoid bodies (EBs). In addition, deprivation of HA resulted in the inhibition of generation of CD31+ cells, stromal fibroblast-like cells and contracting myocytes in EBs. RT-PCR and immunocytochemistry revealed that HA deprivation did not influence the dynamics of OCT4 expression, but decreased the expression of BRY, an early mesoderm marker, and BMP2, a later mesoderm marker in differentiating EBs. In addition, the endoderm markers α-FP and SOX17 were decreased, whereas the expression of the ectoderm markers GFAP and

[*] Corresponding Author: Sophia K. Khaldoyanidi, M.D., PhD, Torrey Pines Institute for Molecular Studies, 3550 General Atomics Court San Diego, CA 92121, USA. Tel.: (858) 597 3879. Fax: (858) 597 3804. E-mail: skhaldoyanidi@tpims.org.

FGF5 was higher in HA-deprived cultures. Our findings indicate that endogenously produced HA contributes to the network that regulates the differentiation of hESC and the generation of mesodermal lineage in general and hematopoietic cells specifically.

Keywords: Embryonic Stem Cells, Differentiation, Hyaluronan, Extracellular Matrix

Abbreviations

2 ME – 2-mercaptoethanol
α-FP – alpha-fetoprotein
AA – amino acids
bHABP – biotin-conjugated HA-binding protein
BMP2 – bone morphogenetic protein-2
BMP4 – bone morphogenetic protein 4
BRY– T-brachyury
CFU – colony forming unit
DAPI – (4,6 diamidino-2-phenylindole)
DMEM - Dulbecco's modified Eagle's medium
EB – embryoid body
ECM - extracellular matrix
FBS – fetal bovine serum
FGF5 – fibroblast growth factor 5
GAG – glycosaminoglycan
GFAP – glial fibrillary acidic protein
GlcA – D-glucuronate
GlcNAc – the disaccharide N-acetyl-D-glucosamine
HA – hyaluronan
HARE – hyaluronan receptor for endocytosis
HAS1– HA synthase 1
HAS2 – HA synthase 2
HAS3 – HA synthase 3
h-bFGF – human basic fibroblast growth factor
hESC – human embryonic stem cell
HLA – human leukocyte antigen
KSR – knockout serum replacement
OCT4 – Octamer-4
RHAMM – hyaluronan-mediated motility receptor
RT-PCR – reverse transcription polymerase chain reaction
SOX17 – sex determining region Y-box 17
SSEA-1 – stage specific embryonic antigen-1

Introduction

The concept of stem cell based therapy implies that damaged tissues can be repaired by tissue-specific stem cells that generate mature functionally active progeny. Among the variety of tissue-specific multipotent stem cells, hematopoietic stem cells (HSCs) have been routinely used in clinical practice for over than 30 years. In currently used protocols, HSCs are isolated either from adult (bone marrow or mobilized peripheral blood) or neonatal (umbilical cord blood) sources.

Despite the obvious success of the HSC transplantation approach, there remain obstacles for effective HSC-based therapy: due to a shortage of HLA-matched donors and the technical limits for in vitro expansion of HSCs only one third of patients receive the required HSC transplantation.

Thus, additional sources for HSCs are needed, and pluripotent human embryonic stem cells (hESCs) theoretically represent an alternative source. Current knowledge on generation of HSCs from hESCs suggests that the properties of hESC-derived HSCs, including self-renewal, multipotency, regenerative capacity and survival, depend on the culture conditions used to differentiate hESCs [1]. The critical issue, which has not been sufficiently addressed, is the efficiency of hESC differentiation into the hematopoietic lineage. The strategy which is most likely to succeed will include a sequence of in vitro treatments that guide the differentiating cell into the desirable lineage.

Thus, treatments that regulate lineage competition between mesoderm, ectoderm and endoderm will constitute the first step. One example of such lineage-specific treatments is BMP-4, a factor that drives ESCs into mesoderm, and subsequently enhances the efficiency of HSC generation [2]. There is a need to identify other molecular pathways that selectively drive hESCs into mesoderm and precludes them from differentiation into ectoderm and endoderm with a view to optimize in vitro differentiation protocols of hESC towards the hematopoietic lineage.

HA, a member of the glycosaminoglycan (GAG) family, is a large negatively charged polymer containing multiple copies of the disaccharide N-acetyl-D-glucosamine (GlcNAc) and D-glucuronate (GlcA). HA is present in all organs, tissues and biological fluids in mammalian organisms. It was initially believed that HA expands and maintains extracellular space by binding salt and water. Later studies demonstrated that HA participates in local extracellular matrix (ECM) assembly [3] by interacting with a variety of extracellular molecules, such as aggrecan, versican, neurocan, etc. Identification of receptors that bind HA demonstrated that HA is also implicated in specific receptor-ligand interactions that consequently influence cell behavior.

These receptors include CD44, RHAMM and HARE, and HA is involved in the regulation of multiple cell functions, including cell proliferation [4, 5], migration [6], cytokine production [7-10] and adhesion molecule expression [11] through receptor-mediated pathways. It was our original observation that HA is a necessary and specific signal-inducing molecule for hematopoiesis [9, 12]. The importance of HA in regulating hematopoiesis was later confirmed by others demonstrating a role for HA in mediating HSC migration [13] and lodgment [14].

The vital role of HA was proven when it was demonstrated that inactivation of the HA synthase 2 gene in mice is embryonically lethal [15]. While the involvement of HA-mediated pathways is generally appreciated in normal cell and tumor biology, its role in the regulation of ESC behavior is not well understood. The results presented here suggest that HA is a critical component of the extracellular microenvironment that is required for the differentiation of hESCs into mesoderm and subsequently into hematopoietic lineage.

Materials and Methods

Cell Lines and Treatments

ESCs (WH09 line) were cultured on a feeder layer established from HS27 human fibroblasts that were grown in Dulbecco's Modified Eagle's Medium (DMEM) supplemented with non-essential amino acids (AA), L-Glutamax and 10% fetal bovine serum (FBS). Prior to use for ESC cultures, the feeder layers were irradiated with 40Gy (4000 rads). Human ESCs were grown on the feeder layers in DMEM/F12 supplemented with 20% knockout serum replacement (KSR), 10mM non-essential amino acids, 1mM L-Glutamax, 10ng/ml h-bFGF and 0.1mM 2-mercaptoethanol (ME) (Invitrogen, Carlsbad, CA). The cultures were fed every two days and passaged by the manual dissection method every 6 days. To induce ESC differentiation, the ESC colonies were removed from the feeder layers and cultured in DMEM/F12 supplemented with 20% FBS, 10mM non essential amino acids, 2 mM L-Glutamax and 0.1 mM 2-ME in suspension as clustered spheroids of cells referred to as embryoid bodies (EBs). Where indicated, the cultures were treated with HA'ase free of other contaminating degrading enzymes (1U/ml, hyaluronidase, Sigma or Seikagaku), 4MU (100μM, 4-methylumbelliferone sodium salt, MP Biomedicals, Solon, OH,) or HA (100μg/ml, umbilical vein, Sigma).

Clonogenic Assays

For colony forming unit (CFU) assays, the cell suspension (10^5 cells/ml of plating mixture) was mixed with semisolid methylcellulose medium supplemented with hematopoiesis-supporting cytokines (StemCell Technologies, Canada). The cultures were incubated in a humidified incubator with 5% CO_2 in air at 37°C for 7-14 days.

Fluorescent Activated Cell Sorter (FACS) Analysis

For cell surface immunostaining, $5x10^5$ cells were stained according to standard procedures [16]. PE-conjugated CD45 and CD31 specific monoclonal antibodies and control isotype-matched PE- or FITC-conjugated IgG were purchased from PharMingen (PharMingen, San Diego, CA). Fluorescence analysis was performed on a FACScan (Becton Dickinson) and analyzed using the CellQuest program.

Immunohistochemistry

EBs were seeded on Matrigel-coated glass-slides, cultured in differentiation media and fixed with 4% paraformaldehyde, permeabilized with 0.2% Triton-X100 and incubated with mouse anti-OCT4, goat anti-BMP2, rabbit anti-FGF-5 (all from Santa Cruz Biotechnology, Santa Cruz, CA), mouse anti-SSEA-1, mouse-anti αFP and goat anti-T-brachyury (all from R&D Systems). Secondary anti-mouse, rabbit or goat antibodies conjugated with Alexa-Fluor 568 (Invitrogen, Carlsbad, CA) or Alexa-Fluor 488 (Invitrogen, Carlsbad, CA) (1:400) were used to visualize the antigens, and DAPI (4,6 diamidino-2-phenylindole) was used to stain nuclei. HA polymers were detected by biotin-conjugated HA-binding protein (bHABP), followed by incubation with PE-conjugated avidin (both from Sigma). Images were captured by confocal microscopy (Olympus FLUOVIEW FV 1000) and analyzed using Open Lab software.

Gene Expression

Triplicate cultures of hESCs and EBs were cultured as described above, harvested and total RNA was isolated using a Qiagen RNA isolation kit. Probe preparation and chip hybridization was performed according to the manufacturer's recommendations (Illumina, San Diego, CA). Genes of interest were defined as detectable if their hybridization signal intensities in all three samples were detected with at least 99% confidence.

RT-PCR

For semiquantitative RT-PCR, RNA was reverse transcribed using the Omniscript Reverse Transcription kit (Qiagen) according to the supplier's instructions including DNase treatment during RNA preparation. PCR was performed with the primers shown in Table 1, and amplification was performed for 35 cycles using straight and 1:10 dilutions of cDNA samples.

Table 1. The primers utilized for RT-PCR of stem cell markers expressed in hESCs

Marker	Forward	Reversed
OCT 4	GGGAAGGTATTCAGCCAAACG	GGTTCGCTTTCTCTTTCGGG
BRY	ACTGGATGAAGGCTCCCGTCTC	CCAAGGCTGGAACCAATTGTCATG
BMP-2	CCCGACACTGAGACGCTGTTC	GGGGAAGCAGCAACGCTAGAA
α-FP	AAATACATCCAGGAGAGCCA	CTGAGCTTGGCACAGATCCT
SOX 17	CAGCTACGCGCAGGTCTCGG	AAATGGCCCCGTGGCTGTCG
FGF-5	AGTCAATGGATCCCACGAAG	TGGGTAGAGATATGCTGGGG
GFAP	TGCTCGCCGCTCCTACGT	CTCAGCAGCCAGCGCCTT
β-actin	GAGCTGCCCGATGGCCAGGTCATCACC	TTAGAAGCATTTGCGGTGGACGATGGA

Statistical Analysis

Statistical analysis was carried out by Student's t-test.

Results

Expression of HA Pathway Components in hESCs

Human ESCs were cultured as described in Materials and Methods (Figure 1A). The pluripotency of hESCs was confirmed by the expression of OCT4 (Figure 1B), which disappeared upon differentiation of hESC in the EB cultures [17].

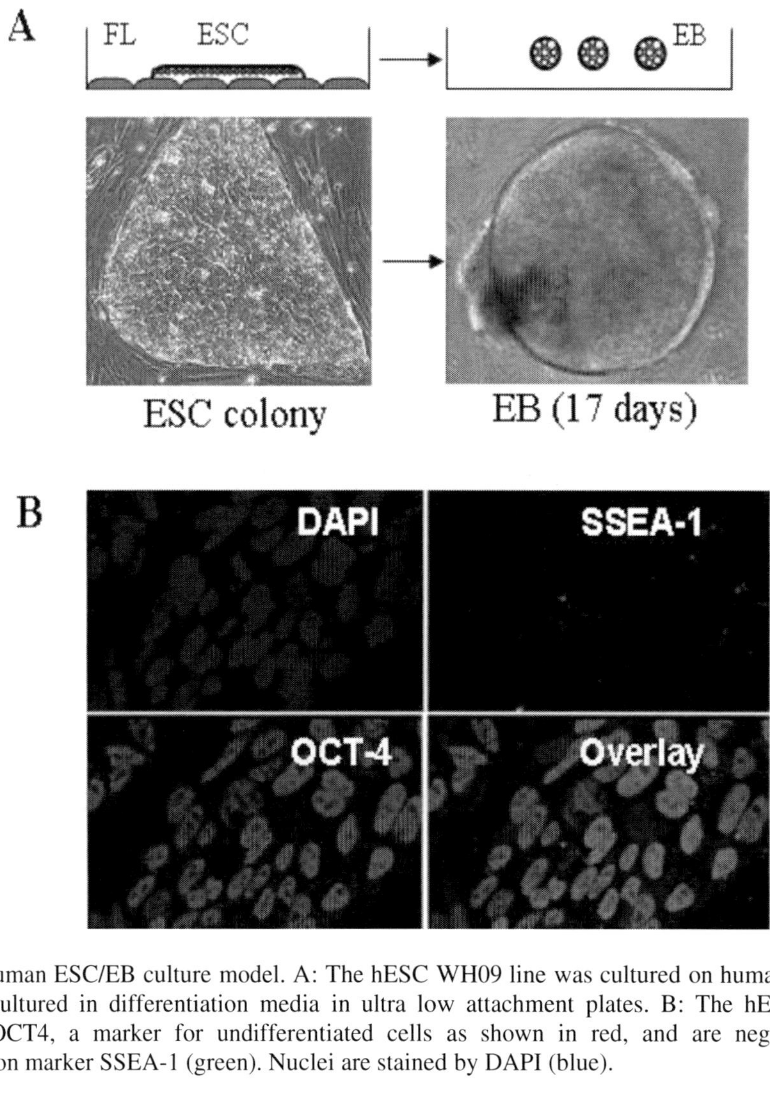

Figure 1. Human ESC/EB culture model. A: The hESC WH09 line was cultured on human fibroblasts. EBs were cultured in differentiation media in ultra low attachment plates. B: The hESCs colonies expressed OCT4, a marker for undifferentiated cells as shown in red, and are negative for the differentiation marker SSEA-1 (green). Nuclei are stained by DAPI (blue).

To address a role of HA in regulation of hESC differentiation, we screened for genes encoding components of the HA pathway. Using gene arrays, we found that HA synthase 2 (HAS2) was expressed in both undifferentiated and differentiating ESCs (Figure 2A). The high level of expression of HAS2 was not dependent on the differentiation status of hESCs. Low but detectable levels of the expression of HA synthase 1 (HAS1) and HA synthase 3 (HAS3) were found in both undifferentiated and differentiating hESCs. The activity of HASs was confirmed by the detection of HA polymers in hESC and EB cultures (Figure 2B and Figure 4A).

Treatment of cultures with highly specific hyaluronidase (HA'ase) resulted in degradation of HA as reflected by undetectable levels of HA (Figure 4A).

The expression of mRNA for the HA receptors including RHAMM, HARE and CD44 was detected in both undifferentiated and differentiated hESC cultures (Figure 2B). Interestingly, while high levels of CD44 mRNA was present in hESC cultures (Figure 2A), barely detectable levels of CD44 protein were detected in undifferentiated hESC (Figure 2B). However, high levels of CD44 protein expression appeared in cell subpopulations of differentiating EBs (Figure 2C).

Similarly, the expression of HARE and RHAMM proteins was detectable in differentiating EBs (not shown).

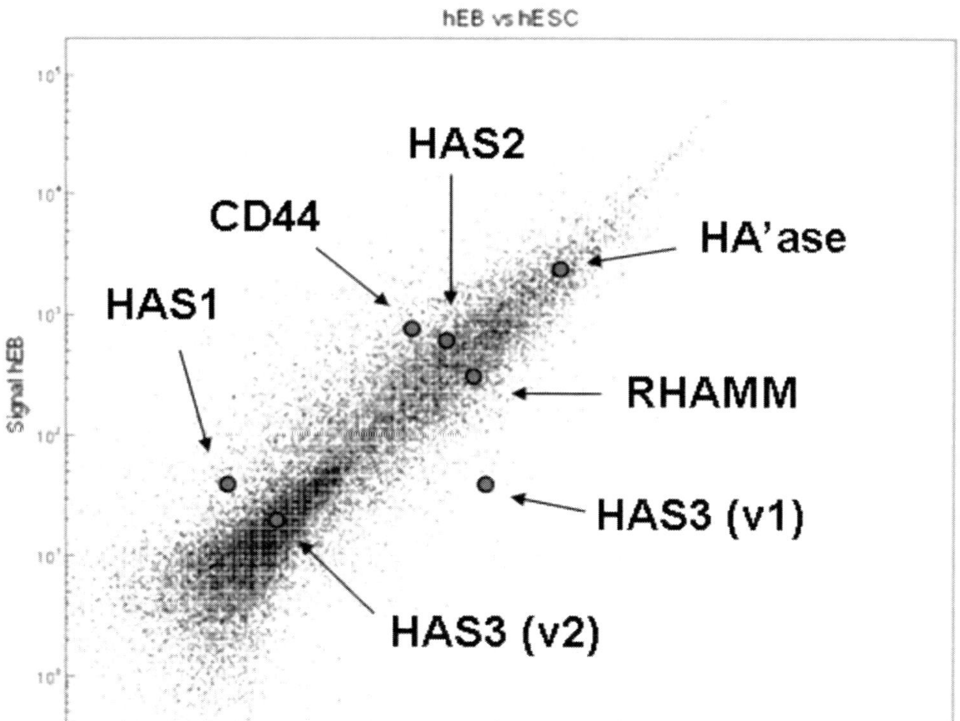

a

Figure 2. (continued).

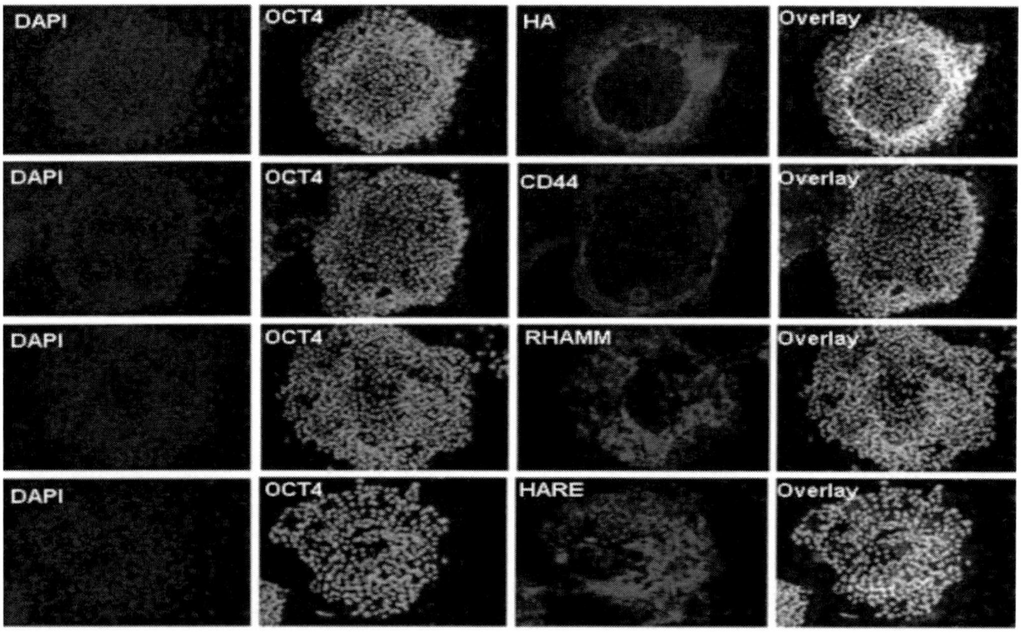

b

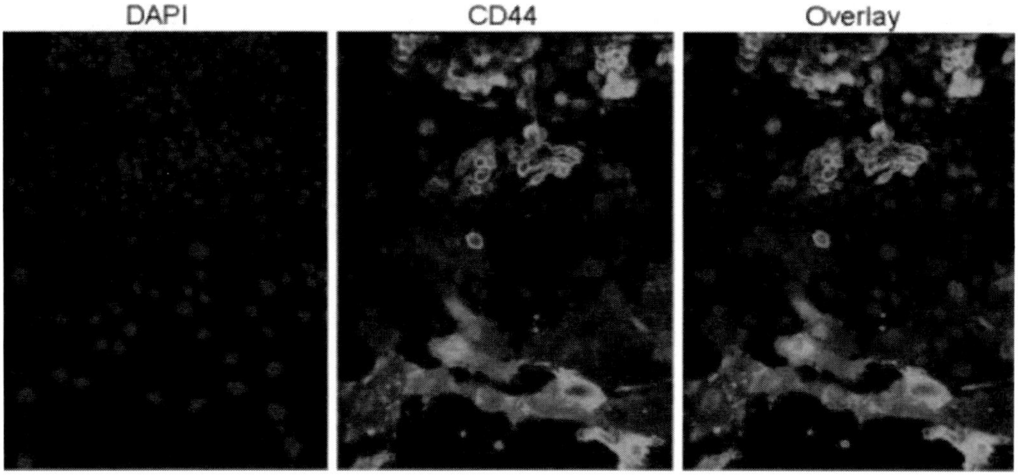

c

Figure 2. The expression of HA pathway related genes in the hESC/EB model. A: Microarray analysis of differential gene expression in hESCs versus EBs is shown. In the log transformed graph the hybridization signals for over 10,000 genes are plotted. Hybridization signals obtained from ESC samples (X-axis) are compared to those from EB samples (day 7, Y-axis). Genes that were statistically significantly expressed in the samples are shown. Each sample was averaged from four biological replicates. Genes of interest are indicated by arrows. B: The expression of HA, CD44, RHAMM and HARE in hESC colonies was detected by immunohistochemistry using bHABP or CD44-, RHAMM- and HARE-specific antibodies. The right panel shows the overlay of HA, CD44, RHAMM or HARE staining (red), nuclear staining (DAPI, blue) and OCT4 (green). Representative images out of two similar experiments are shown. C: Expression of CD44 differentiated EB cultures (day 17) was detected by immunohistochemistry using CD44-specific antibodies (× 60) and is shown in green. Nuclear staining (DAPI) is shown in blue. Representative images out of eight similar experiments are shown.

Degradation of HA Results in a Decreased Generation of Hematopoietic Cells in EBs

Since HA is expressed in hESC colonies and because it is involved in regulation of adult hematopoiesis [9, 12], we investigated whether the deprivation of HA in hESCs before they differentiate into the major germ layers would influence the ability of hESC to generate cells of hematopoietic lineage. To address the role of endogenously produced HA a method of enzymatic degradation of HA by HA'ase was used. Cell viability tests which were performed prior to these experiments showed that HA'ase was not toxic to cells at the used concentrations (not shown). We used two experimental approaches: 1) HA'ase was added in undifferentiated hESC cultures and withdrawn during spontaneous differentiation in EB cultures; 2) HA'ase was added only during spontaneous differentiation in EB cultures. In the first set of experiments, the decreased levels of HA did not change the morphology of hESC colonies: the colonies remained flat with sharp edges (Figure 3A). On day 6, HA'ase treatment of hESC cultures was discontinued and EB cultures were set up.

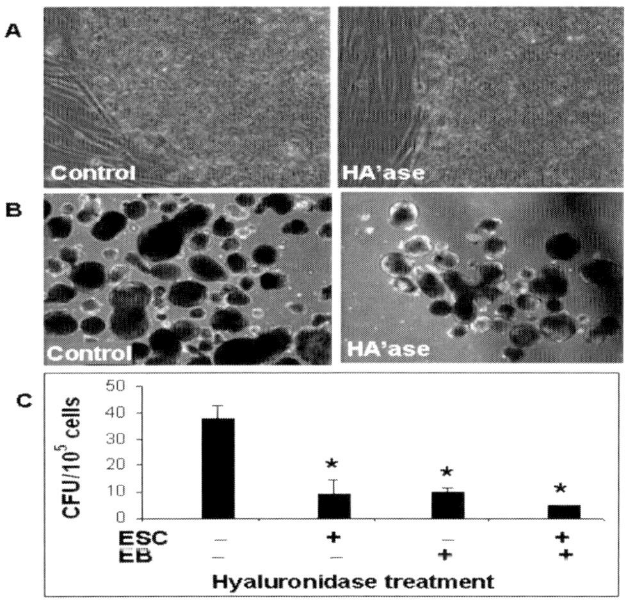

Figure 3. The effect of HA deprivation in hESCs. A: Images of control and HA'ase-treated hESC colonies. B: EBs established from control and HA'ase-treated hESC colonies. C: HA'ase (1U/ml) was added into the hESC and EB cultures (indicated by (+)) or withdrawn (indicated by (-)). At day 17, the cells prepared from EBs were counted and examined for the number of progenitors using the CFU assay. Cells were cultured in triplicates and mean values and S.D. of one out of five similar experiments are shown. (*indicates $p<0.01$).

While HA'ase-treated hESCs were capable to form EBs (Figure 3B), the total number of EBs and the total number of recovered cells was 1.5-fold lower in cultures established from HA'ase treated hESCs (ESC(+)/EB(-)), as compared to controls (ESC(-)/EB(-)). This pretreatment of ESCs with HA'ase correlated with a 4-fold (ESC(+)/EB(-) cultures) or 8-fold (ESC(+)/EB(+) cultures) decrease in the number of total hematopoietic progenitors measured by a CFU assay (Figure 3C). In the second set of experiments, the EB cultures were treated with HA'ase to reduce the extracellular HA concentration during hESC differentiation starting from day 1 of EB culture. HA'ase-induced degradation of HA was confirmed by immunocytochemistry (Figure 4A). The enzymatic degradation of HA in EBs resulted in a significant decrease in the total number of cells generated in HA'ase-treated cultures compared to control ($18.6 \pm 1.7 \times 10^5$/culture *versus* $31.3 \pm 2.9 \times 10^5$/culture respectively, p=0.0008).

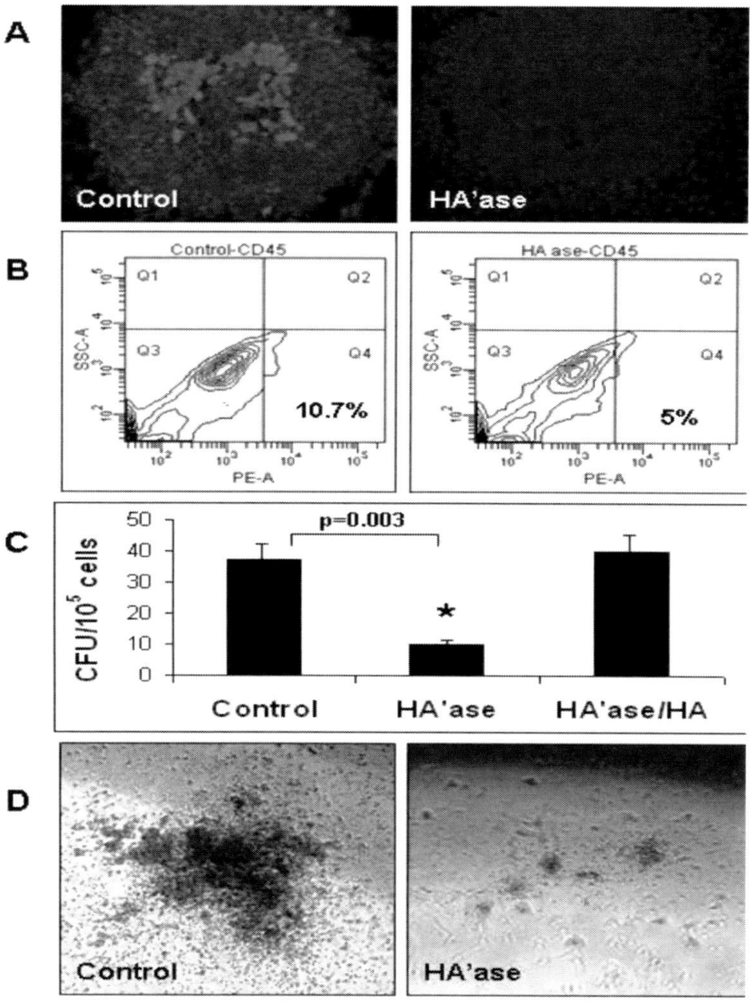

Figure 4. The effect of HA deprivation in EBs. A: Expression of HA in control and HA'ase-treated EBs was detected using bHABP. The overlay of stained nuclei (DAPI, blue) and HA (red) is shown (× 10). B: Cells derived from the control and HA-treated EBs were collected on day 17, a single cell suspension was prepared and the expression of CD45 was evaluated by FACS. Contour plots are shown where the CD45-positive cells are in Q4. In negative controls, cells were stained with isotype-matched PE-conjugated IgG with 1-2% cells in Q4 (not shown). For each sample 10,000 events were collected. C: Cells collected from control and HA'ase treated EBs were counted and 10^5 cells/culture were used in the CFU assay. Where indicated, exogenous HA (100 μg/ml) was added into the EB cultures treated with HA'ase (1U/ml). D: An image of a hematopoietic colony grown from control and HA'ase-treated EBs is shown. Each experiment was performed in triplicates and mean values and S.D. of one out of five similar experiments are shown.

The percent of hematopoietic cells in differentiated EBs was evaluated using the expression of the CD45 pan-leukocyte marker. The number of CD45+ cells generated in HA'ase-treated EBs was 2-fold lower as compared to control (Figure 4B). This correlated with a 4-fold decrease in the relative number of committed progenitors (per 10^5 cultured cells) evaluated by the CFU assay (Figure 4C). The total number of hematopoietic progenitors per culture was 7-fold lower in HA'ase-treated cultures as compared to non-treated cultures. The addition of exogenous HA polymers into the HA'ase-treated EB cultures restored the number of progenitors generated in EBs (Figure 4C) indicating the specificity of the treatment. In addition, the cells derived from HA'ase treated EBs gave rise to hematopoietic colonies of a smaller size as compared to control in the CFU cultures (Figure 4D).

HA is Required for Generation of Cells of Mesodermal Origin

In addition to the decreased production of hematopoietic cells, degradation of HA inhibited generation of other cell types in differentiating EBs.

In particular, generation of CD31-positive cells, which include endothelial cells, was 1.6-fold lower in EBs cultured with HA'ase as compared to control (Figure 5A). In addition, cells derived from the HA'ase-treated EBs showed a decreased ability to establish a monolayer of stromal-like fibroblast cells (Figure 5B). Finally, spontaneous differentiation of hESCs into contracting myocytes in the EB cultures treated with HA'ase was decreased (Figure 5C). While 3-5% of EBs in control cultures were contracting, no contracting EBs were observed in HA'ase treated cultures. Since these cell types are of mesodermal origin, we next investigated whether HA plays a role during mesodermal differentiation of hESCs.

HA is Required for Mesodermal Differentiation of hESCs

Differentiation of hESCs was monitored by the expression of differentiation markers in EBs.

To prevent HA synthesis and avoid the presence of HA degradation products in cultures, EBs were cultured in the presence of the HAS inhibitor 4MU [18]. 4MU was tested for its toxicity to cells prior to experiments and did not show any toxicity at the used concentration (not shown). Treatment with 4MU showed no obvious effect on the expression of the pluripotency marker OCT4 in EBs as determined by RT-PCR (Figure 6A) and immunofluorescence (Figure 6B).

Similar results were observed for NANOG and SOX2 expression (results not shown). In contrast, the expression of the mesodermal marker T-Brachyury (BRY) was significantly lower in the HA-deprived EBs. Lower levels of BRY mRNA in 4MU-treated EBs were detected starting from day 4 of EB culture and remained lower than control throughout the whole culture period (Figure 6A). In line with this observation Bry protein expression was also decreased in 4MU-treated EBs as compared to controls (Figure 6C). In addition, the production of BMP2, a late mesoderm marker, was lower in 4MU-treated cultures as compared to control (Figure 6A and D).

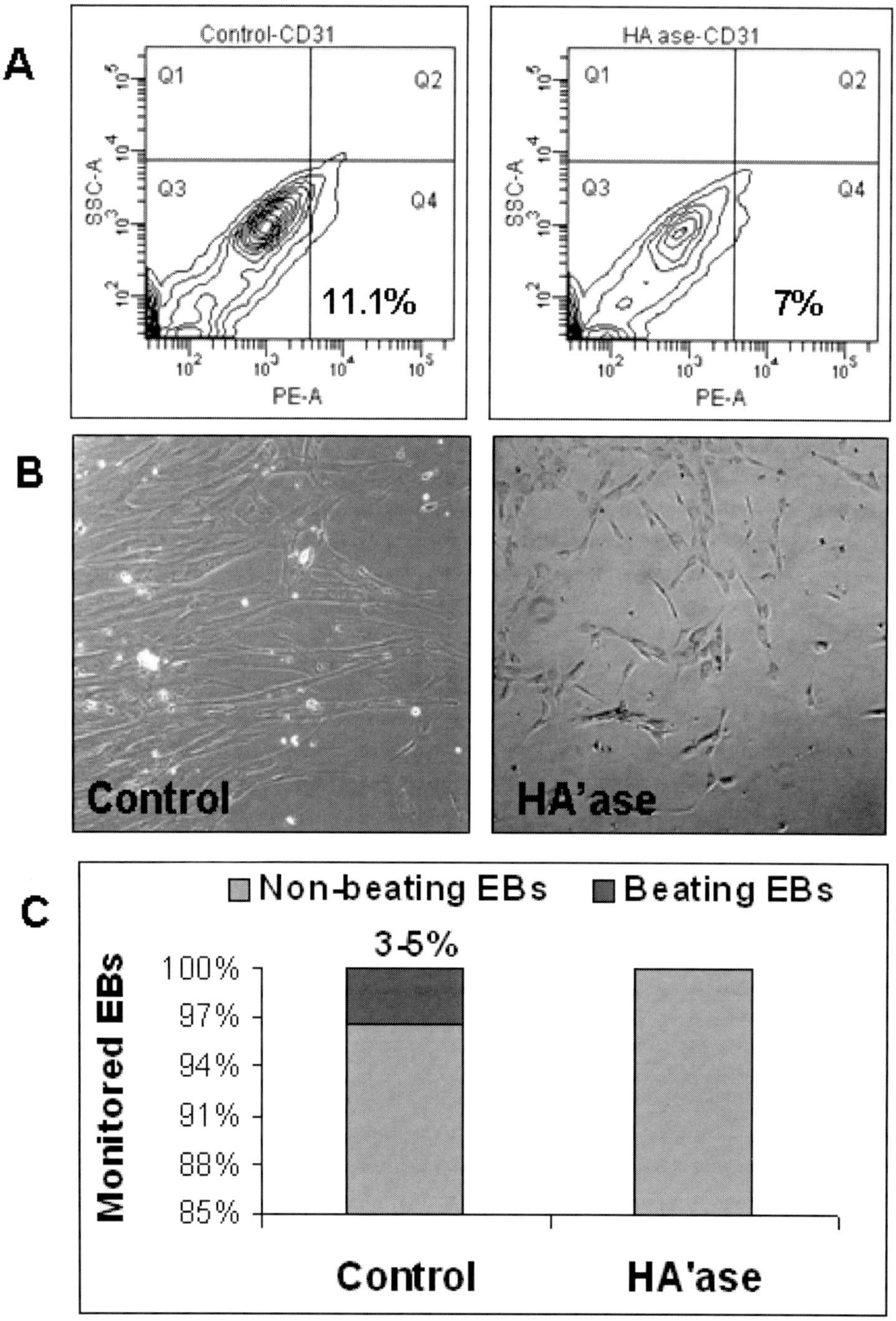

Figure 5. The effect of HA deprivation on generation of non-hematopoietic cells of mesodermal origin. A: Cells derived from the control and HA-treated EBs were collected on day 17, a single cell suspension was prepared and the expression of CD31 was evaluated by FACS. B: The single cell suspension obtained from control and HA'ase (1U/ml) treated EBs was cultured in MSC media. The image shows the formation of the stromal layer after 7 days of culture. C: The number of beating EBs (cultured with or without HA'ase) was evaluated under the microscope and expressed as a percentage of total EBs. Each experiment was performed in triplicates and mean values and S.D. of one out of four similar experiments are shown ($p<0.01$).

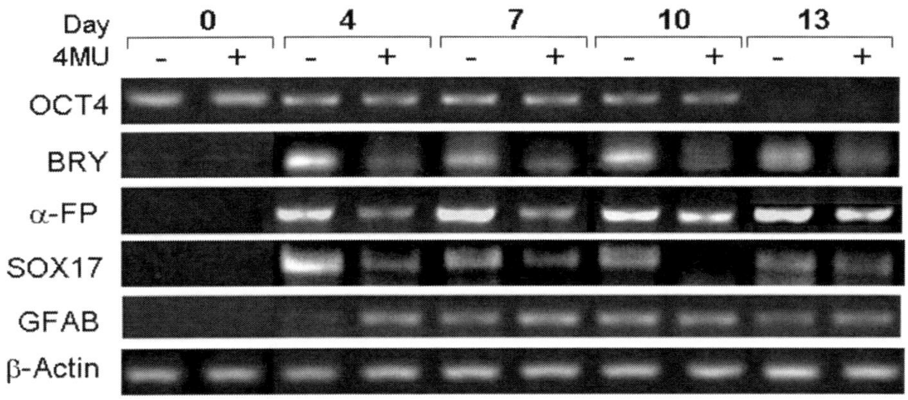

a

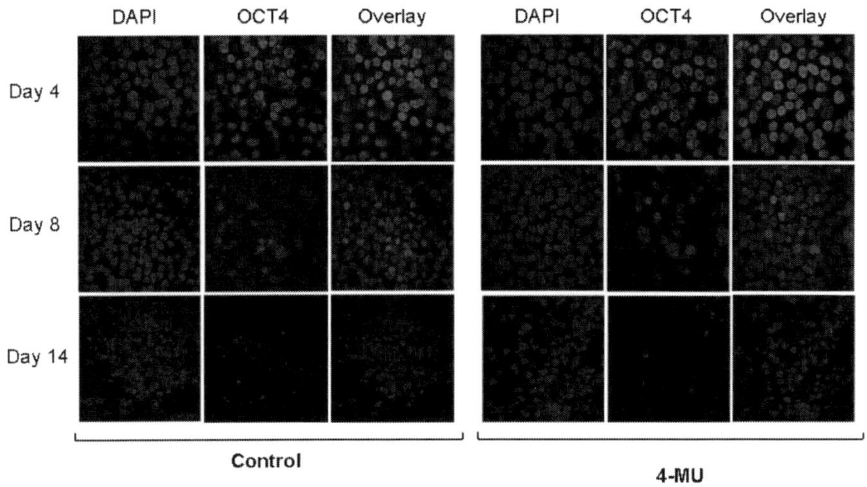

b

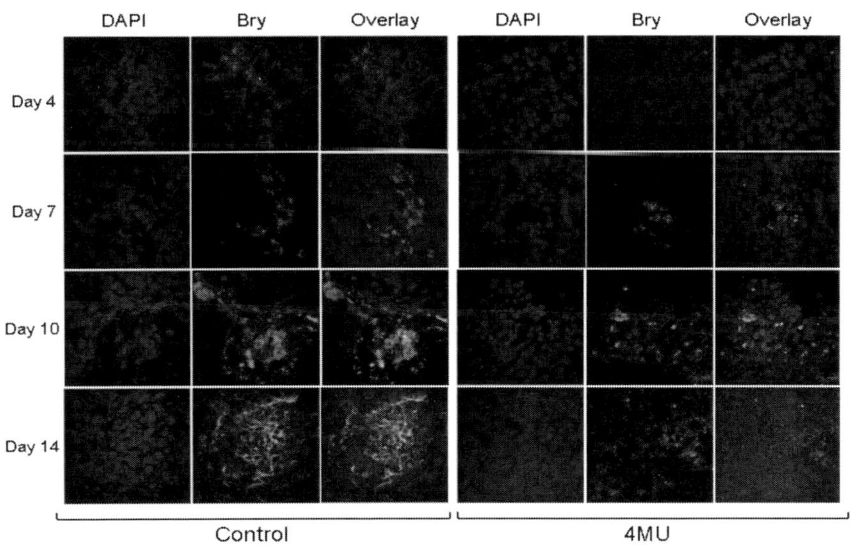

c

Figure 6. (continued).

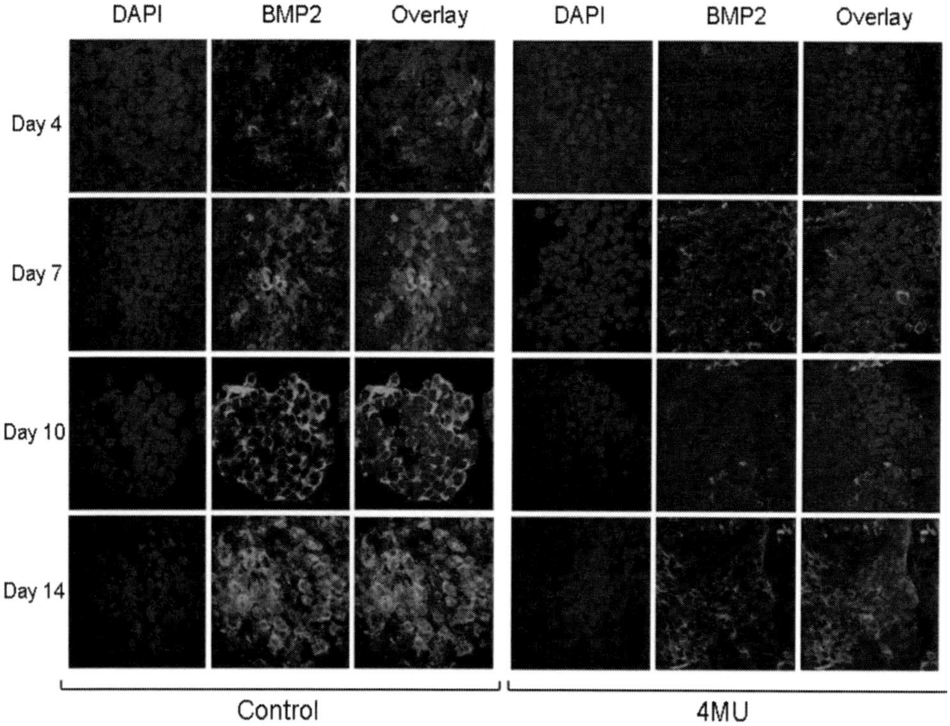

d

Figure 6. The effect of HA deprivation on the gene expression of stem cell markers and differentiation markers in EBs. A: The expression of marker specific mRNA in hESCs was detected by RT-PCR. RNA was purified from four separate sets of hESCs cultures and reverse transcribed. The sequences of primers used to amplify mRNA from each sub-unit are shown in Table 1. Products for the OCT4, BRY, α-FP, SOX 17 and FGF5 were consistently detected as shown on representative gels, one out of four similar experiments. β-Actin was used as control. The expression of proteins of specific markers in differentiating EB cultures was detected by immunofluorescence. The expression of Oct4, a pluripotency marker, shown in red (B), Bry, a marker for early mesoderm (C) and BMP2, a marker for late mesoderm (D) shown in green were tested in EBs on the indicated days. Nuclei are stained with DAPI (blue). Where indicated, the cultures were grown in the presence of 4MU. Representative images out of four similar experiments are shown.

Importantly, the addition of exogenous HA polymers into the 4MU-treated cultures resulted in restoration of BRY and BMP2 mRNA expression (Figure 7A). This correlated with increased levels of Bry and BMP2 proteins produced in 4MU/HA cultures as compared to cultures treated with 4MU alone (Figure 7A and B). HA itself did not increase the expression of these markers in EBs grown in the absence of an HA synthesis inhibitor. The effect of 4MU on the expression of ectodermal and endodermal markers was investigated next.

At early stages of differentiation (days 4 and 7) the expression of the ectodermal markers FGF5 and GFAP was increased in the 4MU-treated EBs as compared to control (Figures 7A and 8A). When exogenous HA polymers were added into the 4MU-treated cultures the expression of FGF5 mRNA was decreased to normal levels (Figure 7A).

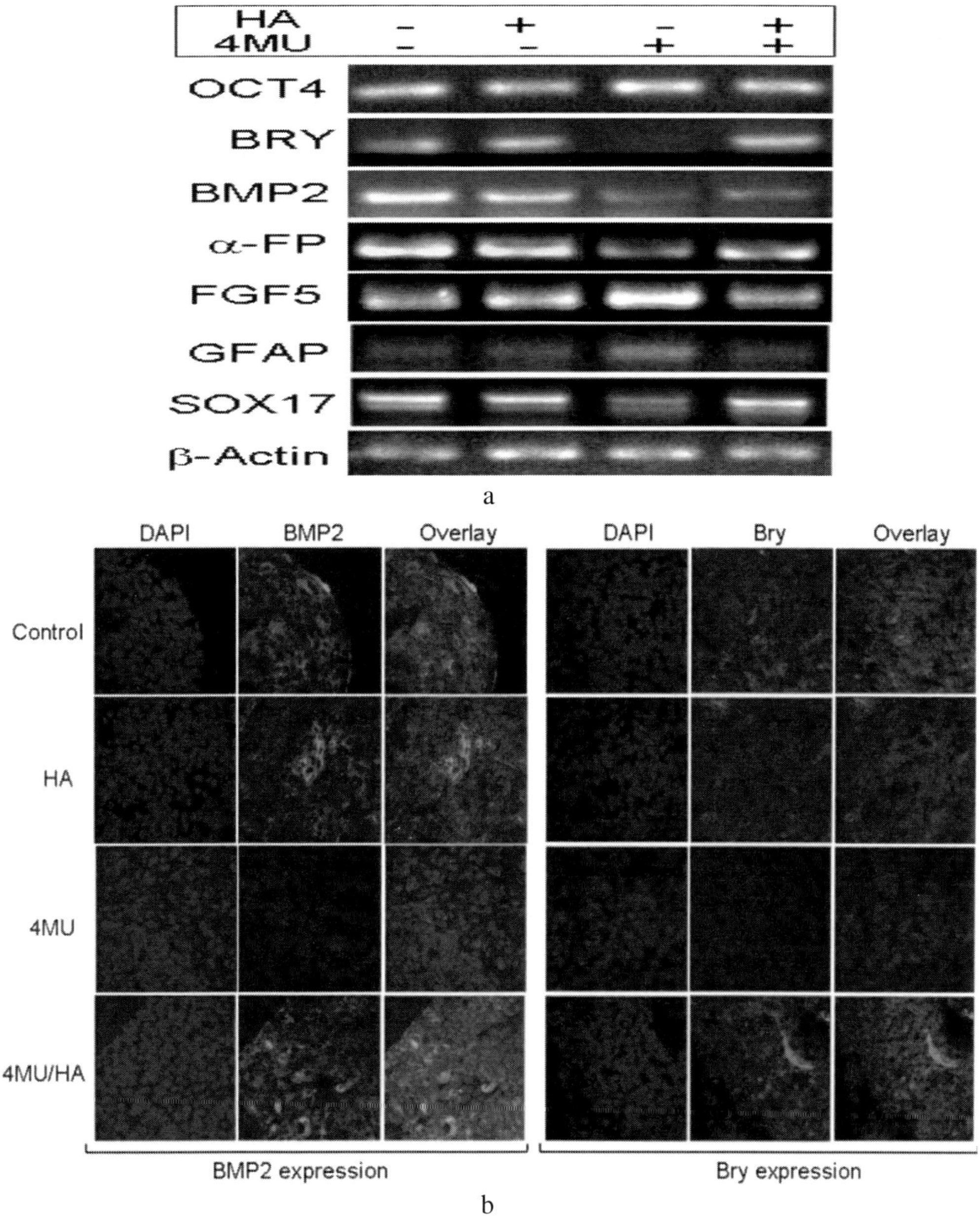

Figure 7. The effect of exogenous HA on the expression of markers in differentiating EBs. EBs were cultured with or without 4MU. Where indicated, exogenous HA polymers were added into the cultures. On day 4 of culture, the EBs were harvested and assayed. A: The expression of marker specific mRNA was detected by RT-PCR. RNA was purified from three separate sets of EB cultures and reverse transcribed as described in the Method section. The sequences of primers used to amplify mRNA from each sub-unit are shown in a Table 1. Products for OCT4, BRY, BMP2, α-FP, SOX17 and FGF5 were consistently detected as shown on representative gels out of three similar experiments. β-Actin was used as control. B: The expression of Bry and BMP2 proteins in 4-day EBs was detected by immunofluorescence. Bry, a marker for early mesoderm and BMP2, a marker for late mesoderm are shown in green and nuclei stained with DAPI are shown in blue. Representative images out of two similar experiments are shown.

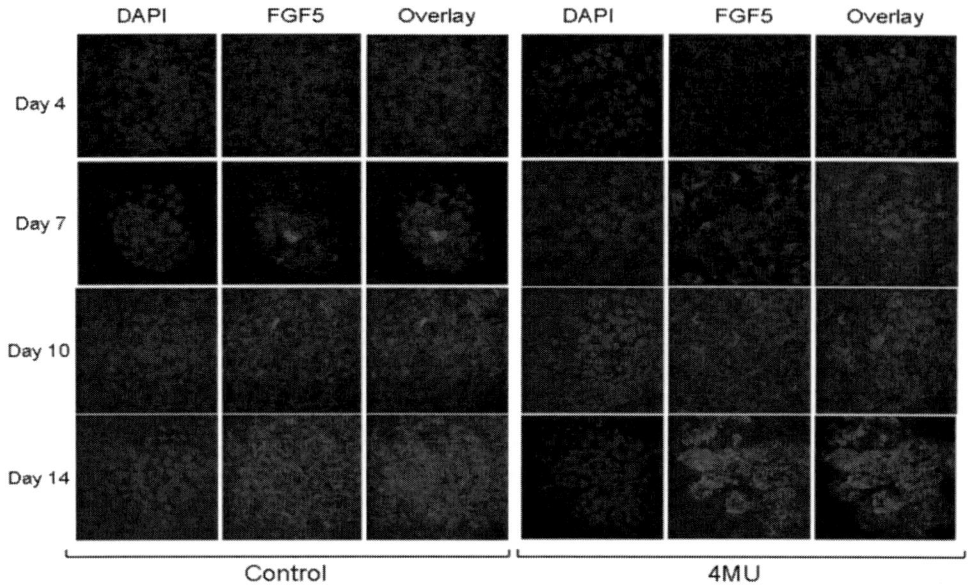

a

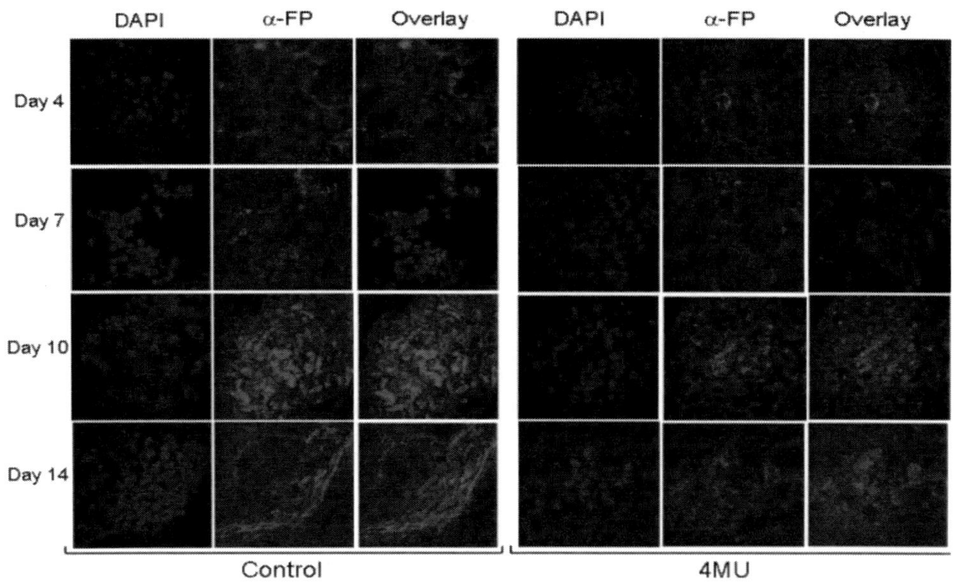

b

Figure 8. The effect of HA deprivation on the expression of stem cells markers in EBs. The protein expression of FGF5 (A), a marker for ectoderm, and α-FP (B), a marker for endoderm, in EBs on indicated days was detected by immune fluorescence. The staining for FGF5 and α-FP is shown in red and nuclei stained with DAPI are shown in blue. Representative images out of two similar experiments are shown.

Investigation of the effect of 4MU on the endodermal markers SOX17 (Figure 7A) and α-FP (Figure 8B) demonstrated decreased levels of their expression under conditions of HA deprivation).

Discussion

In this study we demonstrated an important role for endogenous HA in the regulation of generation of hematopoietic cells from hESCs. Our findings indicate that both undifferentiated and differentiated hESCs express detectable levels of HA synthases (HAS1, HAS2 and HAS3), HA receptors including CD44, RHAMM and HARE and produce HA polymers. Deprivation of HA induced by enzymatic degradation by hyaluronidase (HA'ase) of by inhibiting HA synthesis (4MU) resulted in the inhibition of differentiation of hESC into the mesodermal lineage and decreased generation of hematopoietic cells.

Our microarray results indicate that the expression of HAS2 is higher as compared to HAS1 and HAS3. We monitored only a slight increase in the expression of HAS2 during hESC differentiation. Our microarray results demonstrated that in contrast to HAS2, the expression of HAS1 appears higher in EBs *versus* undifferentiated hESC. Also, an increase in CD44 mRNA and protein expression can be detected during hESC differentiation. One important observation from our microarray results is a constantly high level of expression of HA'ase, which is independent of the stage of hESC differentiation. This indicates the presence of a flexible system that regulates production and degradation of HA in both undifferentiated and differentiated hESCs suggesting an important role of HA in hESC function.

There is evidence that HA is important for cardiac development in mice [15]. Unfortunately, due to embryonic lethality, these HAS2 knockout mice were not investigated for the efficiency of hematopoiesis. Using hESCs, Choudhary and co-workers demonstrated that knockdown of HAS2 results in decreased expression of CD34 cells in differentiated EBs [19]. Since CD34 is a marker for both hematopoietic and endothelial cells, the decrease of CD34 expression in EBs does not indicate specific inhibition of hematopoietic differentiation. Our immunofluorescent and clonogenic assays demonstrate for the first time that degradation of endogenous HA by HA'ase results in lower numbers of mature CD45+ hematopoietic cells and their progenitors providing evidence that HA is important for the generation of hematopoietic cells during hESC differentiation. Since we monitored a decreased generation of cells of other lineages of mesodermal origin including endothelial cells, contracting myocytes and stromal cells, we suggest that HA is important for mesodermal differentiation of hESCs.

To determine whether HA is involved in regulation of the process of hESC differentiation into mesoderm, we selected to test the effect of HA deprivation on the dynamics of expression of two mesodermal markers: BRY as a marker of the early mesoderm and BMP2 as a marker of the late mesoderm. In these series of experiments we selected to deprive hESC cultures from HA by using 4MU, an inhibitor of HA synthesis. While enzymatic degradation of HA is an effective approach to test the number of differentiated cells, it might not be sufficient to test the expression of markers due to possible sensitivity of the gene expression to the products of enzymatic degradation including low molecular weight HA polymers [20, 21]. Furthermore, it is conceivable that the flexible system present in hESC might compensate for the degradation of HA by increased levels of HAS activity. Another possible approach to decrease the levels of HA in hESC cultures is to use an RNAi approach to silence HASs. However, if only HAS2, a major HAS in hESC, is knocked down [19], HA might still be synthesized by HAS1 the expression of which is increased during differentiation resulting in relatively normal levels of HA production. Thus, it appears that blocking HAS activity might be a better approach to test the effect of HA deprivation on gene expression. As expected, treatment of differentiating hESCs with 4MU resulted in decreased expression of both BRY and BMP2 suggesting that HA is required for mesodermal differentiation of hESCs.

In situations when the pluripotent cell does not undergo apoptosis (due to culture conditions or other reasons), it has only two choices: 1) to remain undifferentiated; or 2) to commit to one of the lineages, i.e. ectoderm, mesoderm or endoderm. If the ability of the pluripotent cell to differentiate is blocked, the cells will remain undifferentiated which will be reflected by the continuous expression of pluripotent markers such as OCT4. In this study we demonstrated that the expression of OCT4 was not changed during 4MU treatment compared to control cultures, suggesting that hESCs are not arrested in their pluripotent stage and their ability to differentiate is not affected. This is in line with the previously published observation in which a HAS2 knockdown approach was selected to deprive hESC from HA [19]. Thus, it can be concluded that under conditions of HA deprivation hESC retain their ability to differentiate. If such, this process of differentiation should be reflected by an increased expression of differentiation markers of at least one of the lineages.

Since we demonstrated that mesodermal differentiation of hESC is decreased in the absence of HA, we hypothesized that the ratio of pluripotent cells that choose endodermal or ectodermal differentiation (or both) will be increased. To test this hypothesis, we investigated the effect of HA deprivation on the expression of the endodermal markers α-FP and SOX17 and the ectodermal markers FGF5 and GFAP. While Choudhary and co-workers demonstrated that in the HAS2 knockdown hESCs the expression of markers of all lineages is decreased during differentiation [19], we found that in HA-deprived EBs the expression of ectodermal markers (FGF5 and GFAP) is increased. In contrast, endodermal markers (α-FP and SOX7) were down-regulated suggesting that HA plays a role at the earliest stages of the germ layer formation. Therefore, based on our results we can conclude that endogenous HA is a part of the network that regulates lineage competition during hESC differentiation.

It remains an important question whether exogenous HA can be used to drive differentiation of hESCs toward mesoderm. Our microarray results indicate that both undifferen-tiated and differentiated hESC express high levels of HA'ase suggesting that any excess of HA polymers undergoes enzymatic degradation. Since HA'ase expression depends on HA levels [22-28], this serves as a system to maintain required levels of HA in the system. This may explain why the addition of exogenous HA into the untreated control cultures did not change the level of expression of the stem cells markers, and the addition of HA into the HA-deprived cultures allowed only restoration of the expression of stem cell markers to the level seen in control untreated cultures. In contrast to our observation, another group claimed that the addition of a natural non-modified exogenous HA into the control cultures changed the differentiation potential of hESC toward mesoderm and subsequently enhanced cardiac differentiation of hESCs [19]. In contrast with this report and in line with our observations, Ventura and co-workers reported that only modified HA (ester of HA linked to butyric and retinoic acid), which cannot be degraded by HA'ase drives differentiation ESCs toward myocardiocytes [29]. These findings suggest that manipulation of HA-mediated pathways in hESCs is possible and may represent a useful approach to direct the differentiation choices of hESCs.

Acknowledgment

This work was supported by National Institutes of Health (grant R21NS062428) and University of California TRDRP (grant 16RT-0134) to SKK.

References

[1] Orlovskaya I, Schraufstatter I, Loring J, Khaldoyanidi S. Hematopoietic differentiation of embryonic stem cells. *Methods*. Jun 2008;45(2):159-167.

[2] Bhatia M, Bonnet D, Wu D, et al. Bone morphogenetic proteins regulate the developmental program of human hematopoietic stem cells. *J. Exp. Med.* Apr 5 1999;189(7):1139-1148.

[3] Fraser JR, Laurent TC, Laurent UB. Hyaluronan: its nature, distribution, functions and turnover. *J. Intern Med.* Jul 1997;242(1):27-33.

[4] Brecht M, Mayer U, Schlosser E, Prehm P. Increased hyaluronate synthesis is required for fibroblast detachment and mitosis. *Biochem J.* Oct 15 1986;239(2):445-450.

[5] Hamann KJ, Dowling TL, Neeley SP, Grant JA, Leff AR. Hyaluronic acid enhances cell proliferation during eosinopoiesis through the CD44 surface antigen. *J. Immunol.* Apr 15 1995;154(8):4073-4080.

[6] Andreutti D, Geinoz A, Gabbiani G. Effect of hyaluronic acid on migration, proliferation and alpha-smooth muscle actin expression by cultured rat and human fibroblasts. *J. Submicrosc Cytol Pathol.* Apr 1999;31(2):173-177.

[7] Hiro D, Ito A, Matsuta K, Mori Y. Hyaluronic acid is an endogenous inducer of interleukin-1 production by human monocytes and rabbit macrophages. *Biochem. Biophys Res. Commun.* Oct 30 1986;140(2):715-722.

[8] Hodge-Dufour J, Noble PW, Horton MR, et al. Induction of IL-12 and chemokines by hyaluronan requires adhesion-dependent priming of resident but not elicited macrophages. *J. Immunol.* Sep 1 1997;159(5):2492-2500.

[9] Khaldoyanidi S, Moll J, Karakhanova S, Herrlich P, Ponta H. Hyaluronate-enhanced hematopoiesis: two different receptors trigger the release of interleukin-1beta and interleukin-6 from bone marrow macrophages. *Blood.* Aug 1 1999;94(3):940-949.

[10] Noble PW, Lake FR, Henson PM, Riches DW. Hyaluronate activation of CD44 induces insulin-like growth factor-1 expression by a tumor necrosis factor-alpha-dependent mechanism in murine macrophages. *J. Clin. Invest.* Jun 1993;91(6):2368-2377.

[11] Oertli B, Beck-Schimmer B, Fan X, Wuthrich RP. Mechanisms of hyaluronan-induced up-regulation of ICAM-1 and VCAM-1 expression by murine kidney tubular epithelial cells: hyaluronan triggers cell adhesion molecule expression through a mechanism involving activation of nuclear factor-kappa B and activating protein-1. *J. Immunol.* Oct 1 1998;161(7):3431-3437.

[12] Moll J, Khaldoyanidi S, Sleeman JP, et al. Two different functions for CD44 proteins in human myelopoiesis. *J. Clin. Invest.* Sep 1 1998;102(5):1024-1034.

[13] Avigdor A, Goichberg P, Shivtiel S, et al. CD44 and hyaluronic acid cooperate with SDF-1 in the trafficking of human CD34+ stem/progenitor cells to bone marrow. *Blood.* Apr 15 2004;103(8):2981-2989.

[14] Nilsson SK, Haylock DN, Johnston HM, Occhiodoro T, Brown TJ, Simmons PJ. Hyaluronan is synthesized by primitive hemopoietic cells, participates in their lodgment at the endosteum following transplantation, and is involved in the regulation of their proliferation and differentiation in vitro. *Blood.* Feb 1 2003;101(3):856-862.

[15] Camenisch TD, Spicer AP, Brehm-Gibson T, et al. Disruption of hyaluronan synthase-2 abrogates normal cardiac morphogenesis and hyaluronan-mediated transformation of epithelium to mesenchyme. *J. Clin. Invest.* Aug 2000;106(3):349-360.

[16] Serobyan N, Orlovskaya I, Kozlov V, Khaldoyanidi SK. Exposure to nicotine during gestation interferes with the colonization of fetal bone marrow by hematopoietic stem/progenitor cells. *Stem Cells Dev.* Feb 2005;14(1):81-91.

[17] Loring JF, Wesselschmidt RL, Schwartz PH. *Human Stem Cell Manual: a laboratory guide*: Elsevier; 2007.

[18] Kakizaki I, Kojima K, Takagaki K, et al. A novel mechanism for the inhibition of hyaluronan biosynthesis by 4-methylumbelliferone. *J. Biol. Chem.* Aug 6 2004;279(32):33281-33289.

[19] Choudhary M, Zhang X, Stojkovic P, et al. Putative role of hyaluronan and its related genes, HAS2 and RHAMM, in human early preimplantation embryogenesis and embryonic stem cell characterization. *Stem Cells.* Dec 2007;25(12):3045-3057.

[20] Fieber C, Baumann P, Vallon R, et al. Hyaluronan-oligosaccharide-induced transcription of metalloproteases. *J. Cell Sci.* Jan 15 2004;117(Pt 2):359-367.

[21] Wolf D, Schumann J, Koerber K, et al. Low-molecular-weight hyaluronic acid induces nuclear factor-kappaB-dependent resistance against tumor necrosis factor alpha-mediated liver injury in mice. *Hepatology.* Sep 2001;34(3):535-547.

[22] Allingham PG, Brownlee GR, Harper GS, Pho M, Nilsson SK, Brown TJ. Gene expression, synthesis and degradation of hyaluronan during differentiation of 3T3-L1 adipocytes. *Arch Biochem Biophys.* Aug 1 2006;452(1):83-91.

[23] Asteriou T, Vincent JC, Tranchepain F, Deschrevel B. Inhibition of hyaluronan hydrolysis catalysed by hyaluronidase at high substrate concentration and low ionic strength. *Matrix Biol.* Apr 2006;25(3):166-174.

[24] Cramer JA, Bailey LC, Bailey CA, Miller RT. Kinetic and mechanistic studies with bovine testicular hyaluronidase. *Biochim Biophys Acta.* Aug 18 1994;1200(3):315-321.

[25] Deschrevel B, Lenormand H, Tranchepain F, Levasseur N, Asteriou T, Vincent JC. Hyaluronidase activity is modulated by complexing with various polyelectrolytes including hyaluronan. *Matrix Biol.* Apr 2008;27(3):242-253.

[26] Deschrevel B, Tranchepain F, Vincent JC. Chain-length dependence of the kinetics of the hyaluronan hydrolysis catalyzed by bovine testicular hyaluronidase. *Matrix Biol.* Jun 2008;27(5):475-486.

[27] Foldvari F, Nekam L. [Significance of balance of hyaluronic acid and hyaluronidase in pathogenesis of certain vesicular diseases.]. *Borgyogy Venerol Sz.* Mar 1955;9(2):38-43.

[28] Foldvari F, Nekam L, Jr. [Role of hyaluronic acid-hyaluronidase balance in the pathogenesis of certain bullous diseases.]. *Arch. Klin. Exp. Dermatol.* 1956;203(5):433-439.

[29] Ventura C, Maioli M, Asara Y, et al. Butyric and retinoic mixed ester of hyaluronan. A novel differentiating glycoconjugate affording a high throughput of cardiogenesis in embryonic stem cells. *J. Biol. Chem.* May 28 2004;279(22):23574-23579.

In: Stem Cells in Disease
Editor: Prasad S. Koka

ISBN: 978-1-62257-169-7
© 2012 Nova Science Publishers, Inc.

Chapter VIII

Effects of Inorganic Arsenic on Bone Marrow Hematopoietic Cells: An Emphasis on Apoptosis and Sca-1/c-Kit Positive Population

Jacintha Archana Pereira, Prosun Das, Malay Chaklader, Sumanta Chatterjee, Pratima Basak, Samaresh Chaudhur and Sujata Law[*]

Stem Cell Research and Application Unit, Department of Biochemistry and Medical Biotechnology, Calcutta School of Tropical Medicine, Kolkata

Abstract

Apoptosis, proliferation and differentiation are balanced molecular processes which may alter their pattern during environmental insults. Arsenic is an environmental pollutant, ranks 20th in abundance in the earth crust, 14th in sea water and 12th in the human body. Millions of people worldwide are chronically exposed to arsenic often due to naturally occurring arsenic in ground water. Hematopoietic stem cells within the bone marrow are the source of all haematopoietic cell lineages and are essential for tissue development throughout the life. In this experimental study, we have evaluated the impact of arsenic, on blood and blood forming cells by the changes in their cellular morphology, immune functional capacity, alteration of bone marrow CD34 positive stem/progenitors and changes in the phenotype of Sca-1, c-Kit dual positive primitive stem cell population. The study revealed that arsenic has a significant effect on bone marrow and hematopoietic stem cells, their immune capacity and upregulation of death process, all indicative of impairment in differentiation suggesting presence of deregulation in their precursors by arsenic toxicity.

[*] Corresponding Author: Dr. Sujata Law, Assistant Professor (Stem Cell Biology), Stem Cell Research and Application Unit, Department of Biochemistry and Medical Biotechnology, Calcutta School of Tropical Medicine, Kolkata-700073, India. Email: msuj2002@yahoo.co.in. Phone No: + 91-33-2241-4900/4065 Ext: 224. Cell Phone: +91 9051259521.

Introduction

Development of hematopoietic cells throughout the adult life is a dynamic process which maintains the cellular turnover within the bone marrow. All the cellular elements of blood including the red blood cells and the white blood cells of immune system derive from hematopoietic stem cells (HSCs) which are multipotent precursors that have self renewal capacity and reside within the bone marrow. The HSCs and their progenitors respond efficiently to different forms of stress such as infection, exposure to cytotoxic agents, drugs or in blood loss to replenish the cellular source [1]. Arsenic a metalloid released from both natural and anthropological sources ranks as number one toxic agent in the ATSDR (Agency for Toxic Substances and Disease Registry) priority list of hazardous substances [2] and classified as Group 1 carcinogen by IARC (International Agency for Research on Cancer) [3]. Millions of people worldwide are chronically exposed to inorganic arsenic often due to naturally occurring arsenic in ground water [4, 5]. Though the WHO guideline value for arsenic in drinking water is 10μg/L, some places in India mainly West Bengal, Bangladesh [6], Taiwan and parts of USA have a very high arsenic concentration in drinking water which have become a great environmental as well as health concern [4].

Along with the broad application of arsenic trioxide in tumor treatment, increasing reports showed that excessive or long term arsenic exposure may cause cancer of a variety of organs and is also associated with increased non-cancer diseases such as cardiovascular disease [7], neurological disorders [8], diabetes mellitus [9], hypertrophy of liver [10] and spleen [11, 12]. In blood, normal arsenic levels are less than 7μg/100ml, a higher level shows arsenic poisoning [13]. For the first time in India, the epidemiological survey of arsenic induced dermatoses from consuming arsenic contaminated water was reported by KC Saha of our institute [14]. Recent studies revealed that arsenic target the hematopoietic organ. Studies by Patlolla and Tchounwou have demonstrated that arsenic trioxide is able to induce damage at the molecular level in rat bone marrow cells [15]. The exposure of hematopoietic system to arsenic is commonly associated with anemia and leucopenia [5]. The earlier studies have observed the presence of binucleated and multinucleated cells, internuclear chromatin bridges, irregular nuclear shapes, anomalies in the nuclear membrane [16, 17] and partial maturation arrest of myelopoietic elements in arsenic victim's bone marrow [18].

The function of immune system is to protect the host cells from cellular damage and invading microbes [19]. The cell death, immune response and disease initiation are complex array of signaling, alteration in any one of these causes imbalance of the other two. The studies have shown that inorganic arsenic is also able to exert immuno-toxic and immuno-disruptive effects on human monocyte and macrophage in the blood [20]. The circulation of HSCs and progenitors in and out of bone marrow, by the circadian activity in the brain is a well studied phenomenon [21, 22] during which they usually get more exposed to cytotoxic agents than any other internal cell type. For this reason the hematopoietic and immune system represent particularly sensitive targets for these cytotoxic agents. In response to cellular loss, a positive feedback loop induces HSCs to cycle and subsequently replenish the hematopoietic system [23]. So, it is important to know the ability of these HSCs in executing their function during which blood and bone marrow cells are severely affected. It is also necessary to know whether the effects of arsenic are limited to mature cells and their function or do these HSCs pose a sensitive target for this notorious agent. Unfortunately, limited evidences are available on this issue. In the light of the above data it was thought worthwhile to investigate the effects of arsenic trioxide in experimental Swiss albino mice for evaluation of its effects on bone marrow haematopoietic cells and their traditional source the "hematopoietic stem cells". Studying the impingement of arsenic on the cellular ability to fight against foreign cells via specific immune responses, initiation of cellular death and the proliferative potential of stem and progenitors are particularly important to understand the toxic effects under the event. These findings suggested that hematopoietic cells and HSCs constitute the sensitive target for inorganic arsenic and have significant toxic effects on immune system development and differentiation which leads to increased apoptosis, dysregulation of self renewal capacity and derangement in the primitive bone marrow compartment.

Materials and Methods

Preparation of Animal Group

Inbred Swiss albino mice (*Mus Musculus*) aging between 8-10 weeks were selected for the experimental purpose. The animals were maintained with standard diet and water *ad libitum* and kept under conventional conditions. The mice received 5μg (0.1ml) of arsenic trioxide solution per gram of body weight daily intra-peritoneally through single use-disposable syringe (30G×0.5") for a period of 30 days [24]. Similarly a group of animals were maintained as sham control by injecting equal volume of saline intra-peritoneally. A total number of 18 healthy mice were included in each group. All animals survived throughout the period of exposure. Arsenic trioxide was purchased from Sigma-Aldrich (Cat no: A1010-25G) of purity 99.0%. All the experiments were conducted under sterile condition and the studies were approved by the Institutional Animal Ethical Committee.

Preparation of Peripheral Blood Smear

After the completion of exposure period, peripheral blood was collected from both arsenic exposed and control mice for the blood smear preparation. Briefly, the animal tail was gently massaged and wiped with 70% alcohol. After drying, blood was collected by tail vein puncture. Blood smears were drawn and air dried. Smears were stained with Leishman's stain using standard procedure and examined under microscope for the cellular morphological study.

Isolation of Bone Marrow

The animals were sacrificed by cervical dislocation and the long bones (tibia and femur) were collected in chilled PBS. The bones were stripped off the adherent muscles. A needle (26g) was used to flush out the bone marrow into a 35mm sterile petridish by RPMI-1640 media (without FBS) (Sigma Aldrich Cat No: R6504-1L). The marrow thus obtained was gently pipetted repeatedly using the pasture pipette and then passed through the cell strainer

(100 mesh per inch stainless steel grid) to achieve bone marrow single cell suspension. The suspension was further washed three times in PBS and finally transferred to RPMI- 1640 (without FBS) media, and low density cell (LDC) population was obtained by 1.050 percoll density gradient and finally washed thrice in PBS [25]. The cell content was then noted by counting the cells for each of the control and experimental groups and kept on ice till the experiment.

Preparation of Bone Marrow Smear

Bone marrow smears were prepared in both experimental and control group of mice on clean glass slides and the smears were then stained with Leishman's stain and observed under binocular microscope (Olympus, India) for the identification of cellular morphology.

Studies on Cell Mediated Immune (CMI) Parameters

To determine the immune functional capacity of above mentioned isolated bone marrow derived cells (LDC), the following parameters have been performed.

a) Nitro Blue Tetrazolium (NBT) Reduction Assay

As described earlier [26, 27], effector: target ratio was maintained at 10:1in presence of NBT. NBT was reduced to blue formazan by superoxide free radicals as phagocytosis proceeds. The preparation was incubated for 18 hours at 37°C and 5% CO_2 humidified atmosphere. Finally, the reaction was stopped by adding 0.1 N chilled HCl and pellet was extracted with boiling pyridine for the reduced formazan to appear in the supernatant. The intensity of color, assayed colorimetrically at 540nm provided a direct measure of the extent of phagocytosis and the results were expressed as percentage.

b) Cytotoxicity Assay

The effector: target ratio has been maintained at 10:1. Approximately, 1×10^6 bone marrow low density cells were incubated with 1×10^5 tumor cells (Sarcoma-180) for 18 hours at 37°C. Finally, after 18 hours of incubation cell suspension was mixed with equal volume of 0.4% trypan blue dye and the tumor cell viability was counted in a Hemocytometer (Rohem, India) [26, 27].

Flow Cytometric Analysis of Fas (CD95) Receptor Expression and 7AAD Binding Pattern

For the estimation of apoptosis of bone marrow stem/progenitor population in control and arsenic exposed mice, 1×10^6 cells were incubated with 2μl of mouse anti-Fas (CD95)-PE monoclonal antibody (mAB) (e-Bioscience, USA) for 30 minutes at 37°C in dark [28].

To investigate the dead cells and cells which were in terminal state of apoptosis, 1×10^6 cells were stained with 7AAD (BD-Biosciences, USA) by the above-mentioned procedure. Cells were then washed with PBS to remove the unbound antibody and samples were analyzed by BD-FACS Calibur (Becton Dickenson, USA), using Cell Questpro software (v 9.1 Becton Dickenson, USA).

Estimation of Primitive HSCs (Sca-1, c-kit) and Stem/Progenitor Cell Population (CD34) by Flowcytometry

The flow cytometry analyses was done to detect the surface receptor expression of primitive HSCs (Scal, c-Kit) and stem/progenitor cell population (CD 34) in control and arsenic exposed animals. Briefly, in one tube, 1×10^6 cells were fixed with 3% para-formaldehyde (PFA), washed and incubated with 2 µl of each of mouse anti-Scal-PE and anti-c-Kit-FITC conjugated monoclonal antibodies (mAbs) (BD-Biosciences, USA) [21].

To the other tube, 2 µl of mouse anti CD 34 FITC (e-Bioscience, USA) was added and incubated in dark at 37°C for 30 minutes. Cells were washed with PBS and flowcytometric analysis was done in BD-FACS Calibur (Becton Dickinson) using CellQuest Pro software (v 9.1 Becton Dickenson, USA).

Statistical Analysis

The statistical analysis of data was performed using Student's t-Test and presented as mean ± standard deviation (SD) for inter-group comparison. A probability of $P < 0.0001$ was considered to be statistically significant.

Results

Peripheral Blood Smear Study

The peripheral blood smear is an important tool for the identification of several diseased conditions by the presence of abnormal cells and their deviated morphology. The blood smears made from arsenic exposed mice showed appearance of blast cells with abnormal features (Figure 1b, 1c and 1d). The control animals showed normal cellularity and normal morphology of blood cells (Figure 1a) and the presence of abnormal cells in the peripheral blood denoted the toxic effects of arsenic in hematopoietic system.

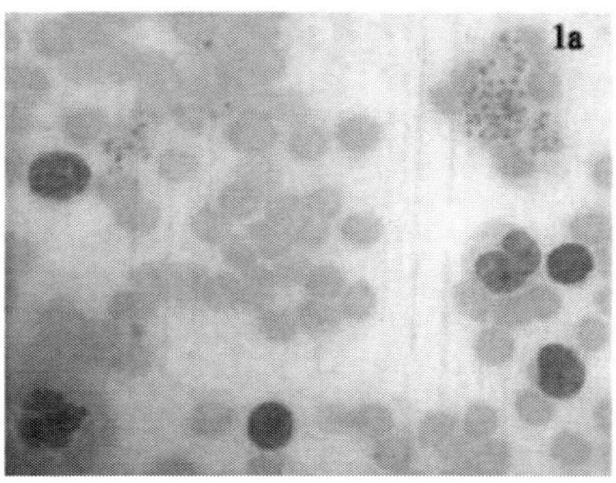

Figure 1a. The peripheral blood smear of the control mice showed normal lymphocytes, neutrophil and eosinophil.

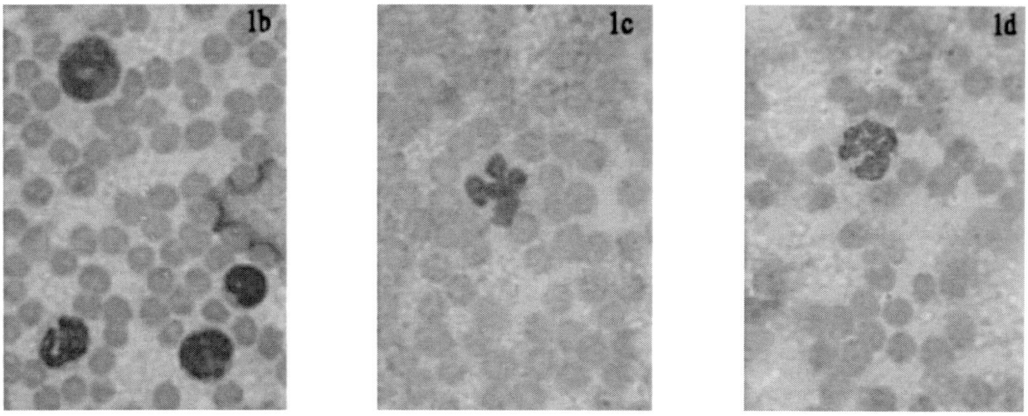

Figure 1b, 1c, 1d. The arsenic exposed mice peripheral blood smear showed abnormal lobulation of neutrophil and presence of immature neutrophil (ring shaped nucleus).

Bone Marrow Smear Study

The bone marrow cellular organization was studied by staining the bone marrow smears of arsenic exposed (Figure 2b and 2c) and control mice (Figure 2a) and it gave a valuable suggestion regarding the morphological abnormality. The smear of arsenic exposed mice showed nuclear fragmentation and abnormal differentiation of the myeloid and lymphoid precursors. The presence of abnormal cells in the bone marrow of arsenic exposed mice raised a question about their functional activity mainly focusing the immune response.

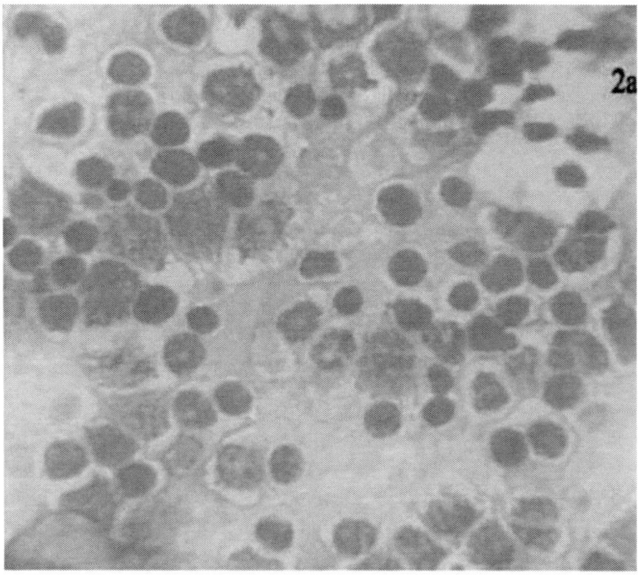

Figure 2a. The Leishman's stained bone marrow architecture of control mice demonstrates a particular cellular organization within the tissue.

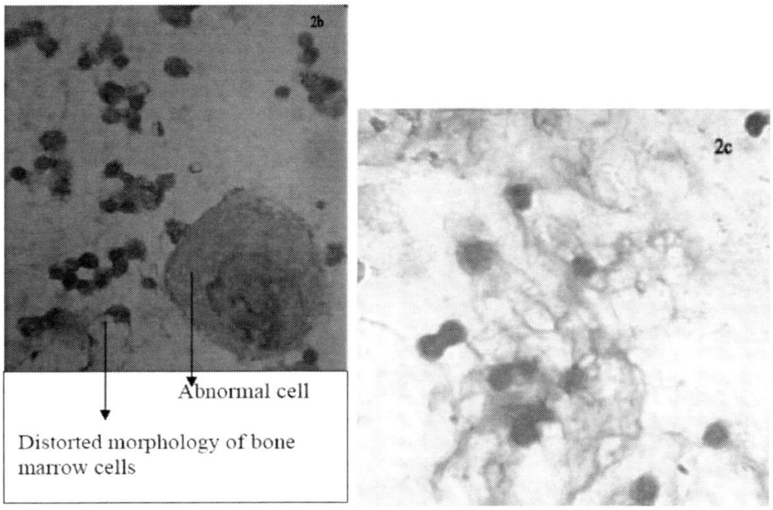

Figure 2b and 2c. The Leishman's stained bone marrow smear of arsenic exposed mice showed morphologically distorted cells in comparison with control.

Cell Mediated Immune Function

The CMI functional parameters of arsenic exposed mice bone marrow LDC showed great deviation from control mice bone marrow LDC. The NBT reduction assay of arsenic exposed mice (4.5±0.97%) and control mice (7.7±0.56%) varied significantly ($P<0.0001$) (Figure 3a). The cytotoxicity efficiency of arsenic exposed mice bone marrow LDC (6.25±0.64%) decreased significantly ($P<0.0001$) in comparison to control mice (13.03±0.74%) (Figure 3b).

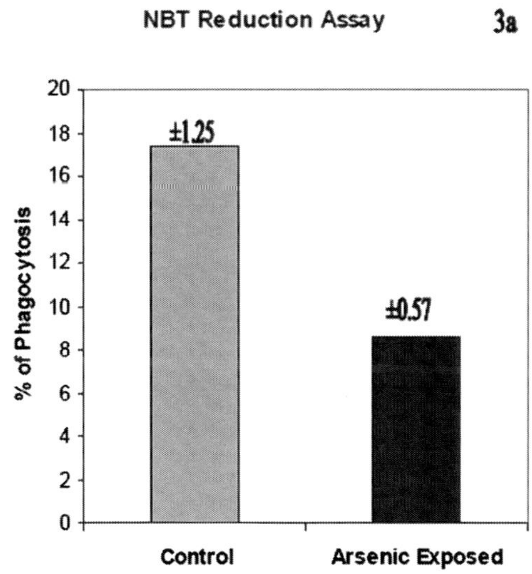

Figure 3a. The phagocytic capacity of bone marrow LDC population of arsenic exposed mice was significantly reduced to 4.5±0.97% in comparison with control mice 7.7 ±0.56% ($P<0.0001$) by NBT reduction assay.

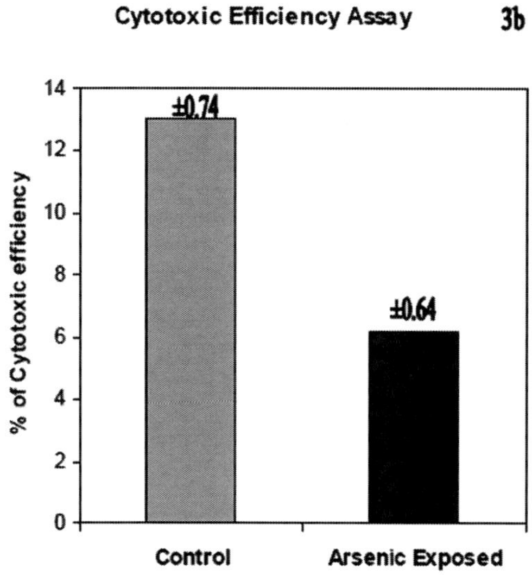

Figure 3b. The cytotoxicity capacity of bone marrow LDC of control mice was 13.03±0.74% whereas in arsenic exposed mice the cytotoxicity capacity was 6.25±0.64% which is significantly lower than the control mice bone marrow cells (P<0.0001).

Flowcytometry Results

Apoptosis study by the expression of Fas (CD95) receptor expression and 7AAD dye binding pattern

The Fas (CD95) receptor expression of arsenic exposed animals stem/progenitor cell population was significantly higher (14.96±1.47%) (Figure 4b) in comparison to control (2.59±1.3%) (P<0.0001) (Figure 4a). The 7-amino-actinomycin D (7AAD) dye binds to the apoptotic or dead cell DNA. The flowcytometric analysis showed 9.0±0.78% (Figure 5b) of arsenic exposed mice stem/progenitor population was positive for 7AAD while 4.4±1.16% (P<0.0001) (Figure 5a) of control mice stem/progenitor population showed 7AAD positivity.

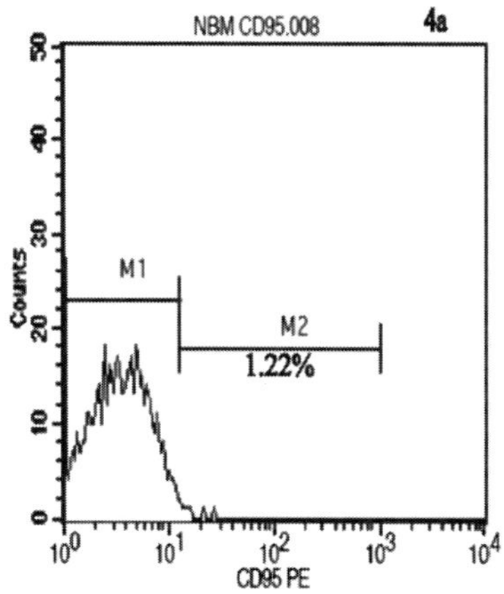

Figure 4a. Flow cytometric analysis of Fas (CD95 PE) receptor expression in control mice stem/progenitor cell population was 2.59±1.3%.

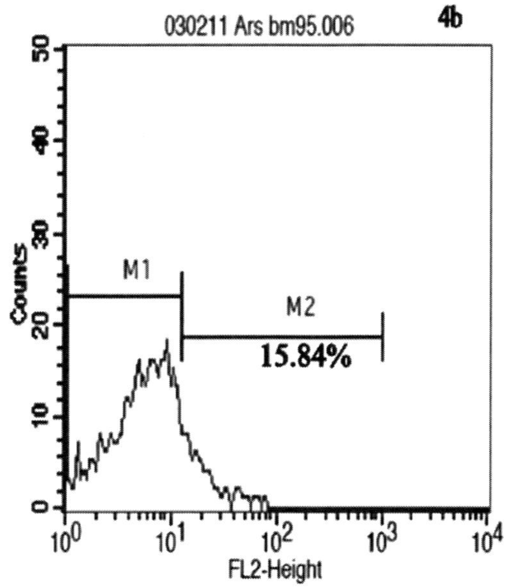

Figure 4b. The Fas (CD95PE) death receptor expression was significantly high in arsenic exposed mice bone marrow stem/progenitor cell population (14.96±1.47%) in comparison to control (P<0.0001).

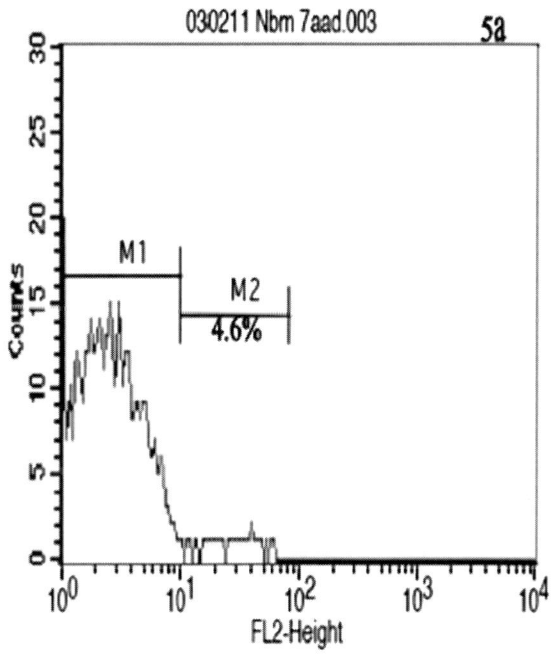

Figure 5a. The Flowcytometric analysis of 7AAD of control mice bone marrow stem/progenitor population showed 4.4±1.16% positivity.

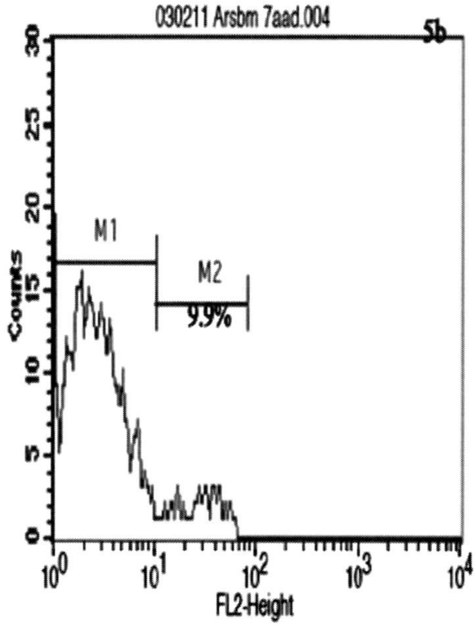

Figure 5b. The 7AAD analysis of arsenic exposed mice bone marrow stem/progenitor cells showed increased 7AAD positive cells (9.0±0.78%) (P<0.0001).

Estimation of stem/progenitor cell population by CD34

The hematopoietic stem/progenitor cells express a sialomucin receptor CD34 on their surface. Arsenic exposed mice showed decreased population of this marker (20.19±3.0%) (Figure 6b) in comparison with control (35.19±3.29%) (P<0.0001) as shown in Figure 6a.

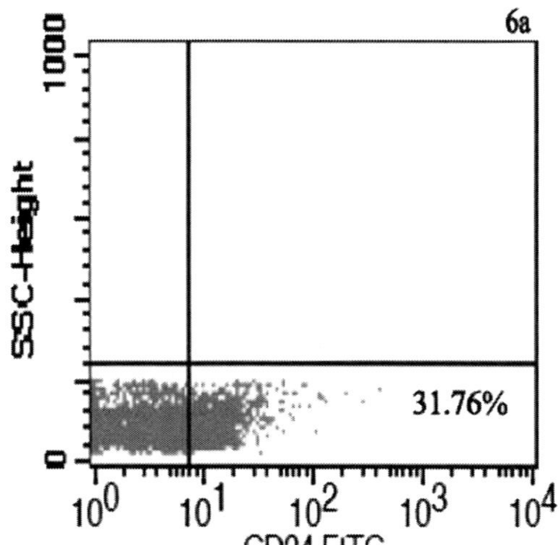

Figure 6a. The phenotypic characterization of CD 34 (FITC) receptor expression in control mice bone marrow cells showed 35.19±3.29% positivity.

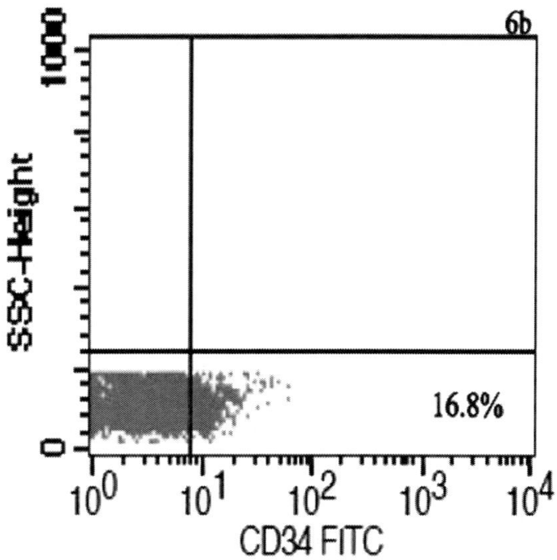

Figure 6b. The phenotypic characterization of CD 34 (FITC) receptor expression in arsenic exposed mice bone marrow cells showed decreased CD 34 (FITC) expression (20.19±3.0%) in comparison to control (P<0.0001).

Analysis of Sca-1, c-Kit positive stem cell population

The stem cells were denoted by Sca1, c-Kit receptor expression on their surface and labeled with Sca-1-PE and c-kit-FITC monoclonal antibodies which showed decreased $Sca1^+$, $c\text{-}Kit^+$ population (3.0±0.41%) (Figure 7b) in arsenic exposed animals in comparison to control (9.2±0.63%) (Figure 7a). The analysis indicated the loss in primitive stem cell population in arsenic exposed mice.

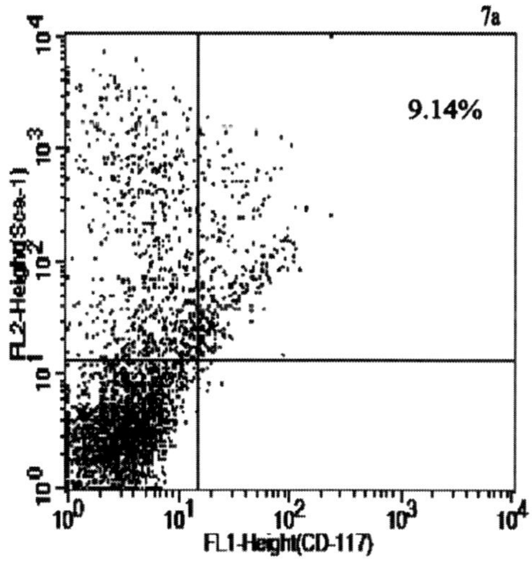

Figure 7a. The phenotypic analysis of Sca-1(PE), c-Kit (FITC) dual positive HSCs in control mice bone marrow cells showed 9.2±0.63 % positivity.

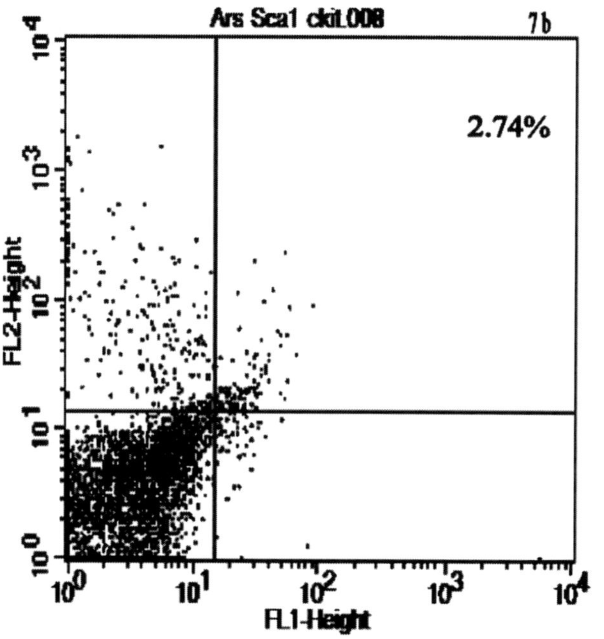

Figure 7b. The Sca-1(PE), c-Kit(FITC) dual positive HSC population in arsenic exposed mice reduced significantly which showed 3.0±0.41% positive cells (P<0.0001).

Discussion

The classic HSC features are self renewal, the capacity to differentiate, resistance to apoptosis and limitless proliferative potential [29]. Exposure to potentially hazardous environmental toxicants like arsenic leads to development of various types of morphological, physiological and biochemical changes in bone marrow hematopoietic cells and suppresses the normal immune response.

In the present study, we have exposed Swiss albino mice to arsenic trioxide by repeated injections to evaluate the effects of arsenic on hematopoietic cells and their precursors-the hematopoietic stem cells, the immune functional efficiency and death pattern to explore novel potential pathological mechanisms involved during arsenic toxicity in the bone marrow stem cell compartment.

The Leishman's stained peripheral blood smear of arsenic exposed mice showed cellular immaturity and morphological abnormalities suggesting the abnormal differentiation and the possible dysregulation in the blood forming compartment i.e. bone marrow. Simultaneously, Leishman's stained bone marrow smears of arsenic exposed mice showed distorted morphology of cells and appearance of abnormal cells in contrast to control mice bone marrow which depicted normal cellular structure and well organized distribution of cells. The typical bone marrow smear during arsenic toxicity showed partial maturation arrest of myelopoietic elements and presence of abnormal myeloid cells with nuclear fragmentation. Presence of these abnormal cells in the bone marrow threw the question about their immune functional capacity during foreign invasion.

The cell mediated immune functional parameters such as, phagocytosis and cytotoxicity revealed the inhibitory effects of arsenic on immune function of the bone marrow low density cells. Similar results were observed by Galicia *et al* [30] where human peripheral blood mononuclear cells were treated with arsenic *in vitro* [5]. The immunotoxicity caused by exposure to arsenicals includes the damages to the humoral and cell mediated immunity which could be a result of premature death [22] or due to presence of functionally inefficient cells. Apoptosis is characterized by certain morphological changes such as nuclear shrinkage, blebbing, nuclear and cytoplasmic fragmentation. A number of reports are available on arsenic as apoptotic agent. The analysis of death receptor Fas (CD95) in the arsenic exposed bone marrow stem/progenitor population revealed high amount of cells were in the pursuit of apoptosis. The cellular DNA which is in the terminal stage of death binds to 7AAD, a fluorescent dye which intercalates between cytosine and guanine bases. Analysis of 7AAD binding pattern showed a higher percentage of positive cells in arsenic exposed group in comparison with control. The types of proteins embedded in the membrane of stem cell are different from those of a fully differentiated adult cell. Thus, the receptor composition varies depending on the differentiation state of the cell. Under normal circumstances, the functionally defective cells and apoptotic cells are quickly replenished by the progenitor and primitive stem cells. The stem/progenitor cells were analyzed by the expression of CD34 [31], a marker of immature cells showed decreased expression suggesting the possible damage to the precursor cell compartment. The precursor devastation in the bone marrow leads to functional incapability which resulted in cellular death of the immune cells. This prompted us to carry the experiment further to analyze the fate of primitive stem cells which are responsible for the production of all the blood cells without seizing and are characterized by Sca-1, c-Kit positivity. The cell surface expression of Sca-1 is involved in regulating the HSC self-renewal. The receptor c-Kit which is expressed on HSCs, thought to be involved in the process of homing and engraftment by allowing HSCs to interact with stroma by binding to stem cell factor. In the healthy adult mouse, the HSC activity is featured by small subset of dual Sca-1$^+$ c-Kit$^+$ bone marrow hematopoietic cells [22] and these are the cells upon which the entire lineage depends. The flowcytometric analysis represented decrease in primitive HSC (Sca-1, c-Kit) population in comparison to control which hints at qualitative and quantitative loss of stem cell population in the bone marrow compartment due to arsenic toxicity. One possible explanation of the stem cell exhaustion is the weaker association between the HSCs and their niche cells resulting in 'evacuation of HSCs' [23].

In conclusion, we found that arsenic potentially impairs the immune response of bone marrow hematopoietic cells, induce apoptosis and cause significant alterations in stem and progenitor cell phenotype. It has been said that bone marrow not only shelters the HSCs, but also other tissue specific stem cells, which reside there. The recent concept of bone marrow stem cell oscillations from bone marrow to different tissue could possibly give a clue on tissue specific disorders in an individual by arsenic toxicity where the phenotypically and functionally deregulated HSCs along with other tissue specific stem cells, can not implement their function of tissue repair properly and results in various organ/tissue diseases.

Acknowledgment

We are thankful to the Department of Science and Technology, Government of India for their sponsorship. We are also thankful to Director, Calcutta School of Tropical Medicine.

References

[1] Salomoni, P. Stemming out of a new PML era? *Cell Death and Differ*, 2009, 16(8), 1083-1092.

[2] Agency for Toxic substances and disease registry CERCLA Priority List of hazardous substances. *Department of Health and Human Services.* 2005.

[3] Overall evaluations of carcinogenicity: an update of IARC monographs on the evaluation of carcinogenic risks to humans,Geneva. *IARC.* 1989, (7), 1-42.

[4] Germolec DR, Spalding J, Yu HS et al. Arsenic enhancement of skin neoplasia by chronic stimulation of growth factors. *Am. J. Pathol*, 1998, 153(6), 1775-1185.

[5] Cheng HY, Li P, David M, Smithgall TE, Feng L, Lieberman MW. Arsenic inhibition of the JAK-STAT pathway. *Oncogene*, 2004, 23(20), 3603-3612.

[6] Mandal AK, Das S, Basu MK, Chakrabarti RN, Das N. Hepatoprotective activity of liposomal flavonoid against arsenite-induced liver fibrosis. *J. Pharmacol. Exp. Ther*, 2007, 320(3), 994-1001.

[7] Chen CJ, Chiou HY, Chiang MH, Lin LJ, Tai TY. Dose-response relationship between ischemic heart disease mortality and long-term arsenic exposure. *Arterioscler. Thromb. Vasc. Biol,* 1996, 16 (4), 504-510.

[8] Chakraborti D, Mukherjee SC, Pati S et al. Arsenic groundwater contamination in Middle Ganga Plain, Bihar, India: a future danger? *Environ. Health Perspect*, 2003, 111(9), 1194-1201.

[9] Mukherjee S, Das D, Darbar S, Mukherjee M, Das AS, Mitra C. Arsenic trioxide generates oxidative stress and islet cell toxicity in rabbit. *Current Science*, 2004, 86(6), 854-857.

[10] Das S, Santra A, Lahiri S, Guha Mazumder DN. Implications of oxidative stress and hepatic cytokine (TNF-alpha and IL-6) response in the pathogenesis of hepatic collagenesis in chronic arsenic toxicity. *Toxicol. Appl. Pharmacol*, 2005, 204(1), 18-26.

[11] Burchiel SW, Mitchell LA, Lauer FT et al. Immunotoxicity and biodistribution analysis of arsenic trioxide in C57Bl/6 mice following a 2-week inhalation exposure. *Toxicol. Appl. Pharmacol,* 2009, 241(3), 253-259.

[12] Szymanska-Chabowska A, Antonowicz-Juchniewicz J, Andrzejak R. Some aspects of arsenic toxicity and carcinogenicity in living organism with special regard to its influence on cardiovascular system, blood and bone marrow. *Int. J. Occup. Med. Environ. Health*, 2002, 15(2), 101-116.

[13] Agency for toxic substances and disease registry. Medical management guidelines for arsenic trioxide (As2O3).

[14] Saha KC. Melanokeratosis from arsenic contaminated tubewell water. *Indian J. Dermatol,* 1984, 29(4), 37- 46.

[15] 15. Patlolla AK, Tchounwou PB. Cytogenetic evaluation of arsenic trioxide toxicity in Sprague- *Dawley rats. Mutat Res.*, 2005, 587(1-2), 126-133.

[16] Feussner JR, Shelburne JD, Bredehoeft S, Cohen HJ. Arsenic-induced bone marrow toxicity: ultrastructural and electron-probe analysis. *Blood*, 1979, 53(5), 820-827.

[17] Westhoff DD, Samaha RJ, Barnes A Jr. Arsenic intoxication as a cause of megaloblastic anemia. *Blood,* 1975, 45(2), 241-246.

[18] Pralle H, Manz F. Influence of chronic arsenic poisoning on bone marrow morphology. A case report. *Blut*, 1985, 50(1), 51-54.

[19] Lage CR, Nayak A, Kim CH. Arsenic ecotoxicology and innate immunity. *Integr.* Comp. Biol, 2006, 46(6), 1040-1054.

[20] Sakurai T, Kaise T, Matsubara C. Inorganic and methylated arsenic compounds induce cell death in murine macrophages via different mechanisms. *Chem. Res. Toxicol*, 1998, 11(4), 273-283.

[21] Scadden DT. Circadian rhythms: Stem cells traffic in time. *Nature*, 2008, 452(7186), 416-417.

[22] Mendez-Ferrer S, Lucas D, Battista M, Frenette PS. Haematopoietic stem cell release is regulated by circadian oscillations. *Nature,* 2008, 452(7186), 442-447.

[23] Trumpp A, Essers M, Wilson A. Awakening dormant haematopoietic stem cells. *Nat. Rev. Immunol,* 2010, 10(3), 201-209.

[24] Rego EM, He LZ, Warrell RP Jr, Wang ZG, Pandolfi PP. Retinoic acid (RA) and As2O3 treatment in transgenic models of acute promyelocytic leukemia (APL) unravel the distinct nature of the leukemogenic process induced by the PML-RARalpha and PLZF-RARalpha oncoproteins. *Proc. Natl. Acad. Sci. USA*, 2000, 97(18), 10173-10178.

[25] Basak P, Chatterjee S, Das M et al. Phenotypic alteration of bone marrow HSC and microenvironmental association in experimentally induced leukemia. *Curr. Stem Cell Res. Ther*, 2010, 5(4), 379-386.

[26] Chatterjee S, Chaklader M, Basak P et al. An animal model of chronic aplastic bone marrow failure following pesticide exposure in mice. *Int.J. Stem Cells*, 2010, 3(1), 54-62.

[27] Law S, Begum B, Chaudhuri S. Pluripotent bone marrow cells in leukemic mice elicit enhanced immune reactivity following sheep erythrocyte administration in-vivo. A possible S-LFA3 interactive immunotherapy. *J. Exp. Clin. Cancer Res*, 2003, 22(2), 213-221.

[28] Chatterjee S, Dutta RK, Basak P et al. Alteration in marrow stromal microenvironment and apoptosis mechanisms involved in aplastic anemia: An animal model to study the possible disease pathology. *Stem Cells Int*, 2010 (PMID: 21048856).

[29] Chumsri S, Matsui W, Burger AM. Therapeutic implications of leukemic stem cell pathways. *Clin. Cancer Res*, 2007, 13(22 pt1), 6549-6554.

[30] Galicia G, Leyva R, Tenorio EP, Ostrosky-Wegman P, Saavedra R. Sodium arsenite retards proliferation of PHA-activated T cells by delaying the production and secretion of IL-2. *Int Immunopharmacol*, 2003, 3(5), 671-682.

[31] Krause DS, Ito T, Fackler MJ, Smith OM, Collector MI, Sharkis SJ, May WS. Characterization of murine CD34, a marker for hematopoietic progenitor and stem cells. *Blood* 1994, 84(3), 691-701.

In: Stem Cells in Disease
Editor: Prasad S. Koka

ISBN: 978-1-62257-169-7
© 2012 Nova Science Publishers, Inc.

Chapter IX

Sulfatide Administration Leads to Inhibition of HIV-1 Replication and Enhanced Hematopoeisis

*I. Birgitta Sundell[1], Ramesh Halder[2], Menghua Zhang[1], Igor Maricic[2], Prasad S. Koka[1] and Vipin Kumar[*2]*

[1]Laboratories of Stem Cell Biology and
[2]Autoimmunity, Torrey Pines Institute for Molecular Studies,
San Diego, California, US

Abstract

The pathogenesis of HIV-1 infection is a complex process in which Natural Killer (NK) and Natural Killer T (NKT) cells play an important role. NKT cells express markers for NK cells and a TCR of the conventional T cells and recognize lipid antigens presented by the non-polymorphic CD1 molecule. CD1d-restricted type I NKT cells express an invariant TCR and can recognize αGalCer, whereas a major subset of type II NKT expressing diverse TCR can recognize a self-glycolipid, sulfatide. It has been shown that CD4+ type I NKT cells are infected by HIV-1 and decreased in HIV-1-infected individuals. However, their exact role in HIV-1 infection as well as the biology and function of the type II NKT cell subset in HIV-1 infection and disease progression are not known. Our earlier studies have shown that activation of CD1d-restricted type II NKT cells by sulfatide and their interactions with plasmacytoid dendritic (pDC) and myeloid dendritic (mDC) cells result in anergy induction in type I NKT cells in several models. Here we used SCID-Hu (Thy/Liv) animals, co-implanted with human fetal liver and thymus, and found that these implants contain both type I and type II NKT cells, CD161+CD3+ NKT cells, NK cells and dendritic cells during HIV-infection. We found that the administration of sulfatide (bi-weekly, 20 μg/animal, i.p.) in SCID-Hu animals inhibits HIV-1 replication more efficiently than treatment with the nucleoside analog reverse transcriptase inhibitor, AZT. Virus replication was lowered significantly up to 4-8 weeks post infection. Furthermore sulfatide administration also resulted in significant

[*] Corresponding Authors: Vipin Kumar, M.S., Ph.D. Tel: 858-597-3870. Email: vkumar@tpims.org.

retention of hematopoeisis that is lost during HIV-1 infection. Advantageously, sulfatide administration itself was not associated with anemia or bone marrow suppression, that are severe side effects of HAART. Since the CD1d-mediated immune pathway is highly conserved between rodents and humans, sulfatide treatment may represent a novel HLA-independent approach for intervention of HIV-1 pathogenesis.

Keywords: HIV-1, Sulfatide, NKT cells, CD1, SCID-Hu, Hematopoiesis

Introduction

The pathogenesis of HIV-1 infection is a complex process dependent upon several factors including host's immune and genetic characteristics. This results in a variable pattern of disease progression among HIV-infected individuals. Innate immune mechanisms are active at the mucosal surfaces that are primary sites for HIV-1 entry. Thus, an alteration in innate immunity mediated by Natural Killer (NK) and type I Natural Killer T (NKT) cells can have important effects on HIV-1 infection and disease progression.

NK cells, as first line of defense against pathogens, are very potent in destroying infected and transformed cells. Two subsets of NK cells (CD161+ and CD56+) can either directly kill infected host cells or rapidly secrete cytokines (e.g., IFN-γ) and chemokines upon activation with type I interferons (IFNα or IFNβ). Interactions between NK cells and dendritic cells (DC) also influence the nature of subsequent immune response [1]. In HIV pathogenesis, NK cells are thought to play an important role [1, 2] and increased NK cell activity (IFN-γ and TNF-α secretion) has been found to be associated with HIV-1 exposed but uninfected subjects [3]. Recently, HLA and killer-cell immunoglobulin-like receptor (KIR) polymorphisms have been reported to significantly influence the progression of AIDS in HIV-infected patients [4]. And a decrease in number and function of NK cells in PBL is associated with rapid disease progression [2].

NKT cells play an important role in autoimmune diseases, anti-tumor immunity and in host defense against foreign microbes and viruses [5-11]. Natural killer T cells (NKT) possess features of NK cells as well as T cells and express corresponding cell surface receptors e.g., NK1.1 or CD56/CD161 and TCR. Most NKT cells recognize lipid antigens bound in the context of CD1 molecules which are non-polymorphic, MHC class I-like and associated with β2-microglobulin [12, 13]. Antigen-presenting cells such as dendritic cells, macrophages and subsets of B cells express CD1 molecules. CD1 proteins are conserved among species and comprised of CD1a, CD1b, and CD1c proteins in human; and the CD1d molecule, present in both mouse and in human.

Based upon their TCR gene usage CD1d-restricted NKT cells can be divided into 2 categories: one using the invariant TCR (iNK T or type I) and the other expressing non-invariant or diverse TCRs (type II NKT) [7, 14]. The invariant TCR used by type I NKT cells is encoded by the germline TCR α chain (mouse Vα14Jα18, human Vα24-JαQ) and diverse mouse Vβ8 or human Vβ11 chains [5, 7, 14]. Most type I NKT cells can recognize α–galactosylceramide (αGalCer), a marine sponge-derived glycolipid, and iGB3, a self-glycolipid. A major subset of type II NKT cells has been shown to recognize a self-glycolipid sulfatide (3'-sulfogalactosyl ceramide) in both mice and in humans [9, 15-21]. In this glycolipid the 3'-OH moiety on the galactose is sulfated and the carbohydrate moiety is attached to the ceramide in a β-linkage. Type I NKT cells display memory or activation markers and upon stimulation, rapidly secrete large quantities of cytokines, including IFN−γ and IL-4 [22]. Furthermore, activation of type I NKT cells with glycolipid results in a cascade of events that includes activation of NK cells, dendritic cells and B cells.

HIV-1 entry into target cells is dependent upon the expression of chemokine receptors, such as CCR5 or CXCR4 in conjunction with CD4 [23]. Additionally, HIV-1 infection is also modulated by cellular signals within the target CD4+ T cells; for example resting T cells are relatively resistant and activation of T cells augments infection. CD1d-restricted type I NKT cells are autoreactive, activated and express memory cells surface markers such as CD69. These cells are also CD4+ and also express co-receptor CCR5. These features collectively make type I NKT cells one of the key targets for HIV-1-infection. Consistently, these cells have been shown to be infected by HIV-1 and are depleted in HIV-infected individuals [24-27]. Indeed R5-tropic HIV-1 replicates well in CD4+ type I NKT cells and induces their rapid destruction in vitro [25]. Based upon these features of type I NKT cells, it has been speculated that CD4+ NKT cells could serve as a gateway for R5-tropic HIV-1 during the initial stages of infection [28]. These cells could also contribute to spread of HIV-1 through bystander activation of other cells. Thus, cytokines and chemokines secreted by activated NKT cells could activate not only NK cells and DC but also resting conventional CD4+ T cells and render them susceptible to HIV infection [28].

Recent studies have shown that the number of type I NKT (Vα24+Vβ11+CD161+CD4+) cells can be significantly restored following early treatment with HAART and IL-2 [29-31]. Furthermore, it was shown that supernatant from activated CD4+ NKT cells isolated from the PBL strongly suppresses HIV-1 replication in vitro [30]. Consistently, expression of CD1d molecules has been shown to be downregulated by HIV-1. Nef and gp120 proteins and HAART-mediated viral suppression restored CD1d expression [32-34]. Thus the immune reconstitution mediated by HAART is not restricted to conventional CD4+ and CD8+ T cells but also involves restoration of an important immunoregulatory axis involving CD1d and NKT cells. Although HIV-specific lipid antigens for CD1d-restricted NKT cells have not yet been identified, HIV-associated alterations in lipid metabolism has been suggested [35].

DC are the key antigen-presenting cells and can influence both innate and adaptive immunity. DC can pick up antigens and migrate into secondary lymphoid organs to initiate antigen-specific adaptive CD4+ and CD8+ T cell responses. They are also effectors of innate immunity: (a) pDC, a subset of DC, are specialized for the production of type I interferons following stimulation; (b) DC secrete IL-12; and (c) they can regulate both NK and NKT cell activities. Qualitative and quantitative changes have been shown to occur in DC populations during HIV-1 infection. Both conventional or myeloid (mDC) and plasmacytoid (pDC) are reduced in PBL especially in patients with advanced disease and with active viral replication (36-39). The mechanism by which DC are lost in HIV-1 infection is not clear and may involve migration, killing due to direct infection, or indirectly by cytotoxic CD8+ T cells. Interestingly, a high frequency of pDC and increased production of IFNα in response to viral infection have been reported in the PBL of long-term nonprogressors and long-term survivors, suggesting a potential key role for this subset of DC in control of HIV-1 infection [40, 41].

Currently, the biology and function of type I vs type II NKT cell subsets and their interactions with DC and NK cells in HIV-1 infection and disease progression is not entirely understood. In this study, using the SCID-Hu (Thy/Liv) model, we show that activation of type II NKT cells by sulfatide administration significantly inhibits HIV-1 replication, even post-infection, and is able to prevent HIV-1 related pancytopenia. As to the highly conserved nature of CD1d-mediated lipid presentation pathway from mouse to human, this study has important implications for the development of novel therapeutic strategies against the virus.

Results

Sulfatide administration inhibits HIV-1 replication and augments hematopoeisis in SCID-Hu Thy/Liv animals: SCID-Hu Thy/Liv mice were treated with sulfatide or AZT at different times in relation to HIV-1 infection and viral load as well as phenotype of cells was determined. Sulfatide was injected i.p. twice a week beginning (a) one day prior, (b) same day, (c) one day later than HIV-1 infection, (d) 4 or 8 weeks post-infection until their sacrifice.

Table 1. Inhibition of HIV-1 replication in infected SCID-Hu mice following treatment with sulfatide. SCID-Hu mice were treated i.p. with 20 μg/animal of sulfatide in PBS/vehicle or AZT or none at indicated time points. Viral load was determined using real-time PCR (42, 43). Multilineage hematopoiesis in vitro was assessed by colony forming assay (CFA) of 5 X 10^6 total cells, not separated from CD34+CD38- population, derived from the implants in methylcellulose (myeloid and erythroid) and in megacult-C (megakaryoid) media. These data are derived from 4-7 animals in each group and are representative of 3 individual experiments. *p values are 0.002.

Infection	Drug Treatment Initiation	Cessation or Biopsy	Viral load (#HIV-1 proviral copies/μg DNA)	% CD4+ Cells	Colony Forming Activity (CFA) Myeloid	Erythroid	Megakaryoid
Mock	None	8 wks (day 56)	0	97 +/- 4	587 +/- 37	685 +/- 51	231 +/- 120
Mock	AZT day 0	8 wks (day 56)	0	84 +/- 2	555 +/- 45	535 +/- 127	151 +/- 37
Mock	Sulfatide day 0	8 wks (day 56)	0	86 +/- 7	590	661	313
HIV-1	None	4 wks (day 28)	4404 +/- 262	51 +/- 5	51	116	11
HIV-1	Sulfatide day -1	4 wks (day 28)	392 +/- 5*	73 +/- 2	406	653	131
HIV-1	Sulfatide day 0	4 wks (day 28)	324 +/- 8*	65 +/- 3	313	174	76
HIV-1	Sulfatide day +1	4 wks (day 28)	379 +/- 8*	62 +/- 8	534	341	108
HIV-1	None	8 wks (day 56)	3981 +/- 145	5 +/- 2	60	72	9
HIV-1	AZT day 28	8 wks (day 56)	941 +/- 8	9 +/- 1	152	220	12
HIV-1	Sulfatide day 28	8 wks (day 56)	488 +/- 6*	42 +/- 4	268	328	144

As shown in Table 1, even at 8 wks post-infection, sulfatide administration alone attenuates HIV-1 replication by about 10-fold compared to only about 4.5-fold by AZT. Whereas AZT treatment of mock infected animals decreased multilineage CFA by about 35%, sulfatide administration inhibits CFA by only about 11%. It is notable that sulfatide injection 4 and 8 weeks post infection significantly lowered virus replication. Our data suggest that cytopenias that occur following HIV-1 infection and HAART therapy may be also circumvented by treatment with sulfatide. We have not found any toxicity associated with sulfatide at the doses used so far. Thus inhibition of virus replication that occurs results in enhanced multi-lineage hematopoiesis of the human CD34+ progenitor stem cells. The SCID-Hu were unaffected by the sulfatide administration and continue to behave like the mock treated animals in the absence of HIV-1 infection.

Sulfatide administration influences different subsets of innate-like lymphocytes, including NKT cell subsets during HIV-1 infection in the SCID-Hu animals. Since activation of type II NKT cells by sulfatide significantly inhibits HIV-1 replication, we studied the role of type II NKT cells and their cellular interactions during HIV-1 infection.

We found that a number of innate-like lymphocytes, including type I NKT (αGalCer /CD1d-tetramer+), type II NKT (sulfatide/humanCD1d-tetramer+) cells and NK cells (CD3-CD56+) are present in Thy-Liv implants in the SCID-Hu animals. To confirm staining of human cells, MNCs were gated on human CD45+ cells to avoid murine cell types. Relative numbers of different cell types in mock infected animals is shown in the Figure 1 below.

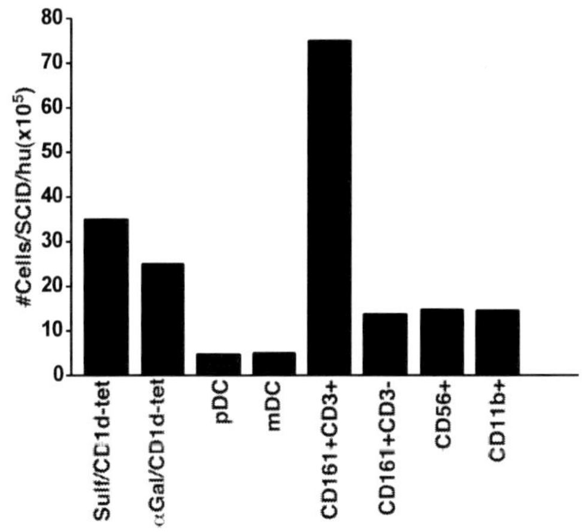

Figure 1. Enumeration of type I and type II NKT cells, NK cells, dendritic cell subsets, and macrophages in SCID-hu-mice. The SCID-hu-mice were sacrificed on day 15 following mock or HIV infection and single cell suspensions were prepared and were stained with several anti-human antibodies and tetramers (see bar graph) and analyzed by flow cytometry. Human lymphocytes were distinguished using CD45-FITC staining. The bar graph represents the absolute numbers of different subsets of leukocytes from mock infected SCID-hu-mice and alterations in different populations following HIV infection is presented in the Table 2. These percent cells are found in the total thymocytes in each human graft. Regularly, we have been able to collect a total of more than 200 million cells from both mock- or HIV-infected SCID-hu grafts around 2.5 weeks. For the enumeration of type II NKT cells, sulfatide/humanCD1d-tetramers and for type I NKT (αGalCerhuman CD1d-tetramers or Vα24+Vβ11+ staining was used. Various combinations of mAbs against human cell surface antigens (BD-Biosciences, Immunotech, eBiosciences and Miltenyi) were used for staining NK cells, plasmacytoid DC (pDC), myeloid DC (mDC) or CD11b+ macrophages. These data are representative of three independent experiments.

Table 2. Different subsets of leukocytes from mock infected SCID-hu-mice and alterations in different populations following HIV infection

Cell subsets	% Positive cells	
	Mock	HIV-infected
$CD4^+$	94.98	95.58
$CD8\beta^+$	73.08	80.87
$CD11b^+$	0.1-0.2	0.6-1.74
CD56+	0.12	0.59
$CD3^+CD161^+$	0.71	3.04
CD161+	0.18	0.14
Type I NKT	0.36	0.29
Type II NKT	0.84	1.12

As shown, sulfatide-reactive type II NKT cells are consistently higher in number than type I NKT cells. More importantly, we found that while the number of type I NKT cells decreases 2-3 weeks following HIV-1 infection in SCID-Hu implants, the number of type II NKT cells remain similar or even slightly increased. A summary of the changes in these different cell subsets is given below in the Table 2. We also found that most of the invariant or type I NKT cells as well as sulfatide/CD1d-tetramer+ type II NKT cells appear to be CD161+ and are CD3+.

Interestingly, following HIV-1 infection both subsets of DC (pDC and mDC) as well as CD11b+ cells are significantly increased in Thy-Liv implants in SCID-Hu animals. Although, total CD56+ cells were significantly increased in HIV-infected animals, CD3-CD56+ NK cells appear to be decreased suggesting expression of CD56 by other cells including NKT.

Discussion

In this study, we show that activation of type II NKT cells by administration of sulfatide, even post-infection, inhibits HIV-1 replication in the SCID-Hu (Thy/Liv) model. Compared to AZT, the antiviral effect of sulfatide is higher and does not involve the side effect of pancytopenia. Furthermore, our data suggest a loss of type I NKT cells and an elevation in the number of type II NKT cells following HIV-1 infection in SCID-Hu animals.

CD1d-restricted type I NKT cells are infected in HIV-1 individuals and also their number is significantly reduced. It is not known whether type II NKT cells are infected and also activated during HIV-1 infection. Type I NKT cells in both mice and in humans in the unmanipulated or "naïve" state, show a memory phenotype, and express co/receptors (CD4+CCR5+) required for HIV-1 infection [23]. In contrast, we have found that murine sulfatide-reactive type II NKT cells identified using sulfatide/CD1d-tetramers are CD69- and do not express other activation/memory markers (17) (75). Our data suggest that sulfatide-reactive type II NKT cells in human PBL also do not express memory or activated phenotype, and thus it is likely that they will not be infected with HIV-1 initially. It is not known whether following HIV infection, NKT subsets are differentially activated and then infected with the virus.

Several features of type I NKT cells suggest important implications for their potential role in HIV pathogenesis. These cells have been shown to be deficient in autoimmune diseases, e.g., IDDM [44]. Also in experimental models for multiple sclerosis, type 1 diabetes, and lupus, both type I and type II NKT cells have been shown to regulate autoimmunity [6-8, 10, 11, 45]. It is therefore possible that loss of type I NKT cells in HIV-infected individuals may lead to hyperactivation of self-reactive T cells. Similarly, since type I NKT cells also have anti-tumor activity, their depletion may contribute to the elevated incidence of tumors in AIDS patients, e.g., sarcoma or lymphomas in AIDS patients. Consistent with the immunoregulatory role of type I NKT cells against tumors and other infections, a higher level of type I NKT cells has been associated with a reduced risk of cancer [46]. Thus HIV-1-induced innate immune dysfunction may contribute to poor immunosurveillance and development of HIV related tumors. On the other hand, type I NKT cells play a key role in protective immunity against bacterial and viral infections. They have been shown to recognize bacterial-derived lipids and mount an immune response [5, 7]. Therefore loss of these cells could result in HIV-infected individuals to become more susceptible to opportunistic mycobacterial infections and perhaps the hepatitis C virus infection.

Since innate lymphocte-mediated immune responses are generated within hours following infection, presentation of either self-glycolipids or viral derived antigens by CD1 molecules may set the stage for subsequent adaptive humoral (antibodies) or celluar immunity (Class I and class II MHC-restricted T cells) against the HIV-1, respectively. It is clear from our studies, in experimental models of autoimmunity and tumor models, that interaction of type I and type II NKT cells with DC populations either tolerizes or activates them depending upon the context and antigens. These interactions eventually influence both T and B cell responses against protein antigens. Therefore it is important to analyze for CD1d expression as well as other activation molecules on DC subsets early following HIV-1 infection. We have already found that CD1d is expressed in most of the cells isolated from Thy/Liv implants during HIV-1 infection. How HIV-I infection influences activation or CD1d expression in two major subsets of DC, pDC vs. mDC is not known. It is likely that both pDC and mDC express CD1d and this becomes upregulated selectively on one or both populations following HIV-1 infection. We have found that pDC express higher levels of CD1d in comparison to mDC or other APCs in the murine models. Also in addition to CD1d expression, capacity to stimulate type I and type II NK T cells will depend upon the expression of other co-stimulatory molecules. Therefore we cannot predict the behavior of these DC in stimulating NKT cells based upon the CD1d levels alone without knowing the expression of co-stimulatory molecules.

The mechanism(s) by which sulfatide administration in SCID-Hu animals inhibits HIV-1 replication is not understood. Is this achieved by the immunological mechanism, or it also involves non-immune mechanisms. Two key experimental observations in murine models suggest that sulfatide-mediated induction of anergy in type I NKT cells and treatment of autoimmunity is mediated by immune cells: (a) type II NKT cell and pDC activation results in anergy induction in type I NKT cells that is absolutely CD1d-dependent [16]; (b) Anergy induction in type I NKT cells in recipients can be transferred by mDC but not pDC from sulfatide-injected animals. These data suggest that both NKT cell subsets and DC subsets are influenced *in vivo* by CD1d-dependent immune regulatory events. Additionally, sulfatide has been shown to have a number of effects on other membrane receptors that are non-immune related. For example, it has been shown earlier, that sulfatide can also bind to gp120 in *in vitro* assays and can inhibit HIV-1 entry into CD4-/CXCR4+ cells [47]. However, concentration of glycolipids required for these membrane-related changes is 2-3 logs higher than the concentrations used in our experiments. Therefore it is unlikely that direct non-immune effects of sulfatide are responsible for the inhibition of viral replication. As mentioned above, in murine models we have found that the effects mediated by the microgram quantities of sulfatide in *in vivo* assays are dependent upon the presence of CD1d molecules that present lipids to type II NKT cells [15-18, 21]. These studies were done using CD1d-/- mice and blocking presentation using anti-CD1d mAb. We have not used blocking anti-CD1d mAbs in SCID-Hu animals injected with sulfatide to determine whether inhibition of HIV-1 replication is reversed, because they have been shown to be agonistic on their own and activates APCs in vivo. Furthermore, it is possible that sulfatide also inhibits HIV-1 entry and thereby infection in SCID-Hu animals.

It is clear from our data that following CD1d-dependent recognition of sulfatide in murine models, it is the pDC and not mDC that are selectively stimulated and express elevated levels of CD40, CD80, CD86, and CD1d molecules. Human pDCs (CD11c-CD123+) have been shown to be one of the targets of HIV-1 and respond to the virus by producing type 1 IFNs (IFNα or IFNβ) [48]. Several studies have also shown that both DC subsets are reduced in numbers in patient's blood [36-39]. It has been shown that activated pDC also lead to maturation of mDC in a bystander fashion during HIV-1 infection [48]. It is not clear at present whether type I IFN secretion following HIV infection is influenced in sulfatide-treated animals. Type I IFNs not only directly inhibit HIV replication [49-51] but also have adjuvant effects on other cells, including NK cells and conventional CD4/CD8 T cells.

It is surprising that despite their low numbers, CD1d-restricted NKT cells may have a profound effect in the conjoint human organ in SCID-Hu animals. Based on the studies in other murine models about sulfatide-reactive type II NKT cells and their interactions with other cells *in vivo*, we can propose a number of ways in which they might influence HIV-1 infection: (a) NKT cells could help B cells to generate neutralizing antibodies against HIV-1 antigens; (b) NKT cells and other activated cells such as DC and NK cells can secrete IFN-□ and type I interferons that have been shown to have strong anti-viral effects; (c) NKT/NK cells could also secrete chemokines, such as RANTES and Mip1β that could block entry of HIV-1 into neighboring CD4+ T cells; (d) Activation of DC and secretion of cytokines can also result in augmentation of conventional CD4+ and CD8+ cytotoxic responses against HIV antigens; (e) NKT cells can also regulate hematopoiesis. Studies are in progress to investigate these possibilities in the SCID-Hu model of HIV-1 infection. A detailed study of the activation, expansion or deletion of CD1d-restricted NKT cells during HIV infection in humans will have important implication for the development of novel intervention strategies for the viral replication as well as for the regulation of hematopoiesis [52].

Materials and Methods

HIV-1 Infection in SCID-Hu Thy-Liv Mice

C.B-17 scid/scid (Balb background) mice were used in these studies as recipients of human fetal tissues or cells and were purchased from The Jackson Laboratory and housed in our institute (TPIMS) vivarium. All mice were maintained in specific pathogen free-conditions in BSL-2 facilities at the TPIMS. Treatment of animals was in compliance with federal and institutional guidelines and approved by the TPIMS Animal Care and Use Committee. SCID mice received transplants of 1-mm^3 pieces of human fetal thymus and liver tissues under the renal capsule. The resulting conjoint organ was allowed to grow for 3 to 5 month, as described previously [53, 54]. The Thy/Liv implants were then infected by intra-implant injection of 100 IU (50-100 ml) of HIV-1_{NL4-3} or the R5-tropic viral strain JR-CSF, which were produced in the CEM or 293T cell lines. Control mock-infected animals were injected with the same volume of mock-infected cell line culture medium alone. At specific time intervals post-infection, sequential wedge biopsies were obtained and processed for flow cytometry and viral loads. Viral loads were determined using real-time RT PCR analysis, as described earlier [42, 55, 56] Real-time PCR was carried out using Brilliant SYBER Green QPCR kit (Stratagene) on a Stratagene Mx3000p machine. The calculation of comparative mRNA expression was performed by the Stratagene software and was designated as relative quantity after normalization against internal control gene and after consideration of amplification efficiency of individual genes.

Glycolipids

Chemically synthesized α–galactosylceramide (αGalCer)dissolved at the concentration of 220 mg/ml in vehicle (0.5% polysorbate 20 and 0.9% NaCl solution) was provided by Pharmaceutical Research Laboratory of Kirin Brewery Co., Japan [57]. Purified myelin-derived sulfatide was purchased from Matreya Inc. and also dissolved in the "vehicle" as above and diluted with PBS for *in vivo* intraperitoneal bi-weekly injections into SCID-Hu animals.

Tetrameric CD1d-Lipid Complexes

PE-labeled αGalCer/CD1d and sulfatide/CD1d tetrameric complexes were generated by loading human PE-labeled CD1d protein (NIH Tetramer Facility) with different glycolipids in a molar ratio of 1:3 over night at room temperature.

Antibodies and Flow Cytometry

Mononuclear cells (MNCs) isolated from Thy-Liv implants were suspended in FACS buffer (1-2 x 10^6/ml) containing PBS in 0.02% NaN_3 (wt/vol) and 2% FBS (vol/vol). In all experiments, cells were first incubated with antibodies against FcR-γ and then labeled and gated on the human CD45+ population to exclude murine cells. FITC-, PE-, Cy-Chrome and allophycocyanin-conjugated mAbs were acquired from BD Biosciences: PE-anti-human CD8β, APC-Anti-human CD8, PE-Anti-human CD1d, PE mouse anti-human CD3, FITC-anti-human CD161, PE-anti-human CD56, PE-Cy7 anti-human CD123, PE-anti-human ILT7, FITC-anti-human CD69; Miltenyi Biotec: FITC-anti-human CD1c (BDCA-1); Immunotech:

PE anti-human TCR Vα24, FITC-anti-human TCR Vβ11; eBioscience: FITC anti-human CD3, purified human FcγR-binding inhibitor. Flow cytometry analysis was performed using FACSCalibur instrument with CellQuest software (Becton Dickinson).

Colony-Forming Assay

The CFA were performed as previously described using the semi-solid methylcellulose medium in Petri dishes with grids in duplicate to facilitate counting of the myeloid and erythroid colonies. The methylcellulose medium consists of the hematopoietic cytokines or growth factors, IL3, IL6, SCF, GM-CSF and Erythropoietin as reported earlier [43]. Megakaryoid colonies were evaluated in the Megacult-C medium. CD34+ cells seeded in these media at 250 or 500 cells/dish are cultured in these media for two weeks prior to counting of the colonies.

Statistical Analysis

Comparison of viral RNA copy numbers in treated vs. untreated samples were performed using a two-sided Wilcoxin rank sum test as earlier [42, 43]. Fisher's exact test was used to determine the significance of the differences in cell number between mock- vs. viral-infected or treated population. In some cases, statistical significance between groups was determined using an unpaired Student's t-test.

Acknowledgments

This work was supported by grants R01HL079846 (PSK) and R01 CA100660, DNRG and MSNRC (VK).

References

[1] Lanier, L. L. 2008. Evolutionary struggles between NK cells and viruses. *Nat. Rev. Immunol* 8:259-268.

[2] Fauci, A. S., D. Mavilio, and S. Kottilil. 2005. NK cells in HIV infection: paradigm for protection or targets for ambush. *Nat. Rev. Immunol* 5:835-843.

[3] Scott-Algara, D., L. X. Truong, P. Versmisse, A. David, T. T. Luong, N. V. Nguyen, I. Theodorou, F. Barre-Sinoussi, and G. Pancino. 2003. Cutting edge: increased NK cell activity in HIV-1-exposed but uninfected Vietnamese intravascular drug users. *J. Immunol.* 171:5663-5667.

[4] Martin, M. P., Y. Qi, X. Gao, E. Yamada, J. N. Martin, F. Pereyra, S. Colombo, E. E. Brown, W. L. Shupert, J. Phair, J. J. Goedert, S. Buchbinder, G. D. Kirk, A. Telenti, M. Connors, S. J. O'Brien, B. D. Walker, P. Parham, S. G. Deeks, D. W. McVicar, and M. Carrington. 2007. Innate partnership of HLA-B and KIR3DL1 subtypes against HIV-1. *Nat. Genet* 39:733-740.

[5] Bendelac, A., P. B. Savage, and L. Teyton. 2007. The biology of NKT cells. *Annu. Rev. Immunol* 25:297-336.

[6] Cerundolo, V., and M. Salio. 2007. Harnessing NKT cells for therapeutic applications. *Curr. Top Microbiol. Immunol.* 314:325-340.

[7] Kronenberg, M. 2005. Toward an understanding of NKT cell biology: progress and paradoxes. *Annu. Rev. Immunol* 23:877-900.

[8] La Cava, A., and F. D. Shi. 2006. Natural and adaptive immune cell-based therapies in autoimmunity. *Curr. Med. Chem* 13:1557-1566.

[9] Terabe, M., and J. A. Berzofsky. 2007. NKT cells in immunoregulation of tumor immunity: a new immunoregulatory axis. *Trends Immunol* 28:491-496.

[10] Van Kaer, L. 2007. NKT cells: T lymphocytes with innate effector functions. *Curr. Opin Immunol.* 19:354-364.

[11] Yamamura, T., K. Sakuishi, Z. Illes, and S. Miyake. 2007. Understanding the behavior of invariant NKT cells in autoimmune diseases. *J. Neuroimmunol.* 191:8-15.

[12] Brigl, M., and M. B. Brenner. 2004. CD1: antigen presentation and T cell function. *Annu Rev Immunol* 22:817-890.

[13] Porcelli, S. A., and R. L. Modlin. 1999. The CD1 system: antigen-presenting molecules for T cell recognition of lipids and glycolipids. *Annu. Rev. Immunol.* 17:297-329.

[14] Godfrey, D. I., J. Rossjohn, and J. McCluskey. 2008. The fidelity, occasional promiscuity, and versatility of T cell receptor recognition. *Immunity* 28:304-314.

[15] Ambrosino, E., M. Terabe, R. C. Halder, J. Peng, S. Takaku, S. Miyake, T. Yamamura, V. Kumar, and J. A. Berzofsky. 2007. Cross-regulation between type I and type II NKT cells in regulating tumor immunity: a new immunoregulatory axis. *J. Immunol.* 179:5126-5136.

[16] Halder, R. C., C. Aguilera, I. Maricic, and V. Kumar. 2007. Type II NKT cell-mediated anergy induction in type I NKT cells prevents inflammatory liver disease. *J. Clin. Invest* 117:2302-2312.

[17] Jahng, A., I. Maricic, C. Aguilera, S. Cardell, R. C. Halder, and V. Kumar. 2004. Prevention of autoimmunity by targeting a distinct, noninvariant CD1d-reactive T cell population reactive to sulfatide. *J. Exp. Med.* 199:947-957.

[18] Roy, K. C., I. Maricic, A. Khurana, T. R. Smith, R. C. Halder, and V. Kumar. 2008. Involvement of Secretory and Endosomal Compartments in Presentation of an Exogenous Self-Glycolipid to Type II NKT Cells. *J. Immunol.* 180:2942-2950.

[19] Shamshiev, A., A. Donda, I. Carena, L. Mori, L. Kappos, and G. De Libero. 1999. Self glycolipids as T-cell autoantigens. *Eur. J. Immunol.* 29:1667-1675.

[20] Shamshiev, A., A. Donda, T. I. Prigozy, L. Mori, V. Chigorno, C. A. Benedict, L. Kappos, S. Sonnino, M. Kronenberg, and G. De Libero. 2000. The alphabeta T cell response to self-glycolipids shows a novel mechanism of CD1b loading and a requirement for complex oligosaccharides. *Immunity* 13:255-264.

[21] Zajonc, D. M., I. Maricic, D. Wu, R. Halder, K. Roy, C. H. Wong, V. Kumar, and I. A. Wilson. 2005. Structural basis for CD1d presentation of a sulfatide derived from myelin and its implications for autoimmunity. *J. Exp. Med.* 202:1517-1526.

[22] Bendelac, A., M. N. Rivera, S. H. Park, and J. H. Roark. Mouse CD1-specific NK1 T cells: development, specificity, and function. *Annu. Rev. Immunol. 1997;15:535-62.*

[23] Moore, J. P., A. Trkola, and T. Dragic. 1997. Co-receptors for HIV-1 entry. *Curr Opin Immunol* 9:551-562.

[24] Montoya, C. J., J. C. Catano, Z. Ramirez, M. T. Rugeles, S. B. Wilson, and A. L. Landay. 2008. Invariant NKT cells from HIV-1 or Mycobacterium tuberculosis-infected patients express an activated phenotype. *Clin. Immunol.* 127:1-6.

[25] Motsinger, A., D. W. Haas, A. K. Stanic, L. Van Kaer, S. Joyce, and D. Unutmaz. 2002. CD1d-restricted human natural killer T cells are highly susceptible to human immunodeficiency virus 1 infection. *J. Exp. Med.* 195:869-879.

[26] Sandberg, J. K., N. M. Fast, E. H. Palacios, G. Fennelly, J. Dobroszycki, P. Palumbo, A. Wiznia, R. M. Grant, N. Bhardwaj, M. G. Rosenberg, and D. F. Nixon. 2002. Selective loss of innate CD4(+) V alpha 24 natural killer T cells in human immunodeficiency virus infection. *J. Virol.* 76:7528-7534.

[27] van der Vliet, H. J., B. M. von Blomberg, M. D. Hazenberg, N. Nishi, S. A. Otto, B. H. van Benthem, M. Prins, F. A. Claessen, A. J. van den Eertwegh, G. Giaccone, F. Miedema, R. J. Scheper, and H. M. Pinedo. 2002. Selective decrease in circulating V alpha 24+V beta 11+ NKT cells during HIV type 1 infection. *J. Immunol.* 168:1490-1495.

[28] Unutmaz, D. 2003. NKT cells and HIV infection. *Microbes Infect* 5:1041-1047.

[29] Moll, M., J. Snyder-Cappione, G. Spotts, F. M. Hecht, J. K. Sandberg, and D. F. Nixon. 2006. Expansion of CD1d-restricted NKT cells in patients with primary HIV-1 infection treated with interleukin-2. *Blood* 107:3081-3083.

[30] Vasan, S., M. A. Poles, A. Horowitz, E. E. Siladji, M. Markowitz, and M. Tsuji. 2007. Function of NKT cells, potential anti-HIV effector cells, are improved by beginning HAART during acute HIV-1 infection. *Int. Immunol.* 19:943-951.

[31] van der Vliet, H. J., M. G. van Vonderen, J. W. Molling, H. J. Bontkes, M. Reijm, P. Reiss, M. A. van Agtmael, S. A. Danner, A. J. van den Eertwegh, B. M. von Blomberg, and R. J. Scheper. 2006. Cutting edge: Rapid recovery of NKT cells upon institution of highly active antiretroviral therapy for HIV-1 infection. *J. Immunol.* 177:5775-5778.

[32] Chen, N., C. McCarthy, H. Drakesmith, D. Li, V. Cerundolo, A. J. McMichael, G. R. Screaton, and X. N. Xu. 2006. HIV-1 down-regulates the expression of CD1d via Nef. *Eur. J. Immunol.* 36:278-286.

[33] Cho, S., K. S. Knox, L. M. Kohli, J. J. He, M. A. Exley, S. B. Wilson, and R. R. Brutkiewicz. 2005. Impaired cell surface expression of human CD1d by the formation of an HIV-1 Nef/CD1d complex. *Virology* 337:242-252.

[34] Hage, C. A., L. L. Kohli, S. Cho, R. R. Brutkiewicz, H. L. Twigg, 3rd, and K. S. Knox. 2005. Human immunodeficiency virus gp120 downregulates CD1d cell surface expression. *Immunol Lett* 98:131-135.

[35] Raulin, J. 2002. Human immunodeficiency virus and host cell lipids. Interesting pathways in research for a new HIV therapy. *Prog. Lipid Res.* 41:27-65.

[36] Barron, M. A., N. Blyveis, B. E. Palmer, S. MaWhinney, and C. C. Wilson. 2003. Influence of plasma viremia on defects in number and immunophenotype of blood dendritic cell subsets in human immunodeficiency virus 1-infected individuals. *J. Infect Dis.* 187:26-37.

[37] Donaghy, H., A. Pozniak, B. Gazzard, N. Qazi, J. Gilmour, F. Gotch, and S. Patterson. 2001. Loss of blood CD11c(+) myeloid and CD11c(-) plasmacytoid dendritic cells in patients with HIV-1 infection correlates with HIV-1 RNA virus load. *Blood* 98:2574-2576.

[38] Pacanowski, J., S. Kahi, M. Baillet, P. Lebon, C. Deveau, C. Goujard, L. Meyer, E. Oksenhendler, M. Sinet, and A. Hosmalin. 2001. Reduced blood CD123+ (lymphoid) and CD11c+ (myeloid) dendritic cell numbers in primary HIV-1 infection. *Blood* 98:3016-3021.

[39] Servet, C., L. Zitvogel, and A. Hosmalin. 2002. Dendritic cells in innate immune responses against HIV. *Curr Mol Med* 2:739-756.

[40] Montoya, C. J., P. A. Velilla, C. Chougnet, A. L. Landay, and M. T. Rugeles. 2006. Increased IFN-gamma production by NK and CD3+/CD56+ cells in sexually HIV-1-exposed but uninfected individuals. *Clin. Immunol.* 120:138-146.

[41] Soumelis, V., I. Scott, F. Gheyas, D. Bouhour, G. Cozon, L. Cotte, L. Huang, J. A. Levy, and Y. J. Liu. 2001. Depletion of circulating natural type 1 interferon-producing cells in HIV-infected AIDS patients. *Blood* 98:906-912.

[42] Koka, P. S., J. K. Fraser, Y. Bryson, G. C. Bristol, G. M. Aldrovandi, E. S. Daar, and J. A. Zack. 1998. Human immunodeficiency virus inhibits multilineage hematopoiesis in vivo. *J. Virol.* 72:5121-5127.

[43] Koka, P. S., C. M. Kitchen, and S. T. Reddy. 2004. Targeting c-Mpl for revival of human immunodeficiency virus type 1-induced hematopoietic inhibition when CD34+ progenitor cells are re-engrafted into a fresh stromal microenvironment in vivo. *J. Virol.* 78:11385-11392.

[44] Wilson, S. B., S. C. Kent, K. T. Patton, T. Orban, R. A. Jackson, M. Exley, S. Porcelli, D. A. Schatz, M. A. Atkinson, S. P. Balk, J. L. Strominger, and D. A. Hafler. 1998. Extreme Th1 bias of invariant Valpha24JalphaQ T cells in type 1 diabetes. *Nature* 391:177-181.

[45] Kukreja, A., G. Cost, J. Marker, C. Zhang, Z. Sun, K. Lin-Su, S. Ten, M. Sanz, M. Exley, B. Wilson, S. Porcelli, and N. Maclaren. 2002. Multiple immuno-regulatory defects in type-1 diabetes. *J. Clin. Invest* 109:131-140.

[46] Nowicki, M. J., C. Vigen, W. J. Mack, E. Seaberg, A. Landay, K. Anastos, M. Young, H. Minkoff, R. Greenblatt, and A. M. Levine. 2008. Association of cells with natural killer (NK) and NKT immunophenotype with incident cancers in HIV-infected women. *AIDS Res. Hum. Retroviruses* 24:163-168.

[47] Fantini, J., D. Hammache, O. Delezay, G. Pieroni, C. Tamalet, and N. Yahi. 1998. Sulfatide inhibits HIV-1 entry into CD4-/CXCR4+ cells. *Virology* 246:211-220.

[48] Fonteneau, J. F., M. Larsson, A. S. Beignon, K. McKenna, I. Dasilva, A. Amara, Y. J. Liu, J. D. Lifson, D. R. Littman, and N. Bhardwaj. 2004. Human immunodeficiency virus type 1 activates plasmacytoid dendritic cells and concomitantly induces the bystander maturation of myeloid dendritic cells. *J. Virol.* 78:5223-5232.

[49] Hartshorn, K. L., D. Neumeyer, M. W. Vogt, R. T. Schooley, and M. S. Hirsch. 1987. Activity of interferons alpha, beta, and gamma against human immunodeficiency virus replication in vitro. *AIDS Res. Hum. Retroviruses* 3:125-133.

[50] Poli, G., J. M. Orenstein, A. Kinter, T. M. Folks, and A. S. Fauci. 1989. Interferon-alpha but not AZT suppresses HIV expression in chronically infected cell lines. *Science* 244:575-577.

[51] Yamamoto, J. K., F. Barre-Sinoussi, V. Bolton, N. C. Pedersen, and M. B. Gardner. 1986. Human alpha- and beta-interferon but not gamma- suppress the in vitro replication of LAV, HTLV-III, and ARV-2. *J. Interferon Res.* 6:143-152.

[52] Kotsianidis, I., J. D. Silk, E. Spanoudakis, S. Patterson, A. Almeida, R. R. Schmidt, C. Tsatalas, G. Bourikas, V. Cerundolo, I. A. Roberts, and A. Karadimitris. 2006. Regulation of hematopoiesis in vitro and in vivo by invariant NKT cells. *Blood* 107:3138-3144.

[53] Aldrovandi, G. M., G. Feuer, L. Gao, B. Jamieson, M. Kristeva, I. S. Chen, and J. A. Zack. 1993. The SCID-hu mouse as a model for HIV-1 infection. *Nature* 363:732-736.

[54] McCune, J. M., R. Namikawa, H. Kaneshima, L. D. Shultz, M. Lieberman, and I. L. Weissman. 1988. The SCID-hu mouse: murine model for the analysis of human hematolymphoid differentiation and function. *Science* 241:1632-1639.

[55] Brooks, D. G., D. H. Hamer, P. A. Arlen, L. Gao, G. Bristol, C. M. Kitchen, E. A. Berger, and J. A. Zack. 2003. Molecular characterization, reactivation, and depletion of latent HIV. *Immunity* 19:413-423.

[56] Korin, Y. D., and J. A. Zack. 1998. Progression to the G1b phase of the cell cycle is required for completion of human immunodeficiency virus type 1 reverse transcription in T cells. *J. Virol.* 72:3161-3168.

[57] Kawano, T., J. Cui, Y. Koezuka, I. Toura, Y. Kaneko, K. Motoki, H. Ueno, R. Nakagawa, H. Sato, E. Kondo, H. Koseki, and M. Taniguchi. 1997. CD1d-restricted and TCR-mediated activation of valpha14 NKT cells by glycosylceramides. *Science* 278:1626-1629.

In: Stem Cells in Disease
Editor: Prasad S. Koka

ISBN: 978-1-62257-169-7
© 2012 Nova Science Publishers, Inc.

Chapter X

Putative Innate Immunity of Antiatherogenic Paraoxonase-2 via STAT5 Signal Transduction in HIV-1 Infection of Hematopoietic TF-1 Cells and in SCID-Hu Mice

***Jinyun Yuan*[1], *Asokan Devarajan*[2], *Rosita Moya-Castro*[1], *Menghua Zhang*[1], *Stella Evans*[1], *Noam Bourquard*[2,3], *Peter Dias*[1], *Catherine Lacout*[4], *William Vainchenker*[4], *Srinivasa T. Reddy*[2,3,*] and *Prasad S. Koka*[1#]**

[1]Laboratory of Stem Cell Biology,
Torrey Pines Institute for Molecular Studies,
3550 General Atomics Court, San Diego, California, US
[2]Department of Medicine,
[3]Department of Molecular and Medical Pharmacology,
University of California, Los Angeles, CA, US
[4] Institut National de la Santé et de la Recherche Médicale U790, Villejuif;
Institut Gustave Roussy, Villejuif; France

Abstract

Paraoxonase-2 (PON2) activity was increased upon *human immunodeficiency virus-1* (HIV-1) infection of the CD34+CD4+ hematopoietic cell line TF-1. Thymocytes derived from the human fetal conjoint thymus/liver hematopoietic organ of SCID-hu mice also exhibited an increase in PON2 activity following HIV-1 infection. Additionally, a remarkable increase of PON2 mRNA expression was also observed in

[*] Srinivasa T Reddy, PhD Tel (310) 206 3915 Email sreddy@mednet.ucla.edu.
[#] Corresponding Authors: *Prasad S. Koka, PhD Tel (858) 597 3886 Fax (858) 597 3804 Email pkoka@tpims.org.

both TF-1 and thymocytes following HIV-1 infection. The phosphorylation of STAT5 was decreased in TF-1 cells upon HIV-1 infection. Interestingly, phosphorylation of STAT5 does not occur in GM-CSF "starved" TF-1 cells; however, PON2 protein, activity, and mRNA expression are increased under these conditions, similar to HIV-1 infection. We conclude that PON2 is induced in HIV-1 infection through a mechanism that may involve STAT5 inactivation.

Keywords: TF-1, Paraoxonase-2, HIV-1, innate immunity, STAT5 phosphorylation, GM-CSF starvation

Introduction

Oxidative stress is thought to play an important role in the progression of HIV infection. Perturbations in antioxidant defense systems, and consequently redox imbalance, are present in many tissues of HIV-infected patients [1]. The PON gene family consists of three members, PON1, PON2, and PON3, located adjacent to each other on the long arm of chromosome 7 in humans and chromosome 6 in mice (23). PON1 and PON3 are high density lipoprotein-associated proteins whereas PON2 is an intracellular membrane associated protein. *In vitro, in vivo* and epidemiological studies documented that all PON proteins protect against oxidative stress (3-9). PON1 activity is lowered whereas PON2 activity is increased during oxidative stress conditions (10). Recent studies have shown that PON1 activity is lowered and treatment with efavirenz (non nucleoside reverse transcriptase inhibitor) improves the PON1 activity in HIV patients (11). In this study, we examined whether intracellular PON2 is upregulated following HIV infection using hematopoietic CD34+CD4+ cell line; TIF 1 cells and *in vivo* in the SCID-hu mouse model.

Materials and Methods

In Vitro Model

TF-1 and TF-1/c-mpl cell lines were cultured with human GM-CSF (2.5 ng/ml) in RPMI 1640 medium containing 10 % FBS. For HIV-1 infection, TF-1 and TF-1/c-mpl cells (3 x 10^6) were incubated with HIV-$_{1NL4-3}$ (100 IU in 50 to 100 μl of RPMI 1640 medium) in the presence of Polybrene (5 μg/ml) at 37°C for 2 hour. For starvation experiments the cells were cultured without GM-CSF.

In Vivo Model

SCID-hu mice received simultaneous transplants of 1-mm^3 pieces of human fetal thymus and liver tissues under the renal capsule, and the resulting conjoint organ of the SCID-hu animals were allowed to grow for 3 to 5 months, as described previously (12-18). The Thy/Liv implants were then infected by intra-implant injection of HIV-1_{NL4-3} (100 IU in 50 to 100 μl), which was produced in CEM cells. Control mock-infected animals were injected with the same volume of mock-infected CEM culture medium alone. At specific time intervals post infection, sequential wedge biopsies (~25% of each implant) were obtained and were processed and analyzed as described below. Viral infectivity of the thymocytes of the Thy/Liv implants was determined by PCR of the proviral DNA, as described previously (12-18).

Real-time PCR

For proviral load, DNA from infected cells was subjected to PCR amplification (ABI) using AA55 and SR primers and FAM probes. Proviral load was measured according to the HIV-1 $_{NL4-3}$ standard (12-18). For mRNA examination, total RNA was purified from uninfected and infected cells using RNeasy mini kit (Qiagen) and was used to generate cDNA using Super ScriptII (Invitrogen, Carlsbad, CA, USA). RT products were subjected to PCR amplification using PON2 and GAPDH primers. Relative expression of PON2 mRNA was normalized to GAPDH.

Western Blotting

Lysates (50 μg protein) from *in vitro* studies and *in vivo* studies were subjected to SDS-polyacrylamide gel electrophoresis and electroblotted onto polyvinylidene difluoride membranes. The blots were blocked with 5% skim milk in Tris-buffered saline (TBS) for 1 hour at room temperature and then incubated with the appropriate concentration of primary antibody p-STAT5, STAT5 (1:2000) (BD pharmingen, New Jersey, USA), PON2 (1: 500) (R&D system, Minneapolis, MN, USA) GAPDH (1:10000) (Santa Cruz, CA. USA) for 1hours at RT.

The blots were washed with TBS containing 0.1% Tween-20, and then probed with appropriate secondary antibodies (1:5000 dilution) conjugated with horseradish peroxidase for 30min at room temperature. After a second washing, the blots were incubated with an enhanced chemiluminescence substrate (ECL, Western blot detection system; Amersham Pharmacia Biotech, Buckinghamshire, England) and exposed to Hyperfilm ECL (Amersham Pharmacia Biotech) to visualize the immunoreactive bands.

PON2 activity assay

The lactonase activity of PON2 was measured using lysates with 50 μg protein and 1 mM *dihydrocoumarin* (DHC) as a substrate dissolved in 50 mM Tris/HCl (pH 8.0) and 1 mM $CaCl_2$. The absorbance increase at 280nm was monitored from 0 to 10 minutes after substrate addition. Measurements were as follows: 1U of lactonase activity=1mol of DHC hydrolyzed/minute.

Results and Discussion

Quantification of HIV Copies

TF-1 And TF-1/c-mpl cells were infected with HIV-1 virus and the HIV-1 copies in the infected cells were quantified. There was no significant difference in HIV–copies between the TF-1 and TF-1/c-mpl groups (Table. 1)

Table 1. HIV-1 copies/100,000 cells were determined by real-time RT-PCR. The data were represented as +/- standard deviation obtained from three independent experiments

Infection	# HIV-1 Copies /100,000 cells		
In vitro/ In vivo	Cells	Mock	HIV-1
In vitro	TF-1	0	2820 ± 790
In vitro	TF-1/c-mp1	0	2453 ±1300
In vivo	Thymocytes	0	25180 ± 4500

PON2 Is Upregulated in HIV-1 Infection

PON2 activity was significantly increased in HIV-1 infected TF-1 and TF-1/ c-mpl cells compared to mock cells (Table 2). Thymocyte from infected SCID-hu mice showed four fold increase in PON2 activity compared to mock treatment. PON2 mRNA was also increased after HIV-1 infection both *in vitro* as well as *in vivo* (Figure 1)

Table 2. PON2 activity assay was carried out as described in the material and methods and error bars represent standard deviation from three independent experiments

PON2 activity (U/µg)			
Infection	*In vitro*		*In vivo*
	TF-1	TF-1/c-mp1	Thymocytes
Mock	1.7 ± 0.11	2.4 ± 0.12	0.098 ± 0.01
HIV-1	4.4 ± 0.19	4.1± 0.13	0.41 ± 0.11

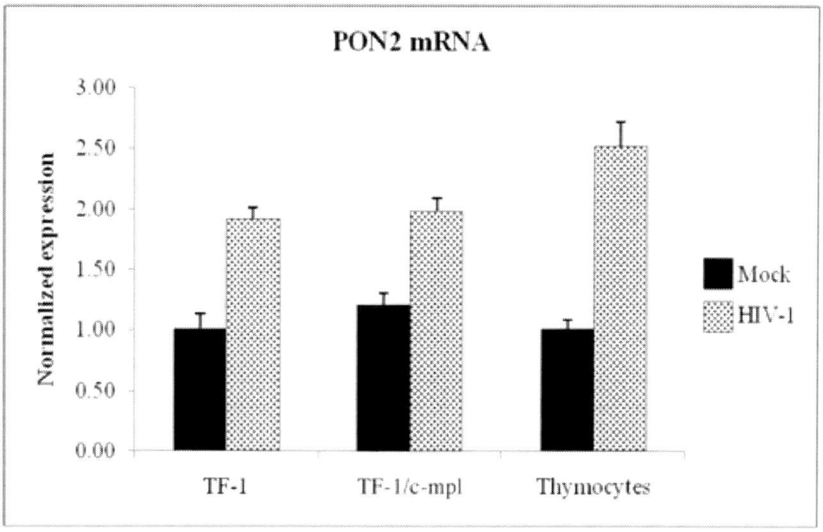

Figure 1. PON2 gene expression was analyzed as described under Materials and methods. TF-1 And TF-1/c-mpl cells were infected with HIV-1 virus. Thymocytes were obtained from Thy/Liv implants of SCID-hu mice. Total RNA was isolated and PON2 gene expression was determined by quantitative RT-PCR. The expression of PON2 mRNA was normalized to GAPDH mRNA.

Decrease of STAT5 phosphorylation in TF-1 and TF-1/C-MPL Cell Lines Following HIV-1 Infection

To study the phosphorylation status of STAT 5 following HIV -1 infection, TF-1 and TF-1/c-mpl cells were infected with or without HIV-1 virus. The phosphorylation of STAT5 was analyzed by Western blotting. HIV infected cells show less STAT5 phosphorylation compared to control cells (Figure 2). There was no difference in phosphorylation status of STAT5 between TF-1 and TF-1/c-mpl cells.

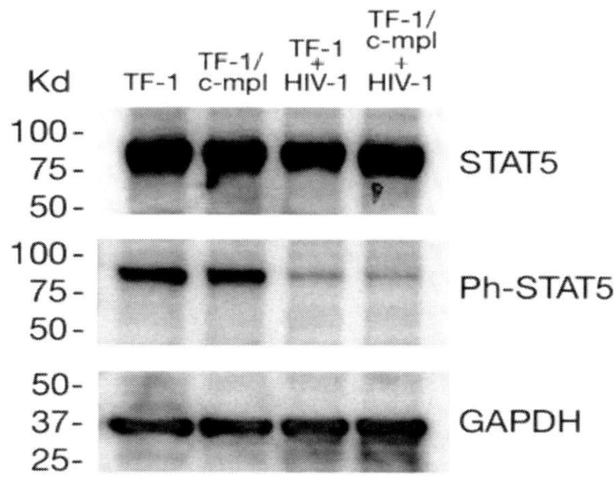

Figure 2. Phospho STAT5 was decreased in HIV-1 infection *in vitro*. 50µg protein of mock and HIV-1 infected TF-1 and TF-1/c-mpl cells lysate was subjected to Western blotting with phospho-STAT5, STAT5, and GAPDH antibodies.

PON2 Is Upregulated under Conditions of STAT5 Dephosphorylation in TF-1 And TF-1/C-MPL Cells

To examine the role of STAT5 signaling on PON2 expression, TF-1 cells and TF-1/c-mpl cells were cultured overnight with or without granulocyte macrophage colony-stimulating factor (GM-CSF) and PON2, STAT5 and phospho STAT5 were analyzed (Figures 3-5). The results show that STAT5 dephosphorylation coincided with increased PON2 expression level compared to control cells that received GM-CSF.

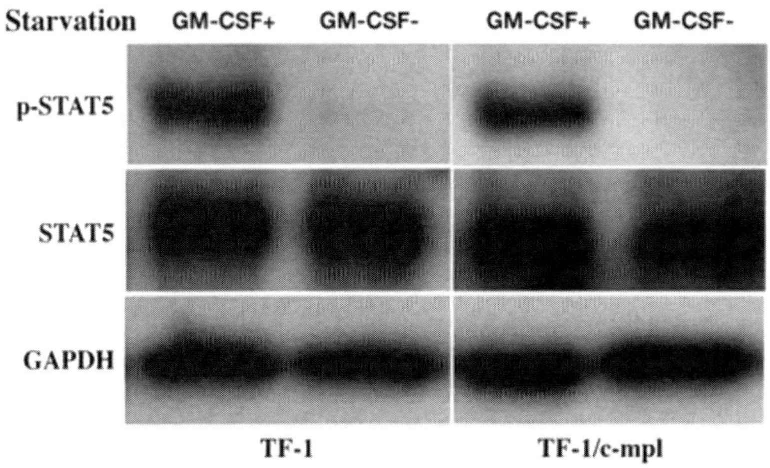

Figure 3. Phosphorylation of STAT5 was blocked in GM-CSF starved cells *in vitro*. TF-1 and TF-1/Cmpl cells were starved without GM-CSF and serum overnight. 50μg of total protein from mock and starved cells was subjected to Western blotting analysis with p-STAT5, STAT5 and GAPDH.

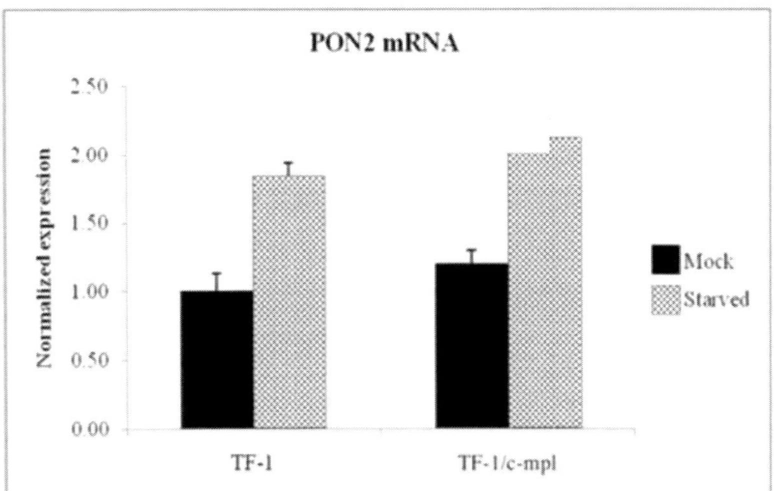

Figure 4. PON2 mRNA was stimulated hen phosphorylation of STAT5 was blocked. Total RNA from control and GM-CSF tarved cells was subjected to real-time RT-PCR. The expression of PON2 mRNA was normalized to GAPDH.

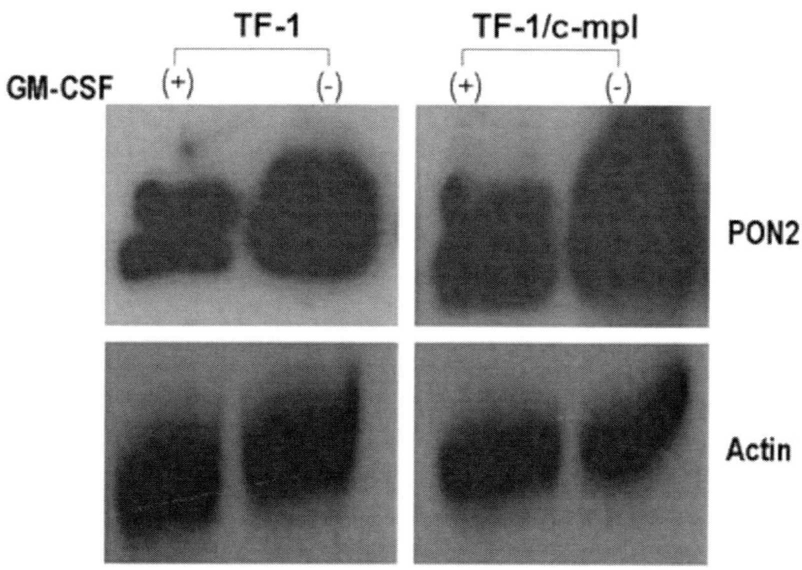

Figure 5. PON2 protein was increased when phosphorylation of STAT5 was blocked. STAT5 phosphorylation was blocked in TF-1 and TF-1/c-mpl cells by serum/GM-CSF starvation. Total lysates were subjected to Western blotting for PON2 and □-actin.

Inflammation and oxidative stress contribute to the etiology of many inflammatory diseases including HIV-1 infection related diseases. Under normal physiological conditions, anti-oxidant systems that comprise intracellular and circulating proteins and enzymes reduce oxidative stress. PON family of proteins has been well characterized for their ability to reduce oxidative stress both *in vitro* and *in vivo* (2,3). Previous studies have shown that PON1 activity is decreased following HIV-1 infection (10). We have previously shown that the intracellular member of PON gene family of proteins, PON2 (in contrast to PON1) is upregulated *in vivo* when challenged with oxidative stress (11). In the present study, we examined the affect of HIV-1 infection both *in vitro* and *in vivo* on PON2 gene expression, protein levels, and activity. Our results demonstrate that PON2 is upregulated following HIV-1 infection.

The role of interferons and the JAK/STAT pathway in innate immunity against viral infections is well established. HIV-1 infection results in STAT5 inactivation (19). Our results show that STAT5 is dephosphorylated in TF-1 cells that were GM-CSF-starved (Figure 3). Interestingly, we observed that PON2 level was elevated (Figures 4-5) under these condition similar to the observations made following HIV-1 infection (Figure 1 and Table 2). Our results demonstrate that the intracellular anti-oxidant enzyme PON2 may be regulated as an innate immune response to viral infections.

Acknowledgments

This work was supported by NIH grant R01HL079846 to PSK and 1R01HL71716 to STR.

References

[1] Suresh DR, Annam V Pratibha K, Prasad BV, Total antioxidant capacity-a novel early bio-chemical marker of oxidative stress in HIV infected individuals. *J Biomed Sci* 2009; 7: 16-61.

[2] Ng CJ, Wadleigh DJ, Gangopadhyay A. Paraoxonase-2 is a ubiquitously expressed protein with antioxidant properties and is capable of preventing cell-mediated oxidative modification of low density lipoprotein. *J Biol Chem* 2001; 276:44444-44449

[3] Reddy ST, Wadleigh DJ, Grijalva VF. Human paraoxonase-3 is an HDL-associated enzyme with biological activity similar to paraoxonase-1 protein but is not regulated by oxidized lipids. *Arterioscler Thromb Vasc Biol* 2001;21: 542-547

[4] Mochizuki, H. Scherer, S.W., Xi, T., Nickle, D.C., Majer, M., Huizenga, J. J, Tsui, L.C., and Prochazka, M. Human PON2 gene at 7q21.3: cloning, multiple mRNA forms, and missense polymorphisms in the coding sequence. *Gene,* 1998; 213:149-157.

[5] Boright A.P., Connelly, P.W., Brunt,J.H., Scherer, S.W., Tsui, L.C., Hegele, R.A. Genetic variation in paraoxonase-2 is associated with variation in plasma lipoproteins in Alberta Hutterties. *Atherosclerosis.* 2005; 139:131-136

[6] Hegele, R.A., Harris, S. B., Connelly, P.W., Hanley, A. J., Tsui, L.C., Zinman, B., and Scherer, S. W. Genetic variation in paraoxonase-2 is associated with variation in plasma lipoproteins in Canadian Oji-Cree. *Clin. Genet.* 1998, 54: 394-399.

[7] Mackness, B., Durrington, P.N., Abuashia, B., Boulton, A. J., Mackness, M. I. Low paraoxonase activity in type II diabetes mellitus complicated by retinopathy. *Clin. Sci.* (Lond.), 2000, 98: 355-363.

[8] Busch,C.P., Ramdath, D.D., Ramsewak, S., and Hegele, R.A. Association of PON2 variation with birth weight in Trinidadian neonates of South Asian ancestry. *Pharmacogenetics,* 1999, 9: 351-356.

[9] Sanghera, D. K., Aston, C. E., Saha, N., and Kamboh, M. I. DNA Polymorphisms in two paraoxonase genes (PON1 and PON2) are associated with the risk of coronary heart disease. *Am. J. Hum.Genet.* 1998, 62: 36-44.

[10] Parra S, Alonso Villaverde C, Coll B, Ferre N, Marsillach J, Coll B, Ferre N, Marsillach J, Aragones G, Mackness M, Mackness B, Masana L, Joven J, Camps J. Serum paraoxonase-1 activity and concentration are influenced human immuno-deficiency virus infection. *Atherosclerosis* 2007; 194(1): 175-180.

[11] Ng CJ, Shih DM, Hama SY, Villa N, Navab M, Reddy ST. The paraoxonase gene family and atherosclerosis. *Free Radic Biol Med.*2005; 5: 38(2):153-

[12] Koka PS, Fraser JK, Bryson Y, Bristol GC, Aldrovandi GM, Daar ES, Zack JA. Human immunodeficiency virus type 1 inhibits multilineage hematopoiesis in vivo. *J Virol* 1998; 72: 5121-5127.

[13] Koka PS, Jamieson BD, Brooks DG, Zack JA. Human immunodeficiency virus type-1 induced hematopoietic inhibition is independent of productive infection of progenitor cells in vivo. *J Virol* 1999; 73: 9089-9097.

[14] Koka PS, Kitchen CM, Reddy ST. Targeting c-Mpl for revival of human immuno-deficiency virus type 1-induced hematopoietic inhibition when CD34+ progenitor cells are re-engrafted into a fresh stromal Microenvironment in vivo. *J Virol* 2004; 78: 11385-11392.

[15] Sundell IB, Koka PS. Chimeric SCID-hu Model as a Human Hematopoietic Stem Cell Host that Recapitulates the Effects of HIV-1 on Bone Marrow Progenitors in Infected Patients. *J Stem Cells* 2006; 1(4): 283-300.

[16] Zhang M, Poh TY, Louache F, Sundell IB, Yuan J, Evans S, Koka PS. Rescue of multilineage hematopoiesis during HIV-1 Infection by human *c-mpl* gene transfer and reconstitution of CD34+ progenitor cells *in vivo*. *J Stem Cells* 2009; 4(3): 161-177.

[17] Zhang M, Evans S, Yuan J, Ratner L, Koka PS. HIV-1 determinants of thrombocytopenia at the stage of CD34+ progenitor cell differentiation in vivo lie in the viral envelope gp120 V3 loop region. *Virology* 2010; in press.

[18] Sundell IB, Halder R, Zhang M, Maricic I, Koka PS, Kumar V. Sulfatide administration leads to inhibition of HIV-1 replication and enhanced hematopoiesis. Accepted for Publication. *J Stem Cells,* Volume 5, Issue 1, 2010.

[19] Selliah N, Finkel TH. HIV-1 NL4-3, but not IIIB, inhibits JAK3/STAT5 activation in CD4(+) T cells. *Virology.* 2001; 286(2):412-21

In: Stem Cells in Disease
Editor: Prasad S. Koka

ISBN: 978-1-62257-169-7
© 2012 Nova Science Publishers, Inc.

Chapter XI

Potential Yoga Modules for Treatment of Hematopoietic Inhibition in HIV-1 Infection

Hemant Bhargav[1*], Nagarathna Raghuram[1], Nagendra Hongasandra Rama Rao[1], Padmini Tekur and Prasad S. Koka[1,2]

[1]Department of Integrative Cell Biology, Division of Yoga and Life Sciences, Swami Vivekanada Yoga Anusandhana Samsthana (SVYASA) University, Gavipuram Circle, Kempegowda Nagar, Bangalore, India
[2]Laboratory of Stem Cell Biology, Torrey Pines Institute for Molecular Studies, San Diego, California, US

Abstract

This article is expected to contribute towards understanding the therapeutic benefits of specific yoga modules on the inhibition of replication and enhancement to normal levels of hematopoiesis in HIV-1 infected subjects. More unique could be the effects of yoga on the indirect effects of HIV-1 induced hematopoietic inhibition of the CD34+ progenitor stem cells, via the CD4+ T lymphocytes. Such indirect effects may be caused by host cellular factors. Yoga practices may also improve the self renewal capacity (a step that precedes commitment of CD34+ progenitor cells to terminal differentiation), via STAT5 gene regulation. This may eliminate the need for constitutive STAT5 gene expression through gene therapy. In this article recent research and ancient Indian literature are reviewed to devise yoga modules for the potential treatment of hematopoietic inhibition in HIV-1 infection. The possible mechanisms through which hematopoietic inhibition may occur in HIV-1 infected patients are first described followed by the role of stress in the progression of HIV where probable involvement of psycho-neuro-immunological axis (PNI) is highlighted. Yoga therapy is introduced and

* Corresponding Authors: Dr Hemant Bhargav, MBBS, MD Email: urs.aatmiya@gmail.com Phone : +91 8762019348. Dr Prasad Koka, PhD. Email: pkoka@tpims.org.

its effectiveness in terms of evidence in relevant area is reviewed. Further, the basic principles of Integrated Approach of Yoga Therapy [IAYT] are described and depending on the potential mechanisms through which yoga therapy may act, both modern scientific research and ancient "scriptural" evidence are provided at all the five levels of existence (body, life force, emotional, intellectual and bliss). This will enable to design comprehensive yoga modules that may intervene in this indirect inhibition of haematopoiesis in HIV-1 infected individuals and potentially restore normal levels of haematopoiesis.

Keywords: HIV-1, Hematopoiesis, Self-renewal, Yoga, Stress

Introduction to Hematopoietic Inhibition in HIV-1 Infected Subjects

Hematopoetic abnormalities which include its inhibition or lineage specific proliferation of CD34+ progenitor cells often lead to hematological disorders [1]. HIV infected patients often suffer from multiple hematopoietic abnormalities which include anemia, thrombocytopenia, lymphocytopenia, monocytopenia, neutropenia, and myelodysplastic / hyperplastic alterations of the bone marrow microenvironment [2]. Evidence of alteration of fetal hematopoiesis including leukopenia, anemia, and thrombocytopenia has also been found in aborted fetuses from HIV-1 seropositive women [3,4]. The factors which play a role in HIV mediated hematopoietic inhibition could include direct intracellular effects of virus infection, interactions with viral proteins at the cell surface, and perturbation of cytokine network due to abnormal lineage specific expression of cellular genes. Such genes can also include growth factor receptors, receptor tyrosine kinases and factors involved in embryonic development or immune mediated effects.

Indirect Effects of HIV in Hematopoietic Inhibition

It has been observed that hematopoietic progenitor cell colony growth and differentiation is inhibited in long-term bone marrow cultures of HIV positive patients [5-8]. In general, investigators have failed to detect HIV infection in hematopoietic progenitor cells isolated from infected individuals, suggesting that HIV might have an indirect effect on hematopoiesis [2]. Infection of CD34+ progenitor cells in vitro has been reported by some investigators [9, 10]. However, Shen et al, found that bone marrow and peripheral blood derived CD34+ progenitor cells are not susceptible to HIV-1 infection in vitro [11]. It has further been reported that primitive hematopoietic cells resist HIV-1 infection via $p21^{Waf1/Cip1/Sdi}$ [12]. We have used the severe combined immunodeficient mouse co-transplanted with human fetal thymus and liver tissues (SCID-hu Thy/Liv) wherein this conjoint hematopoietic organ that develops is a very useful small chimeric animal model to investigate the mechanisms and therapies for HIV induced hematopoietic inhibition [15]. This model system not only mimics HIV infection but also recapitulates functional human hematopoiesis in vivo, in the absence of confounding factors found in humans. Thus the effects of HIV that are seen in this model are the direct result of virus mediated phenomena. Using the SCID-hu model, we and others have found that HIV-1 inhibits multilineage hematopoiesis in vivo without direct infection of the CD34+ progenitor cells, and presumably via indirect effects of the infected microenvironment [13, 14]. We noted that HIV-1 infection rapidly and severely decreases the ex vivo recovery of human progenitor cells capable of differentiation into both erythroid and myeloid lineages. However, the total CD34+ cell population is not depleted. Combination antiretroviral therapy administered well after loss of multilineage progenitor activity reverses this inhibitory effect, establishing a causal role of viral replication [14]. Taken together, the results suggest that pluripotent stem cells are not killed by HIV-1; rather, a later stage important in both myeloid and erythroid differentiation is affected. HIV possibly alters the stromal/progenitor cell microenvironment that supports hematopoiesis.

We used SCID-hu model to find that HIV-1 mediates hematopoietic inhibition in vivo, as assessed by multilineage colony forming activity (CFA) of the CD34+ progenitor hematopoietic stem cells (HSC) derived from the Thy/Liv implants, through a decrease in their cytokine receptor (c-Mpl) expression [16]. We further noted that these CD34+ cells that experienced the indirect effects of HIV-1 infection in the SCID-hu Thy/Liv implants in vivo can reacquire c-Mpl expression, when engrafted into a fresh stromal microenvironment in irradiated secondary recipient SCID-hu animal implants. Our results have established a correlation between CFA and c-Mpl expression, and that CFA segregates with c-Mpl expression.

Effects of HIV-1 on Self Renewal of CD34$^+$ Cells

Several transcription factors (Notch1, HOXB4, STAT) are possibly involved in self-renewal of hematopoietic precursors that precedes their terminal differentiation [17, 18, 19]. However, STAT5 (signal transducer and activator of transcription-5) proteins are shown to be particularly relevant in self-renewal of the hematopoietic progenitor cells. STAT5 protein A and B isoforms are involved in thrombopoietin (Tpo) receptor proto-oncogene, c-mpl, mediated signaling and regulation of multilineage hematopoiesis [20-23].

In addition, possible mechanisms for HIV induced hematopoietic inhibition in infected individuals most likely include the involvement of both c-mpl and STAT5A. This cytokine receptor (c mpl) and transcription factor (STAT5A), respectively, play a role in stem cell self-renewal and differentiation into multiple lineages, through activation of signaling pathways [24, 41].

Limitations and Shortcomings of Conventional Pharmacological Agents

Although great advances have been made in antiretroviral (ART) treatment of HIV-1 infection, there is still variability in treatment outcome [25], and HIV disease course, that is, the length of time before an acquired immune deficiency syndrome (AIDS) diagnosis and mortality. Cytopenias are also induced by continued drug treatment or HAART (highly active anti-retroviral therapy) of HIV infected patients [15, 26, 27] with thrombocytopenia more persistent than the other cytopenias [28, 29]. Among these cytopenias, thrombocytopenia in particular contributes to cardiac dysfunction [30, 31]. In HIV infected individuals receiving HAART and those who also require cardiovascular surgery, thrombocytopenia can present a greater risk [30]. It has been observed that hematopoietic growth factors such as granulocyte macrophage-colony-stimulating factor (GM-CSF), Epo, and stem cell factor (SCF) can reduce HIV or zidovudine related cytopenias [32, 33]. Miles et al reported in a review that hematopoietic growth factors, along with reduction in dose of zidovudine and ganciclovir, are used to reduce the impact of bone marrow failure in AIDS patients. In spite of these strategies, due to haematologic toxicity of zidovudine approximately 30% of patients with AIDS become transfusion-dependent [34]. Studies using the protease inhibitor, ritonavir, indicate that this drug relieves hematopoietic inhibition and promotes colony formation through a reduction of FAS and ICE (caspase-1) dependent apoptosis [35, 36]. However, ritonavir treatment during HIV infection can give rise to drug resistant virus mutants which can defeat the purpose of increasing hematopoiesis by the appearance of other viral strains *in vivo*. Thus use of such drugs may offset any balance to contain apoptosis related cytopenias in HIV infection, possibly by the evolution of viral strains that can be more severe on hematopoietic inhibition. Higher cost and significant side effects of HAART further supports the need to find simple, low cost, well-tolerated interventions that slowdown the decline of CD4 cell count, decrease viral load and have the potential to be effective in reversing the hematopoietic inhibition. Such low cost interventions, if effective, can additionally be useful to developing nations, where the vast majority of the world's HIV infected population live.

Stress and Progression of HIV

As discussed by Hand et al in a review [37], psychoneuroimmunology theory proposes that the reduction of perceived stress and increased immunity are interrelated. It is interesting to note that the above relation is not found for the reduction of the stressors themselves. Studies suggest that neural, endocrine and immune systems communicate with each other through multidirectional pathways. Immune cells have been found to have specific receptors for catecholamines released during sympathetic nervous system (SNS) activation and for corticosteroids (primarily cortisol) released by the limbic-hypothalamic-pituitary-adrenal axis (LHPA) respectively [38, 39]. Both these pathways of stress response (SNS and LHPA), when activated, inhibit immune functions like natural killer cell number and activity, percentage of circulating B and T lymphocytes, levels of various immunoglobulins, etc.

Most patients with AIDS have elevated basal cortisol levels [40], and a chronic increase in the basal endogenous cortisol levels may provoke an imbalance in cytokine production, with decreased production of type 1 and increased production of type 2 [41]. This type 1 to type 2 shift as well as raised cortisol levels may enhance viral replication and lead to HIV disease progression [41]. Another study indicates that a stressful exposure is associated with down regulation of Th1 cytokines (IFN-gamma and IL-2) and a selective up regulation of Th2 cytokines (IL-4, IL-5, and IL-6) [42]. Nair et al have further demonstrated that cortisol synergizes with gp120 (exterior envelope glycoprotein on HIV-1 which sequentially binds to CD4+ T lymphocytes) and induces apoptosis of CD4+ T lymphocytes [43]. Also, through animal and human studies, it has been reported that immune reactivity to viral challenge is inhibited due to stress [44]. There is substantial evidence that depression and stress are associated with more rapid CD4+ T cell declines and HIV disease progression [45, 46]. A study by Burack and colleagues found that in a cohort of men with HIV, those who scored as depressed on the Center for Epidemiologic Studies Depression Scale (CES-D) had a 38% greater decline in CD4+ T cells compared with men who were not depressed [46]. In a large cohort study of women with HIV by the HIV Epidemiology Research Study (HERS), women with chronic depressive symptoms had more rapid declines in CD4+ T cell counts, and were two times more likely to die compared to women with little or no depressive symptoms, after controlling for other prognostic factors [47]. In a prospective study of up to 7.5years, Leserman et al showed that psychosocial factors such as stressful life events, coping by means of denial, lower satisfaction with social support is associated with accelerated HIV disease progression to AIDS [48]. Further, Leserman concluded in a couple of reviews that chronic depression, stressful events, and trauma may decrease CD4+ T lymphocytes, increase viral load, and may lead to greater risk for clinical decline and mortality in HIV patients [49, 50]. Several psychosocial dimensions like stressors, depression, anxiety and distress, coping, social support, disclosure, emotional expression and adherence may account for the variability in treatment outcome with ART [51, 52]. Further, animal and human studies have demonstrated that stress accelerates HIV-1 disease pathogenesis and impairs the biological impact of ART [53, 54, 55]. Theoretically, stress could adversely affect the progression of HIV infection in a number of ways. Antoni et al. [56] have proposed a working model which provides a framework for the pathways that may be involved, a simplified version of which is presented in Figure 1.

Stress Management Therapies in HIV

A randomized clinical trial by Antoni et al on HIV infected gay men showed that cognitive behavioral stress management as an adjuvant to ART lead to significant decrease in viral load with reduction in depressive symptoms over 15 month period as compared to the control group taking ART only [57]. Experimentally manipulated aerobic exercise training intervention had been shown to attenuate concurrent changes on some affective and immunologic measures such as natural killer cell decline in response to an acute stressor in HIV patients [58]. Stress management therapies have also been reported to decrease HIV-related symptoms and increase CD4 cell number [59].

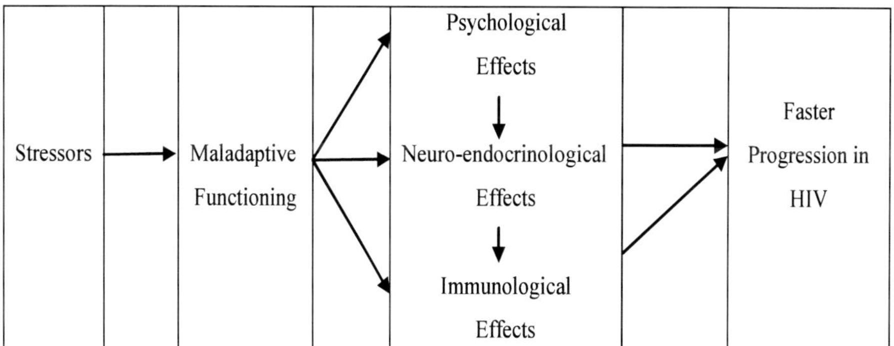

Figure 1. Stressors which result in maladaptive functioning can elicit a series of psychological, neuro-endocrinological and immunological events which may result in faster progression in HIV Infection [56].

Introduction to Yoga Therapy

People living with HIV often use alternative or complementary therapies to manage side-effects of HIV or ART [60-64]. Surveys estimate that 47–74% of HIV-infected individuals in the U.S. have used some form of alternative-complementary therapy to improve general health and well being [64].

One such potentially safe, effective, low cost, and popular intervention that has shown its efficacy its efficacy on HIV infected individuals by reducing psychological distress [65], anxiety and depression [66], increasing T cell count [66], natural killer cell activity [67] and buffering CD4+ T lymphocyte declines [68], is the practice of yoga, which incorporates which incorporates bodily postures, breathing techniques, meditation, mindfulness, spiritual *mantram* repetition and relaxation techniques etc.

The term "yoga" originates from *Samskrit* root "*yuj*" which means union. Madanmohan defines yoga as a psycho-somatic-spiritual discipline to achieve union and harmony between mind, body and soul and to ultimately unite individual consciousness with the Universal consciousness [69].

As described in an ancient yogic scripture called *Patanjali Yoga Sutra* (P.Y.S. 1.2) [70], yoga is a holistic science, that chiefly deals with gaining mastery over the mind through various mind-body techniques such as *āsanas* (postures done with awareness), *Prāṇāyāma* (voluntarily regulated nostril breathing), and meditations along with *kriyās* (purificatory practices) and *yoga nidrā* (guided relaxation with imagery) [71]. Being holistic, it has the potential to bring about a state of complete physical, mental, social and spiritual well being in the practitioners.

Yoga techniques not only bridge psychosocial and somatic aspects of care but also address the subject's spiritual needs. Practitioners have to be actively involved in the practice with a sense of self-control and awareness.

Such awareness combined with relaxation and attention of mental phenomena will alter the perceptions and mental responses to both external and internal stimuli, reduces hyper-reactive responses to such stimuli and instills a greater sense of control over situations, thereby causing reduction in the levels of stress.

Clinical Efficacy of Yoga Therapy

Yoga has been shown to have therapeutic benefits for individuals with a wide range of health conditions, including hypertension [72, 73] and diabetes [74, 75]. The therapeutic benefit of yoga have also been evidenced in numerous other health care concerns such as asthma [76], cardio respiratory illnesses [77], musculoskeletal disorders [78] and cancer [79], in which mental stress is believed to play a role. Yoga techniques were found to be effective in treating obsessive-compulsive disorder, phobias, major depressive disorders, dyslexia, grief, insomnia and other sleep disorders [80] and posttraumatic stress disorder [81]. *Hatha Yoga* (a form of yoga which chiefly focuses on dynamic body postures, cleansing practices and breathing techniques) practices have also been shown to reduce perceived stress, negative affect and salivary cortisol levels [82].

In lymphoma patients, yoga sessions conducted weekly once for 7 weeks produced lower sleep disturbances [83]. Reduced sleep disturbances may also lead to enhanced immune functions. Kochupillai et al measured natural killer cell counts in cancer patients who had completed their standard therapy, to study the effects of *Sudarshan Kriya* (SK) and *Prānāyāma* (*P*), which are rhythmic breathing processes. They found that natural killer (NK) cells increased significantly (P <0.001) at 12 and 24 weeks of the practice compared to baseline. And there was a significant increase in NK cells at 24 weeks (P <0.05) compared to controls [84]. In a randomized control trial, eighty eight stage II and III breast cancer outpatients were randomly assigned to receive yoga (n = 44) or brief supportive therapy (n = 44) prior to radiotherapy treatment. Integrated yoga was used as daily intervention with each session lasting 60 min. Salivary cortisol levels were measured 3 days before and after radiotherapy along with self-ratings of anxiety, depression, and stress collected before and after 6 weeks of radiotherapy. Results showed significant decrease in anxiety, depression, perceived stress, 6 am salivary cortisol and pooled mean cortisol in the yoga group as compared to the control [85]. Similarly, Integrated Yoga has also been found to decrease psychological distress, fatigue, insomnia and loss of appetite over time in early breast cancer patients [86]. Another study demonstrated beneficial effect of integrated yoga on post-chemotherapy-induced nausea frequency and intensity [87]. Still another study showed that following a yoga protocol for eight week, there was lesser pain and fatigue and higher levels of invigoration, acceptance, and relaxation in metastatic breast cancer patients [88].

Yoga Therapy for Hematopoietic Inhibition in HIV: Potential Mechanisms

Stress, a psychophysiological process, causes various biological effects via the pathway of immune-neuroendocrine axis which may lead to a greater replication and faster progression of HIV in the infected subjects [See Figure 1]. Such an increased proviral burden depletes the CD4 counts and also inhibits hematopoiesis [14]. Yoga has been proven to reduce stress levels via decreasing sympathetic activity and causing a state of parasympathetic dominance. Also, by reducing cortisol levels in HIV patients, yoga may prevent switching of cytokines from type 1 to type 2 (as discussed under section stress and progression of HIV) and thereby affect HIV replication in a positive manner, which may decrease viral loads in circulation and consequently improve CD4 counts and restore more normal levels of hematopoiesis. Although it may be logical to expect that the proposed yoga modules may reduce HIV-1 infection, it may also be likely that the yoga therapies may bypass the route of interference with HIV-1 replication and yet enhance hematopoiesis by other unknown mechanisms. As HIV-1 induces hematopoietic inhibition of the CD34+ progenitor stem cells indirectly, via the CD4+ T lymphocytes, yogic techniques may favourably alter the stromal / progenitor cell microenvironment of CD34+ progenitor stem cells to revive the hematopoietic inhibition. Such favourable changes in stromal microenvironment may also help CD34+ cells reacquire normal levels of cytokine receptor (c-Mpl) expression. Yoga may also have a role on the maintenance of quiescence or self-renewal capacity and lineage specificity of differentiation of CD34+ cells, by potential regulation of the cellular transcription factor and STAT5 gene expression, in HIV-1 infected patients. Yoga practices may cause stabilization of STAT5 gene expression to alleviate the need for exogenous introduction (gene therapy through autologous bone marrow transplantation) of a mutant STAT5 (1*6) into the CD34+ cells using lentiviral transduction. This will then maintain the quiescence or self renewal capacity of the CD34+ cells despite the indirect influence of HIV-1 infection and thus may contribute to maintaining close to normal levels of hematopoiesis as assessed by colony forming activity of the CD34+ cells that are exposed to the HIV-1 infected CD4+ T cells.

Among the cytopenias, thrombocytopenia in particular is associated with cardiac dysfunction [90, 91, 92]. Whereas yoga lifestyle intervention has been reported to improve cardiovascular functioning, reduce cardiovascular risk factors, and retard coronary artery disease [93-96].

Further, the poor response of HIV for a lowering of its replication and slower CD4 cell increase in some HIV infected individuals after initiation of HAART is associated with higher autonomic nervous system activity as measured by a series of physiological parameters like palmar skin conductance and EKG inter-beat interval [89]. Hence interventions that reduce autonomic nervous system activity could have beneficial effects in HIV persons who are on antiretroviral treatment.

Principles of Integrated Approach of Yoga Therapy (IAYT)

The Unique contribution of Yoga to therapeutic sciences is the *Panća Kośa* (Five Body) model of existence. Found in *Taittarīya Upanisad*, this concept is unique in providing us a depth to the understanding of human existence. The *Upanisad* describes that every individual has five layers of existence, which are *Annamaya Kośa* (Physical Body), *Prānamaya Kośa* (Body of life force), *Manomaya Kośa* (Mental body), *Vijñanamaya Kośa* (Body of Intellect) and *Ānandamaya Kośa* (Body of bliss) [97].

Concept of IAYT says that man is in perfect health in *Vijñanamaya Kośa* and *Ānandamaya Kośa*. All diseases are manifestation of '*ādhi*' (mental conflicts) which develops as a response to demanding situations in the mental sheath of existence (*manomaya kośa*) resulting in wrong life style. The four components of life style namely diet, lack of exercise, bad habits (alcohol, smoking, uncontrolled desires) and emotional stress are all traceable to the mind. In the mind all these responses have one common factor i.e. these are distressful emotions such as depression, anxiety or anger. When one gets stuck in any of these emotions due to repeatedly demanding situations, he gets into a loop of habituated response. Yoga looks at these problems as uncontrolled speeded up repetition of thoughts in the mind. Hence the entire concept of IAYT is based on reducing the speed of the mind and deep rest to each and every cell of the body to promote normalcy. IAYT techniques point to the fact that gross techniques such as dynamic or slow physical practices and breathing techniques are all useful in reducing the speed of the mind. An ancient yoga text [98] goes on to explain that '*ādhi*' percolates in to *prānamaya kośa* as excessively speeded up flow of *prāna* (life force) that blocks the *prāna* channels. This further manifests as uncontrolled speed at the *annamaya kośa* that can be perceived as functional and structural abnormalities at the cellular level. Thus, in HIV also it is to be understood that the Psycho-Neuro-Immunological (PNI) pathway working through HPA axis is uncontrolled speed at the *annamaya kośa*. Correction of these imbalances by the trick of slowing down is the remedy. Relaxation at *annamaya kośa*, slowing down the rate of breathing at *prānamaya kośa* and calming down the mind at *manomaya kośa* to establish in *ānandamaya kośa*, forms the basis of IAYT [99].

Though, individual *āsanas*, *Prānāyāma*, relaxation and meditative practices can selectively affect sympathetic or parasympathetic nervous system. The overall ability of IAYT to reduce sympathetic activity and bring about a state of parasympathetic dominance forms the rationale for its use in stress management. Thus these principles may provide the logical basis for designing the following techniques of IAYT for containment of HIV infection leading to its reduced replication and in turn rescue of hematopoiesis in these subjects.

Evidence for Efficacy from IAYT

Annamaya Kośa: Scriptural Evidence

Several social behavioral norms are prescribed in an ancient yogic text [70] as preparatory lifestyle changes for a healthy living. These include *yamās* and *nīyamās*. *Yamā* is a set of 'don'ts' and *Nīyamā*: a set of 'dos'. *Yamā* is abstention from harming others, from falsehood, from theft, from incontinence, and greed (P.Y.S.2.30). *Nīyāma* includes cleanliness, contentment, austerity, self-study and resignation to God. (P.Y.S. 2.32). The basis of *yamā* and *nīyama* is to build congenial atmosphere - mandatory for success in any work and they also are basic prerequisites to perform any kind of yogic practices.

A healthy yogic diet, cleansing techniques *(kriyās)*, loosening exercises and *yogāsanas* are used to operate at the *Annamaya Kośa* level and to remove the physical symptoms of the ailments. *Sāttvic* diet which is easy on the system is recommended in the *Gita* [100] by *Śri Kriśna* in a verse -"The foods which increase life, purity, strength, health, joy and cheerfulness, which are savoury and oleaginous, substantial and agreeable, are dear to *Sāttvic* (pure) ones." (B.G. 17.8).

Other yogic texts such as *Hathyoga Pradipika* (H.Y.P.) [101], *Gheranda Samhita* (G.S.) [102] and *Hath Ratnāvali* (H.R.) [103] describe beneficial effects of various *āsanas* and *kriyās* as follows: Steady and comfortable should be the posture (*āsana*) (P.Y.S. 2.46), by loosening of effort and by meditating on infinity, āsana is mastered (P.Y.S.2.47). *Śavāsana* wards off fatigue and brings *ćittaviśranti* (calms down the mind) (H.Y.P. 1.32). *Śavāsana* pacifies the agitations of the mind (G.S.2.28). *Siddhāsana* purifies all 72000 *prānic* channels (*nādis*) (H.Y.P.1.35). *Padmāsana* destroys all the diseases of Yogis (H.Y.P.1.44).

Kriyās : They are purificatory practices described in *hatha yoga* to enhance inner healing potentials. For e.g., *Neti* is a technique to purify and sensitise nasal mucosa, it destroys disorders of *kapha dośa* (imbalances of the phlegm) (G.H. 1.51). *Basti* is another purificatory technique to cleanse the intestines which destroys all the accumulated diseases, dropsy caused by all three *dośas* (basic humors according to *ayurvedic* science) (H.Y.P. 2.28,29).

Annamaya Kośa (Āsanas and Yoga-Based Lifestyle Modifications): Scientific Evidence

Several studies suggest that stress reduction interventions such as relaxation and exercise may have beneficial effects on CD4 count and other measures of immune status in HIV [104, 105, 106]. A recent study by Gopal et al measured physiological parameters like heart rate, respiratory rate, and blood pressure, psychological variables like Global Assessment of Recent Stress Scale and Spielbergers State Anxiety score and biochemical markers like serum cortisol levels, IL-4, and IFN-γ levels at baseline and during the examination, as an indicator of exam stress, in 60 first year medical undergraduate students. The yoga group practiced integrated yoga for 35 minutes daily in the presence of trained yoga teacher for 12 weeks, control group followed daily routine. At the end, they concluded that yoga resists the exam-stress induced autonomic changes and impairment of cellular immunity, as yoga group showed significant improvement compared to the control group in physiological, psychological as well as biochemical parameters. The yoga group showed less significant increase in serum cortisols and decrease in IFN-γ as compared to the control group during the exam [107]. Todd Cade et al [108] randomly assigned sixty pre-hypertensive HIV-infected adults with mild-moderate CVD risk factors to 20 wks of supervised yoga practice or standard of care treatment. Yoga group practiced *āsanas* and breathing techniques 2–3 times/wk for ~60 min/session for a total duration of 20 weeks. They found significant reduction in blood pressure in the yoga group at the end of program as compared to those on standard care. Each session included: alignment of muscle locks (*bandhās*) and controlled breathing (*ujjayī*), Sun Salutations *(Surya Namaskāra),* Standing, Seated and Supine physical postures *(āsanas)* and cooling down (restorative breathing). Our randomized control trial on 70 seropositive HIV patients randomly assigned to either yoga (36) or waitlist control (34) groups, demonstrated the efficacy of 3 month daily 1 hour integrated yoga intervention in improving quality of life and positive affect in HIV positive individuals [109]. In a study on 7 yoga instructors, it was found that alpha waves increased and serum cortisol decreased during the yoga exercise [110]. Another study reported the beneficial effects of two 1-hour Iyengar Yoga classes each week for 5 consecutive weeks on young adults with elevated symptoms of depression. The yoga session specifically focussed on yoga postures particularly back bends, standing poses, and inversions, which are thought to alleviate depression. Results showed significant decreases in self-reported symptoms of depression and trait anxiety [111]. A study by Schmidt et al reported significant increase in urinary excretion of cortisol as well as reduction in the excretion of various hormones like adrenaline, nor adrenaline, dopamine and aldosterone, they also found a decrease in serum testosterone and luteinizing hormone levels in participants after a comprehensive 3 month yoga-based lifestyle program which included yoga, meditation and vegetarian diet [112], suggesting the modulatory effect of yoga on neuro-endocrinal axis. Further, yadav et al found that a 9 day comprehensive yoga-based lifestyle modification (YLMP) program significantly reduced oxidative stress in 104 subjects. They measured thiobarbituric acid reactive substances (TBARS) in blood as an indicator of oxidative stress at the beginning and at the end of YLMP and found significant reduction in the levels [113]. The YLMP consisted of *āsanas, Prānāyāmas*, meditation, lectures and films on yoga, stress management and individual counseling.

Prānamaya Kośa: Scriptural Evidence

Prāna is the basic life principle. *Prānāyāma* is a process for gaining control over *prāna. Maharśi* Patanjali defines *Prānāyāma* as cessation of movement of inhalation and exhalation after having attained mastery over *āsana* (P.Y.S.2.49). The five manifestations of *prāna* and the corresponding most comprehensive definition of *Prānāyāma* in the human system are described in *Praśnopanisad* [114]. Suitable types of *Prānāyāma* and breathing help to remove the random agitations in *prānic* flows in the *prānamaya kośa*. Thus, the ailments are handled at this *prānamaya kośa* level [98, 99].

Other *hathayoga* texts describe usefulness of specialised breathing techniques: Wherever there is affliction due to disease, filling that region with *Prāna* one should hold it there. (H.Y.P. 5.23) Lying supine on even ground and extending the body one should practice *Prānāyāma* for alleviation of every kind of disease. (H.Y.P. 5.21) *Bhastrikā* removes imbalances of all three *dośas* (basic humors according to ayurvedic science); *vāta, pitta* and *kapha*. It also improves body fire (H.Y.P.2.65) and those who do it thrice daily, they shall never suffer from any disease (G.S. 5.77). *Nādishuddhi* is useful in balancing *vāta* (H.Y.P. 2.7, 2.10). *Ujjayī Prānāyāma* should form the core, as it destroys all the diseases of the *nādis*, dropsy, and diseases of the *dhātus* (sevenfold structural components that support the body according to ayurvedic science) and increases gastric fire (H.Y.P. 2.52).

Prānamaya Kośa (Breathing Practices and Prānic Healing): Scientific Evidence

Yogic breathing is a unique method for balancing the autonomic nervous system and influencing psychological and stress-related disorders. *Sudarshan Kriyā Yoga* (SKY), a sequence of specific breathing techniques (*ujjayī, bhastrikā* [99] and *sudarshan kriyā*) can alleviate anxiety, depression, everyday stress, post-traumatic stress, and stress-related medical illnesses [115]. Mechanisms contributing to a state of calm alertness include increased parasympathetic drive, calming of stress response systems, neuroendocrine release of hormones, and thalamic generators. Relaxation and breathing techniques utilize awareness of breathing rate, rhythm, and volume. Most often breathing techniques are used to minimize physiologic responses to stress, possibly by increasing parasympathetic response [116]. In a study, Telles et al checked the effect of breathing exclusively through one nostril on autonomic functions. 48 male subjects were divided randomly into three groups (viz. right nostril breathing, left nostril breathing or alternate nostril breathing). 27 respiratory cycles were repeated 4 times daily for one month. At the end of one month it was observed that right nostril breathing lead to increase in metabolism as shown by the enhancement of 37% in baseline oxygen consumption. This could be due to increased sympathetic discharge to the adrenal medulla. Whereas left nostril breathing caused reduction in sympathetic nervous system activity through significant increase in volar galvanic skin resistance. Thus, breathing selectively through either nostril can have a marked activating effect or a relaxing effect on the sympathetic nervous system [117]. Shannahoff-Khalsa claimed that ancient yogic technique of unilateral forced nostril breathing (UFNB) that employs forced breathing through only one nostril while closing off the other is a non-invasive technique that seems to selectively activate the ipsilateral branch of the sympathetic nervous system [118]. He further found that forced right nostril breathing increases heart rate compared to left forced nostril breathing whereas forced left nostril breathing leads to rise in end diastolic volume and stroke volume [119]. In a single blind control study, Jain et al [120] compared the effect of *Prānic* healing, a non-touch non pharmacological method of treatment, in chronic musculoskeletal pain with a placebo session of random hand movements. Fifty patients with chronic non-malignant continuous musculoskeletal pain of more than 6 months duration were assigned to two groups of 25 each. One group received *prānic* healing for 25 min and another group underwent a placebo session for 25 min. The results showed highly significant reduction in pain and sympathetic activity in *prānic* healing group (student's t- test $p < 0.001$) and non-significant change in placebo group. They concluded that *Prānic* healing when performed in the standardized method by a trained healer is effective in reducing continuous chronic pain of musculoskeletal origin, within 25 minutes as compared to placebo random hand movements which appears similar to the standard method of *prānic* healing.

Manomaya Kośa: Scriptural Evidence

According to Patanjali [70] , the culturing of mind is accomplished by focusing of the mind (*Dhāranā*) initially, followed by relaxed dwelling of the mind in a single thought (*Dhyāna*) for longer and longer durations leading ultimately to superconsciousness (*Samādhi*) (P.Y.S. 3.1, 3.2, 3.3).

For various meditative techniques to be used we can have following scriptural references:

Prānic Energisation Technique [121]: With concentrated mind one should meditate upon the *Vāyu* (life force) and should fill the lungs by inhaling. Then a complete exhalation should effortlessly be performed according to one's capacity (H.Y.P. 5.10) do repeated exhalations and inhalations (H.Y.P 5.11). Whenever any region is afflicted with disease one should concentrate on the *Vāyu* stuck up in that region (H.Y.P. 5.9).

Om Meditation [114]: The three *mantrās* (A U M), when employed separately, leads to fruits that are mortal and finite, but when they are strung together they are not in any sense of the term 'wrongly employed'. But when they are 'properly employed' in all their internal, external and midway functions, the knower thereafter trembles not.

Cyclic Meditation [122]: 'In a state of mental inactivity awaken the mind; when agitated, calm it; between these two states realize the possible abilities of the mind. If the mind has reached states of perfect equilibrium, do not disturb it again' [123, 124].

Mind Sound Resonance Technique [125]: (*Nādānusandhāna)*- 'Senses cannot function without cooperation of the mind and *prāna*, which in turn cannot function without underlying life activities. Life activities, and with them the mental, sensory and motor activities are stopped by yoga. This is called *Layā*. In this state, the yogis hear a centrally aroused sound and lose themselves in that sound (*nāda*); and this suspension of life activity in yoga is not a vacuum. It is a higher state of consciousness (*samādhi*).

After becoming indifferent to the world, a controlled person should fix his mind on the (inner) sound which he hears while his ears are closed at the root, until he attains a state of perfect steadiness (H.R.4.4-6, 4.8) [103]. In the state of *Samādhi*, when *kundalinī* (mystic energy at the root of spine) is at equilibrium and moves up from the middle path, by making internal sound yogi is freed from diseases [H.R. 2.114-115].

Manomaya Kośa (Relaxation Techniques and Meditations): Scientific Evidence

Koar and William found a significant increase in T-cells and a decrease in anxiety and depression in HIV infected individuals following the practice of meditation in their pilot study [66]. Mindfulness meditation is the practice of bringing an open and receptive awareness of the present moment to experiences, avoiding thinking of the past or worrying about the future. It is thought to reduce stress and improve health outcomes in a variety of patient populations. A randomized controlled trial in a diverse community sample of HIV-1 infected adults indicated that 8-week mindfulness meditation and stress reduction program can buffer CD4+ T lymphocyte declines [68]. A quasi-experimental study tested the effect of a structured 8 week Mindfulness-Based Stress Reduction (MBSR) program on HIV infected individuals and reported significant increase in natural killer cell activity and number in the MBSR group compared to the comparison group [67]. In another randomized controlled trial, Bormann et al examined the effect of psycho-spiritual intervention of *mantram* repetition, "a word or phrase with spiritual associations repeated silently throughout the day" on psychological distress, quality of life enjoyment and satisfaction, and existential spiritual well-being, in 93 HIV infected adults randomly assigned to *mantram* (n = 46) or attention control group (n = 47). Results showed significant improvement in *mantram* group as compared to the control in reducing trait anger and increasing spiritual faith and connectedness. *Mantram* practice was positively associated with quality of life and total existential spiritual wellbeing and inversely associated with HIV-related intrusive thoughts [65]. As Madanmohan discussed in a review [126], a study by Maini on 60 young medical students tested the effect of *Sahaj* yoga meditation on lipid peroxidation and found significant decrease in malonyl dialdehyde levels and increase in RBC count, packed cell volume, total leucocyte count, and mean corpuscular fragility [127]. They concluded that *Sahaj* yoga practice decreases lipid peroxidation levels in the blood and levels of stress as well. Further, Tooley et al demonstrated the ability of meditation to affect plasma melatonin levels, as they observed significantly higher levels of plasma melatonin in experienced meditators in the period immediately following meditation. They suggested that facilitation of higher physiological melatonin levels at appropriate times of day might be one avenue through which the claimed health promoting effects of meditation occur [128]. In another study, Harinath et al noted significant improvement in cardiorespiratory performance and increase in plasma melatonin levels following a 3 month practice of *hatha* yoga and *Omkār* meditation in healthy subjects [95]. Oswal et al defined yogic *prānic* energization technique (YPET) as an advanced yoga relaxation practice that involves breath regulation, chanting, and visualization, which according to yogic science revitalizes the tissues by activating the subtle energies (*prāna*) within the body [129]. They performed a randomized control trial in 30 patients randomly divided into yoga (n=15) and control groups (n=15) to test the add-on effect of YPET on healing of fresh fractures, and found significant improvement in pain and tenderness reduction, fracture line density and number of cortices united. They concluded that add-on yoga-based YPET accelerates fracture healing [129]. Cyclic Meditation (CM) is a yoga-based relaxation technique based on a statement from Indian *vedic* text [123], which suggests that combination of "stimulating" and "calming" practices may be especially helpful to reach a state of mental equilibrium. In a study, the oxygen consumption, breath rate and breath volume of 50 male volunteers were assessed before, during, and after sessions of CM and sessions of supine rest in the corpse posture (*Śavāsana*, SH). The results showed that a combination of yoga postures with supine rest (CM) reduces the oxygen consumption more than resting supine alone does [130]. Cyclic Meditation has also been shown to reduce sympathetic activity and bring about a state of parasympathetic dominance [131], to reduce occupational stress [132] and to improve quality of sleep [133].

Vijñanamaya Kośa: Scriptural Evidence

Questioning attitude and logical thinking is the key to operate from *vijñanamaya kośa. Upanisads* are the treasury of such knowledge which is the redeemer of all miseries and obsessions. It is the lack of inner *jñana* (knowledge) which is responsible for many wrong habits, agitations, etc. The secret for happiness, therefore, is conquering of the agitation of mind through knowledge. Once the mind is calm through the logic of knowledge, the understanding becomes deeper and goes beyond the logic and one is able to handle the stressors in a healthy way. Different *Upanisad s* describe different models *(prakriyās)* and techniques *(upāsanās)* to purify and prepare the mind for this knowledge (*Jñana*). Which can be achieved using Yogic counseling based on ancient scriptures (*Upanisad* s, *Bhagavad Gita, Brahmasutras*), Lectures on *Jñana* Yoga, concept of death according to *Vedas* etc., to bring about the notional corrections [134].

Vijñanamaya Kośa (Yogic Counseling, Lectures and Notional Corrections): Scientific Evidence

A study tested the effect of yoga practices on stress induced effects in first year medical undergraduates. The results pointed to the beneficial role of yoga in not only causing reduction in basal anxiety level but also attenuating the increase in anxiety score in stressful state such as exams.

The yoga group also reported improvement in sense of well being, feeling of relaxation, improved concentration, self confidence, improved efficiency, good interpersonal relationship, increased attentiveness, lowered irritability levels, and an optimistic outlook in life as indicated by feedback score [135]. Satyapriya et al randomized healthy pregnant women to practicing yoga and deep relaxation or standard prenatal exercises 1-hour daily, to assess the effect of integrated yoga on perceived stress and autonomic response. The results showed reduction of perceived stress in the yoga group (by 31.57%) and rise of perceived stress in the control group by 6.60% (P=0.001).

Yoga also improved adaptive autonomic responses to stress in healthy pregnant women in the same study [136]. Suggesting that yoga with its vast wisdom base in Indian *vedic* literature, through notional corrections, can favorably change the perception of individuals towards stressful life events.

Ānandamaya Kośa (Laughter Yoga, Action in Blissful Awareness): Scriptural Evidence

The Happiness Analysis model: Search for happiness is instinctive to sustain creation and to avoid fear and death. It is essential to move towards bliss and overcome misery. An ancient *vedic* text describes that this analysis systematically leads the student to that substratum from which *prāna* and mind emerge - the *Ānandamaya Kośa* [97]. It leads to the realization that happiness is within and 'each one of us' in our causal state is '*Ānanda*' (bliss) embodied. As a result, life changes occur in person's outlook.

Knowledge burns the strong attachments, obsessions, likes and dislikes which are the basic reasons for the agitations of mind. Happiness is an inner state. It is an inner silence that is a state of being. Sense objects only give temporary glimpse of our own nature, *Ānanda* [134].

Action in blissful awareness (*Karma yoga*), is a technique where work is enjoyed with mindfulness without caring for fruits.

Routine activities are done with relaxed but aware mind. One lives in the present moment while performing his duties with an attitude of universal well being. As Śri Kriśna tells in *Bhagavad Gita* - 'Whosoever, controlling the senses by the mind, O Arjuna, engages his organs of action in *Karma yoga* (action for universal well being without attachment), he excels.' (B.G. 3.7) [100].

Ānandamaya Kośa (Laughter Yoga, Action in Blissful Awareness): Scientific Evidence

Laughter is basically stimulation and physiological arousal and when combined with yoga practice it leads to a hypo-metabolic state [137]. Relaxation techniques also lead to reduction of metabolic rate and sympathetic activity thereby reducing stress. Laughter has shown different physiological and psychological benefits [138].

A pilot study demonstrated benefits at the biochemical level, in terms of reduction in the serum levels of cortisol, dopac, epinephrine, and growth hormone after a 60 min session of mirthful laughter [139].

Takashi et al tested the effect of Laughter by watching a comic video, on gene expression in type-2 Diabetic patients and observed an up-regulation of about 39 genes at 1.5hr and 27 gene up-regulations were sustained till 4hr after watching the video. Among the up-regulated genes, 14 were related to natural killer cell activity. They concluded that Laughter influences the expression of many genes classified into immune responses [140]. Masahiro et al investigated the effect of Laughter on endocrinological stress marker chromogranin-A (CgA) in 11 healthy males. Saliva samples were collected before and after watching a comic film. They found significant increase in CgA levels, although subjective stress score on visual analog scale was reduced [141].

Laughter Yoga International commissioned a scientific research project involving 200 IT professionals in Bangalore (India), to determine the effect of laughter yoga on stress at the work place. Participants were divided into two groups, laughter yoga (LY) and control. LY group received LY sessions every 2-3 days for 18 days (Total of 7 sessions) while other group was wait listed.

Physiological (autonomic and respiratory variables), biochemical (early morning-salivary cortisol) and psychological (Positive and Negative Affect Scale, Perceived Stress Scale and Toronto Alexythemia Scale) parameters were assessed.

The results showed significant reductions in systolic and diastolic blood pressures, significant reductions in early morning salivary cortisol levels in the LY group as compared to control. There was also a reduction in negative affect, perceived stress and alexithymia [137].

IAYT Module for Reversal of Hematopoietic Inhibition in HIV-1 Infected Patients

Based on Primary (Scriptural) and Secondary (Scientific) Sources of References, the Following Yoga Modules are Devised

The yoga sessions would be standardized to optimize consistency between participants. Two basic Yoga modules, one for intensive residential practice at our health home (IP) [Table 1], *Ārogyadhāma*, for first four weeks and second for regular practice at home as out-patient (OP) [Table 2] for next 16weeks with the help of CD's, books, and printed material are devised, a total of 20 week intervention. Each session would begin with feedback from the participants about their previous session.

Table 1. The Schedule During Intensive Residential Intervention for Initial 4 weeks (Yoga Module 1) (IP)

Time	Activity	Time	Activity
5.00 AM	Ablution	2:00 PM	Yogic Relaxation Technique [99] (Yoga nidrā, Nādānusandhāna)
5:30 AM	Om Meditation [99, 123]	3:00 PM	Cyclic Meditation[122, 124]
6:00 AM	Special Yoga Technique1 (see Table 3) [99] (Āsanas/ Kriyās twice a week)	4:30 PM	Evening snacks (milk or juice)
7:00 AM	Karmayoga [100] (work with mindfullness)	5:00 PM	Evening Walk (Tuning to nature)
8:00 AM	Bhagavad Gita chanting and discourse on yoga philosophy	6:00 PM	Devotional Sessions, Chanting
8:45 AM	Breakfast (sāttvic yoga diet)	6:30 PM	Mind Sound Resonance Technique[125]
9:30 AM	Prānic Energisation Technique [121]	7:30 PM	Dinner
10:30 AM	Yogic Counselling/ Notional Corrections	8:30 PM	Happy Assembly (Laughter Yoga, Yoga games)
11:00 AM	Prānāyāma (see Table 5)[99]	9:30 PM	Rest / Introspection
12:00 Noon	Special Yoga Techique2 (see Table 4) [99]	10:00 PM	Lights Off
1:00 PM	Lunch (sāttvic yoga diet)		

Table 2. The Schedule During Home Practice Intervention for next 16 weeks (Yoga module 2) (OP)

S.N.	NAME OF PRACTICE	TIME AND DURATION	SOURCE
1.	Om Meditation [99, 123]	From 5:30 AM to 6:00 AM (30min)	Om meditation CD
2.	Special Technique 1 [99] (see Table 3)	From 6AM TO 7AM (1 hr)	As Taught During IP And As Per The Printed Material Given
3.	Prānāyāma [99] (see Table 5)	7AM TO 7:45AM (45min)	As Taught During Ip And As Per The Printed Material Given
4.	Prānic Energisation Technique (PET) [121]	9 AM TO 10 AM	PET CD

S.N.	NAME OF PRACTICE	TIME AND DURATION	SOURCE
4.	Karmayoga [100]	While doing daily routine activities or job	As per the lectures taken during IP
5.	Cyclic Meditation [122, 124]	Afternoon 3:00 TO 4:00PM	Cyclic Meditation CD
6.	Special Technique 2 [99] (see Table 4)	Evening 6:00PM TO 7:00PM	As Taught During IP And As Per The Printed Material Given
7.	Mind Sound Resonance Technique (MSRT) [125]	Either Evening 7:00PM TO 8:00PM OR After Dinner Before Sleeping Between 9:00PM TO 10:00PM	MSRT CD

Note: Yogic counselling given once in a fortnight for one hour.
Kriyās to be practiced once a week (as learnt during IP).
Diet as per yogic concepts of sāttvic diet at proper time.

Table 3. Special Technique 1 [99] Duration of Special Technique 1: 1 hour

Sl. No.	Name of practices	Number of rounds	Duration
	Starting prayer		2 mins
Loosening Practices			
1	Jogging	5 rounds	2 mins
2	Forward and backward bending	5 rounds	2 mins
3	Twisting	5 rounds	2 mins
4	Side bending	5 rounds	2 mins
5	*Pavanmuktāsana* stretch	5 rounds	2 mins
Surya namaskāra		5-10 rounds	15 mins
Breathing Practices			
1	Hands in and out Breathing	5 rounds	2 mins
2	Ankle stretch breathing	5 rounds	2 mins
3	*Bhujangāsana* Breathing	5 rounds	2 mins
4	Straight Leg Raise Breathing	5 rounds	2 mins
5	Both Leg Raising	5 rounds	2 mins
Āsanas			
1	*Ardhakati Ćakrásana*	1 round	2 mins
2	*Uśtrāsana*	1 round	2 mins
3	*Paśćimottanāsana*	1 round	2 mins
4	*Bhujangāsana*	1 round	2 mins
5	*Śalabāsana*	1 round	2 mins
6	*Setubandhāsana*	1 round	2 mins
7	*Śavāsana*/Deep Relaxation Technique (DRT)		5 mins
Closing prayer			2 mins

Table 4. Special Technique 2 [99] Duration of Special Technique 2: 1 hour

Sl. No.	Name of practices	Number of rounds	Duration
	Starting prayer		2 mins
Loosening Practices			
1	Jogging	5 rounds	2 mins
2	Forward and backward bending	5 rounds	2 mins
3	Twisting	5 rounds	2 mins
4	Side bending	5 rounds	2 mins
Surya namaskāra		5-10 rounds	15 mins
Breathing Practices			
1	Hands in and out Breathing	5 rounds	2 mins
2	Ankle stretch breathing	5 rounds	2 mins

Table 4. (Continued)

Sl. No.	Name of practices	Number of rounds	Duration
3	*Bhujangāsana* Breathing	5 rounds	2 mins
4	Straight Leg Raise Breathing	5 rounds	2 mins
5	Both Leg Raising	5 rounds	2 mins
Āsanas			
1	*Ardha Ćakrásana/ Ćakrāsana*	1 round	2 mins
2	*Paśćimottanāsana*	1 round	2 mins
3	*Uśtrāsana*	1 round	2 mins
4	*Dhanurāsana*	1 round	2 mins
5	*Sarvāngāsana/Halāsana*	1 round	2 mins
6	*Śirśāsana*	1 round	2 mins
7	*Śavāsana/* Deep Relaxation Technique (DRT)		5 mins
Closing prayer			2 mins

Table 5. Prāṇāyāma (Duration of Prāṇāyāma: 45min)

PRĀṆĀYĀMA [99]			
S. No.	Breathing Practices	ROUNDS	DURATION
Starting prayer			3 mins
1	Kapālabhāti	60-80 rounds/min	5min
3	Sectional breathing: abdominal breathing in supine with AAA chanting thoracic breathing – UUU chanting clavicular breathing in sitting –slow with MMM chanting	5 rounds 5 rounds 5 rounds	5mins
3	Nādishuddhi	27 rounds	10 min
4	Bhastrikā	3 rounds 20 strokes each	6mins
5	Bhrāmari		5min
6	Ujjayī (with Bandhās)		5min
Closing prayer			2 min

These modules include preparatory breathing and loosening practices, *āsanas*, *Prāṇāyāma*, different types of meditations i.e., *om* meditation, *nādānusandhāna* meditation and cyclic meditation, deep relaxation technique (DRT), advanced yoga techniques like *prānic* energisation technique and mind sound resonance technique, interactive lectures on concepts of IAYT, *jñana yoga*, *karma yoga*, etc.

Other practices include healthy yogic diet based on concepts of *triguṇa* (three basic attributes of activity, inertia and balance in the individual personality), devotional sessions and practice of *karma yoga* in the daily routine with mindfulness as selfless service and individual yoga counseling using these concepts.

Conclusion

Thus this article is a unique blend of cellular and molecular biology in biomedical and life sciences and ancient *vedic* prescriptions of Indian (South Asian) treatments for disease.

This literature survey suggests that Integrated Approach of Yoga Therapy [IAYT] modules may have clinical utility in treating HIV-related cytopenias.

Acknowledgments

PSK is a Ramalingaswami Fellow (Dept of Biotechnology, Govt of India). HB is a Junior Research Fellow supported by the Ramalingaswami Fellowship Grant awarded to PSK.

References

[1] Hitchcock IS, Chen MM, King JR, Kaushansky K. 2008. YRRL motifs in the cytoplasmic domain of the thrombopoietin receptor regulate receptor internalization and degradation. *Blood.* 112: 2222-2231.

[2] Moses A, Nelson J, Bagby Jr GC. 1998. The influence of human immunodeficiency virus-1 of hematopoiesis. *Blood.* 91: 1479-1495.

[3] Burstein Y, Rashbaum WK, Hatch WC, Calvelli T, Golodner M, Soeiro R, Lyman WD. 1992. Alterations in human fetal hematopoiesis are associated with HIV infection. *Pediatr Res.* 32: 155-159.

[4] Sugira K, Oyaizn N, Pahwa R, Kalyanaraman VS, Pahwa S. 1992. Effect of human immunodeficiency virus-1 envelope glycoprotein on in vitro hematopoiesis of umbilical cord blood. *Blood.* 80: 1463-1469.

[5] Geissler RG, Ottmann OG, Kleiner K, Mentze IU, Bickelhaupt A, Hoelzer D, Ganser A. 1993. Decreased hematopoietic colony growth in long-term bone marrow cultures of HIV-positive patients. *Res. Virol.* 144: 69-73.

[6] Davis BR, Zauli G. 1995. Effect of human immunodeficiency virus infection on hematopoiesis. *Bailliers Clin. Hematol.* 8: 113-130.

[7] Re MC, Zauli G, Furlini G, Rarieri S, Monari P, Ramazzotti E, LaPlaca M. 1993. The impaired number of circulating granulocyte / macrophage progenitors (CFU-GM) in human immunodeficiency virus type 1 infected subjects correlates with an active HIV-1 replication. *Arch. Virol.* 129: 53-64.

[8] Calenda V, Chermann JC. 1992. The effects of HIV on hematopoiesis. *Eur. J. Hematol.* 48: 181-186.

[9] Chelucci, C., I. Casella, M. Federico, U. Testaa, G. Macioce, E. Pelosi, R. Guerriero, G. Mariani, A. Giampaolo, H. J. Hassan, and C. Peschle. 1999. Lineage-specific expression of human immunodeficiency virus (HIV) receptor/coreceptors in differentiating hematopoietic precursors: Correlation with susceptibility to T- and M-tropic HIV and chemokine-mediated HIV resistance. *Blood.* 94:1590-1600.

[10] Ruiz ME, Ciala C, Arthos J, Kinter A, Catanzaro AT, Adelsberger J, Holmes KL, Cohen OJ, Fauci AS. 1998. Peripheral blood-derived CD34+ progenitor cells: CXC chemokine receptor 4 aand CC chemokine receptor 5 expression and infection by HIV. *J. Immunol.* 161: 4169-4176.

[11] Shen H, Cheng T, Preffer FI, Dombkowski D, Tomasson MH, Golan DE, Yang O, Hofmann W, Sodroski JG, Luster AD, Scadden DT. 1999. Intrinsic Human

immunodeficiency virus type 1 resistance of hematopoietic stem cells despite coreceptor expression. *J. Virol*. 73: 728-737.

[12] Zhang J, Scadden DT, Crumpacker CS. 2007. Primitive hematopoietic cells resist HIV-1 infection via p21. *J. Clin. Invest*. 117:302-304.

[13] Jenkins M, Hanley MB, Moreno MB, Wieder E, McCune JM. 1998. Human immunodeficiency virus-1 infection interrupts thymopoiesis and multilineage hematopoiesis in vivo. *Blood*. 91: 2672-2678.

[14] Koka PS, Fraser JK, Bryson Y, Bristol GC, Aldrovandi GM, Daar ES, Zack JA. 1998. Human immunodeficiency virus type 1 inhibits multi-lineage hematopoiesis in vivo. *J. Virol* .72: 5121-5127.

[15] Sundell IB, Koka PS. 2006. The SCID-hu mouse model as a stem cell host to recapitulate human hematopoiesis in HIV infection and serves as a tool for development of therapies for virus induced cytopenias. *J. Stem Cells*. 1(4): 283-300.

[16] Koka PS, Kitchen CM, Reddy ST. 2004. Targeting c-Mpl for revival of human immunodeficiency virus type 1-induced hematopoietic inhibition when CD34+ progenitor cells are re-engrafted into a fresh stromal microenvironment in vivo. *J. Virol*. 78: 11385-11392.

[17] Schuringa JJ, Chung KY, Morrone G, Moore MAS. 2004. Constitutive activation of STAT5A promotes human hematopoietic stem cell self-renewal and erythroid differentiation. *J. Exp. Med*. 200: 623-635.

[18] Stier S, Cheng T, Dombkowski D, Carlesso N, Scadden DT. 2002. Notch1 activation increases hematopoietic stem cell self-renewal in vivo and favors lymphoid over myeloid lineage outcome. *Blood*. 99: 2369-2378.

[19] Wierenga ATJ, Vellenga E, Schuringa JJ. 2008. Maximal STAT5-induced proliferation and self-renewal at intermediate STAT5 activity levels. *Molec. Cell Biol*. 28: 6668-6680.

[20] Pestina TI, Jackson CW. 2003. Differential role of Stat5 isoforms in effecting hematopoietic recovery induced by Mpl-ligand in lethally myelosuppressed mice. *Exp. Hematol*. 31: 1198-1205.

[21] Schulze H, Ballmaier M, Welte K, Germeshausen M. 2000. Thrombopoietin induces the generation of distinct Stat1, Stat3, Stat5a and Stat5b homo- and heterodimeric complexes with different kinetics in human platelets. *Exp. Hematol*. 28: 294-304.

[22] Zeng H, Masuko M, Jin L, Neff T, Otto KG, Blau CA. 2001. Receptor specificity in the self-renewal and differentiation of primary multipotential hematopoietic cells. *Blood*. 98: 328-334.

[23] Bradley HL, Couldrey C, Bunting KD. 2004. Hematopoietic-repopulating defects from STAT5-deficient bone marrow are not fully accounted for by loss of thrombopoietin responsiveness. *Blood*. 103: 2965-2972.

[24] Miyakawa Y, Drachman JG, Gallis B, Kaushansky A, Kaushansky K. 2000. A structure-function analysis of Serine/Threonine phosphorylation of the thrombopoietin receptor, c-Mpl. *J Biol Chem*. 275: 32214-32219.

[25] May, M. T., Sterne, J. A., Costagliola, D., Sabin, C. A., Phillips, A. N., Justice, A. C., et al. 2006. HIV treatment response and prognosis in Europe and North America in the first decade of highly active antiretroviral therapy: a collaborative analysis. *Lancet*. *368*(9534), 451-458.

[26] Miles SA, Mitsuyasu RT, Moreno J, Baldwin G, Alton NK, Souza L, Glaspy JA. 1991. Combined therapy with recombinant granulocyte colony-stimulating factor and erythropoietin decreases hematologic toxicity from zidovudine. *Blood.* 77: 2109-2117.

[27] Miles SA, Lee S, Hutlin L, Zsebo KM, Mitsuyasu RT. 1991. Potential use of Human stem cell factor as adjunctive therapy for Human immunodeficiency virus-related cytopenias. *Blood.* 78: 3200-3208.

[28] Fauci AS. 1996. Host factors and the pathogenesis of HIV-induced disease. *Nature.* 384: 529-534.

[29] Harbol AW, Liesveld JL, Simpson-Haidaris PJ, Abboud CN. 1994. Mechanisms of cytopenia in human immunodeficiency virus infection. *Blood Rev.* 8: 241-251.

[30] Utley JR. 1990. Pathophysiology of cardiopulmonary bypass: current issues. *J. Card. Surg* 5: 177-189.

[31] Jakobs D. 2001. Heparin induced thrombocytopenia, left ventricular thrombus aand cerebraal embolism during an acute myocardial infarction. *Med. Klin.* 96: 101-104.

[32] Ruiz ME, Ciala C, Arthos J, Kinter A, Catanzaro AT, Adelsberger J, Holmes KL, Cohen OJ, Fauci AS. 1998. Peripheral blood-derived CD34+ progenitor cells: CXC chemokine receptor 4 aand CC chemokine receptor 5 expression and infection by HIV. *J. Immunol* 161: 4169-4176.

[33] Shen H, Cheng T, Preffer FI, Dombkowski D, Tomasson MH, Golan DE, Yang O, Hofmann W, Sodroski JG, Luster AD, Scadden DT. 1999. Intrinsic Human immunodeficiency virus type 1 resistance of hematopoietic stem cells despite coreceptor expression. *J. Virol.* 73: 728-737.

[34] Miles SA, Lee S, Hutlin L, Zsebo KM, Mitsuyasu RT. 1991. Potential use of Human stem cell factor as adjunctive therapy for Human immunodeficiency virus-related cytopenias. *Blood* 78: 3200-3208.

[35] Soland EM, Maciejewski J, Kumar P, Kim S, Chaudhuri A, Young N. 2000. Protease inhibitors stimulate hematopoiesis and decrease apoptosis and ICE expression in CD34+ cells. *Blood* 96: 2735-2739.

[36] Silvestris F, Cafforio P, Tucci M, Dammacco F. 2002. Negative regulation of erythroblast maturation by Fas-L+/TRAIL+ highly malignant plasma cells: a major pathogenic mechanism of anemia in multiple myeloma. *Blood.* 99: 1305-1313.

[37] Hand Gregory A., Kenneth D. Phillips, Wesley D. Dudgeon, William D. Skelton. 2005 Stress Reduction as a Means to Enhance Oral Immunity in HIV-Infected Individuals. *The Journal of the Association of Nurses in AIDS Care: JANAC. 16(5):58-63.*

[38] Borboni, P., Di Cola, G., Sesti, G., Marini, M. A., Del Porto, P., Saveria, M. et al. 1989. Beta-endorphin receptors on cultured and freshly isolated lymphocytes from normal subjects. *Biochemical and Biophysical Research Communications,* 163, 642-648.

[39] De Souza, Webster, Grigoriadis, and Tracey, De Souza, E. B, Webster, E. L., Grigoriadis, D. E., and Tracey, D. E. 1989. Corticotropin-releasing factor (CRF) and interleukin-1 (IL-1) receptors in the brain-pituitary-immune axis. *Psychopharmacology Bulletin*, 25, 299-305.

[40] A Bhansali, RJ Dash, A Sud, S Bhadada, S Sehgal, BR Sharma. 2000. A preliminary report on basal and stimulated plasma cortisol in patients with acquired immunodeficiency syndrome patients. *Indian J. Med. Res.* 112: 173-7.

[41] Tarcisio Vago, Mario Clerici and Guido Norbiato. 1994. 5 Glucocorticoids and the immune system in AIDS. *Baillière's Clinical Endocrinology and Metab.*8(4):789-802.

[42] Kang DH, Fox C. 2001. Th1 and Th2 cytokine responses to academic stress. *Res. Nurs. Health.* 24(4):245-57.

[43] Nair MPN, Mahajan S, Hou J, Sweet AM, Schwartz SA. 2000. The stress hormone, cortisol, synergizes with HIV-1 gp-120 to induce apoptosis of normal human peripheral blood mononuclear cells. *Cell Mol. Biol.* (Noisy-le-grand). 46(7):1227-38.

[44] Mcewen, B. S., Biron, C. A., Brunson, K. W., Bulloch, K., et al. 1997. The role of adrenocorticoids as modulators of immune function in health and disease: Neural, endocrine and immune interactions. *Brain Research Reviews.* 23, 79-133.

[45] Leserman, J., Jackson, E., Petitto, J., Golden, R., Silva, S., and Perkins, D et al. 1999. Progression to AIDS: The effects of stress, depressive symptoms and social support. *Psychosomatic Medicine.* 61: 397-406.

[46] Burack et al., 1993 Burack, JH., Barrett, DC., Stall, RD., Chesney, MA., Ekstrand, ML and Coates, TJ. 1993. Depressive symptoms and CD4 lymphocyte decline among HIV-infected men. *Journal of American Medical Association.* 270, 2568-2573.

[47] Ickovics et.al, 2001 Ickovics, J., Hamburger, M., Vlahov, D., Schoenbaum, E., Schuman, P., Boland, R., and Moore, J. 2001. Mortality CD4 cell count decline and depressive symptoms among HIV-seropositive women: Longitudinal analysis from HIV Epidemiology Research Study. *Journal of American Medical Association.* 285: 1460-1465.

[48] Leserman, J, John M. Petitto, Robert N. Golden, et al. 2000. Impact of Stressful Life Events, Depression, Social Support, Coping, and Cortisol on Progression to AIDS. *Am. J. Psychiatry.* 157:1221-1228.

[49] Leserman, J. 2008. Role of Depression, Stress, and Trauma in HIV Disease Progression. *Psychosomatic Medicine.* 70:539–545.

[50] Leserman, J. 2003. HIV disease progression: depression, stress, and possible mechanisms. *Biol. Psychiatry.* 54(3):295-306.

[51] Eller, L.S. 2006. Depressive symptoms in HIV/AIDS. *Nursing Clinics of North America.* 41, 437-453.

[52] Antoni MH, S. N., Fletcher MA, Goldstein DA, Ironson G, LaPerriere A. 1990. Psychoneuroimmunology and HIV-l. *J. Consult Clin Psychol. 1*(58), 38-49.

[53] Cohen, S., Janicki- Deverts, D., Miller, G.E. 2007. Psychological stress and disease. *JAMA.* 298, 1685–1687.

[54] Cole, S. W., Naliboff, B. D., Kemeny, M. E., Griswold, M. P., Fahey, J. L., and Zack, J. A. 2001. Impaired response to HAART in HIV-infected individuals with high autonomic nervous system activity. *Proc. Natl. Acad. Sci. USA.* 98(22), 12695-12700.

[55] Ironson, G., Balbin, E., Stuetzle, R., Fletcher, M. A., O'Cleirigh, C., Laurenceau, J. P., et al. 2005. Dispositional optimism and the mechanisms by which it predicts slower disease progression in HIV: proactive behavior, avoidant coping, and depression. *Int. J. Behav. Med.* 12(2), 86-97.

[56] Antoni MH, S. N., Fletcher MA, Goldstein DA, Ironson G, LaPerriere A. 1990. Psychoneuroimmunology and HIV-l. *J. Consult. Clin. Psychol. 1*(58), 38-49.

[57] Antoni, M. H., Carrico, A. W., Duran, R. E., Spitzer, S., Penedo, F., Ironson, G., et al. 2006. Randomized clinical trial of cognitive behavioral stress management on human immunodeficiency virus viral load in gay men treated with highly active antiretroviral therapy. *Psychosom. Med. 68*(1), 143-151.

[58] LaPerriere AR, Antoni MH, Schneiderman N, Ironson G, Klimas N, Caralis P, et al. 1990. Exercise intervention attenuates emotional distress and natural killer cell decrements following notification of positive serologic status for HIV-1. *Biofeedback Self Regul.* 15(3):229-42.

[59] Eller, L. S. 1999b. Effects of two cognitive-behavioral interventions on immunity and symptoms in persons with HIV. *International Journal of Nursing Studies, 36*, 223-233.

[60] de Visser R, Ezzy D, Bartos M. 2000. Alternative or Complementary? Nonallopathic Therapies for HIV/AIDS. *Altern. Ther. Health Med.* 6:44–52.

[61] Duggan J, Peterson WS, Schutz M, Khuder S, Charkraborty J. 2001. Use of Complementary and Alternative Therapies in HIV-Infected Patients. *AIDS Patient Care STDS.* 15:159–167.

[62] Knippels HM, Weiss JJ. 2000. Use of alternative medicine in a sample of HIV-positive gay men: an exploratory study of prevalence and user characteristics. *AIDS Care.*12:435–446.

[63] Ozsoy M, Ernst E. 1999. How effective are complementary therapies for HIV and AIDS? - a systematic review. *Int. J. STD AIDS.* 10:629–635.

[64] Cho M, Ye X, Dobs A, Cofrancesco J. 2006. Prevalence of complementary and alternative medicine use among HIV patients for perceived lipodystrophy. *J. Altern. Complement Med.* 12(5):475–482.

[65] Bormann JE, Gifford AL, Shively M, Smith TL, Redwine L, Kelly A et al. 2006. Effects of spiritual mantram repetition on HIV outcomes: a randomized controlled trial. *J Behav Med.* 29(4):359-76.

[66] Koar, William. 1995. Meditation, T-cells, anxiety, depression and HIV infection. *Subtle Energies and Energy Medicine Journal.* 6(1).

[67] Robinson, F. P., Mathews, H. L., and Witek-Janusek, L. 2003. Psycho-endocrine-immune response to mindfulness-based stress reduction in individuals infected with the human immunodeficiency virus: a quasiexperimental study. *J. Altern. Complement Med, 9*(5), 683-694.

[68] Creswell, J. D., Myers, H. F., Cole, S. W., and Irwin, M. R. 2009. Mindfulness meditation training effects on CD4+ T lymphocytes in HIV-1 infected adults: a small randomized controlled trial. *Brain Behav Immun, 23*(2), 184-188.

[69] Madanmohan (2008). *Introducing Yog to Medical Students The JIPMER Experience:* Advanced Centre for Yoga Therapy, Education and Research.

[70] *Four Chapters on Freedom.* Commentary on the Yoga Sutras of Patanjali by Swami Satyānanda Saraswati. 2002. Yoga Publications Trust. Munger, Bihar. India.

[71] Innes KE, Vincent HK. 2007. The influence of yoga-based programs on risk profiles in adults with type 2 diabetes mellitus: a systematic review. *Evid. Based Complement Alternat Med.* 4:469–486.

[72] Innes KE, Bourguignon C, Taylor AG. 2005. Risk indices associated with the insulin resistance syndrome, cardiovascular disease, and possible protection with yoga: a systematic review. *J. Am. Board Fam. Pract.* 18:491–519.

[73] Sainani, G. S. 2003. "Non-drug therapy in prevention and control of hypertension." *J Assoc Physicians* India 51: 1001-1006.

[74] Sahay, B. K. and R. K. Sahay. 2002. "Lifestyle modification in management of diabetes mellitus." *J. Indian Med. Assoc.* 100(3): 178-180.

[75] Yang K. 2007. A review of yoga programs for four leading risk factors of chronic diseases. Evid Based *Complement Alternat Med.*4:487–491.

[76] Nagarathna, R. and H. R. Nagendra. 1985. "Yoga for bronchial asthma: a controlled study." *Br. Med. J.* (Clin Res Ed) 291(6502): 1077-1079.

[77] Jayasinghe, S. R. 2004. Yoga in cardiac health (a review). *Eur. J. Cardiovasc Prev. Rehabil, 11*(5), 369-375.

[78] Raub, J. A. 2002. Psychophysiologic effects of Hatha Yoga on musculoskeletal and cardiopulmonary function: a literature review. *J Altern. Complement Med. 8*(6), 797-812.

[79] Bower, J. E., Woolery, A., Sternlieb, B., and Garet, D. 2005. Yoga for cancer patients and survivors. *Cancer Control. 12*(3), 165-171.

[80] Khalsa, S. B. 2004. Yoga as a therapeutic intervention: a bibliometric analysis of published research studies. *Indian J. Physiol Pharmacol.,* 48(3), 269-285.

[81] Descilo T, Vedamurtachar A, Gerbarg PL, Nagaraja D, Gangadhar BN, Damodaran B, et al. 2010. Effects of a yoga breath intervention alone and in combination with an exposure therapy for post-traumatic stress disorder and depression in survivors of the 2004 South-East Asia tsunami. *Acta Psychiatr Scand.* 121(4):289-300.

[82] West, J., Otte, C., Geher, K., Johnson, J., and Mohr, D. C. 2004. Effects of Hatha yoga and African dance on perceived stress, affect, and salivary cortisol. *Ann. Behav. Med. 28*(2), 114-118.

[83] Cohen L, Warneke C, Fouladi RT, Rodriguez MA, Chaoul-Reich A. 2004. Psychological adjustment and sleep quality in a randomized trial of the effects of a Tibetan yoga intervention in patients with lymphoma. *Cancer.* 15:2253e60.

[84] Kochupillai V, Kumar P, Singh D, Aggarwal D, Bhardwaj N, Bhutani M, Das SN. 2005. Effect of rhythmic breathing (*Sudarshan Kriya* and *Prānayam*) on immune functions and tobacco addiction. *Ann. N Y Acad. Sci.* 1056:242-52.

[85] Vadiraja HS, Raghavendra RM, Nagarathna R, Nagendra HR et al. 2009. Effects of a yoga program on cortisol rhythm and mood states in early breast cancer patients undergoing adjuvant radiotherapy: a randomized controlled trial. *Integr Cancer Ther.* 8(1):37-46.

[86] Vadiraja HS, Raghavendra RM, Nagarathna R, Nagendra HR et al. 2009. Effects of yoga on symptom management in breast cancer patients: A randomized controlled trial. *Int. J. Yoga.* 2(2):73-9.

[87] Raghavendra RM, Nagarathna R, Nagendra HR, Gopinath KS et al. 2007. Effects of an integrated yoga programme on chemotherapy-induced nausea and emesis in breast cancer patients. *Eur. J. Cancer Care (Engl).* 16(6):462-74.

[88] Carson J, Carson K, Porter L, Keefe F, Shaw H, Miller J. Yoga for women with metastatic breast cancer: results from a pilot study. 2007. *J Pain Symptom Manage.* 33:331e41.

[89] Cole, SW., Naliboff BD., Kemeny, ME., Griswold, MP., Fahey JL., Zack, JA . 2001. Impaired response to HAART in HIV-infected individuals with high autonomic nervous system activity. *Proc. Natl. Acad. Sci. USA*. 98:12695-12700.

[90] Jakobs, D. 2001. Heparin induced thrombocytopenia, left ventricular thrombus and cerebral embolism during an acute myocardial infarction. *Med. Klin.* 96:101-104.

[91] Podolsky, S. H., A. Zembowicz, F. J. Schoen, R. J. Benjamin, and L. A. Sonna. 1999. Massive myocardial necrosis in thrombotic thrombocytopenic purpura: a case report and review of the literature. *Arch. Pathol. Lab. Med.* 123:937-940.

[92] Daszynski, J., and T. Ciszewski. 1989. Blood component therapy in open heart surgery. *Master Med. Pol.* 21:207-211.

[93] Bharshankar JR, Bharshankar RN, Deshpande VN, Kaore SB, Gosavi GB. 2003. Effect of yoga on cardiovascular system in subjects above 40 years. *Indian J. Physiol Pharmocol.* 47:202–206.

[94] Bijlani RL, Vempati RP, Yadav RK, et al. 2005. A brief but comprehensive lifestyle education program based on yoga reduces risk factors for cardiovascular disease and diabetes mellitus. *J. Altern Complement Med.* 11:267–274.

[95] Harinath K, Malhotra AS, Pal K, et al. 2004. Effects of Hatha Yoga and Omkar meditation on cardiorespiratory performance, psychologic profile and melatonin secretion. *J. Altern Complement Med.* 10:261–268.

[96] Manchanda SC, Narang R, Reddy KS, et al. 2000. Retardation of coronary atherosclerosis with yoga lifestyle intervention. *J. Assoc. Physicians India.* 48:687–694.

[97] Taittarīya *Upanisad.* With the commentary of Sankaracharya translated by swami Gambhirānanda. 1986. Published byAdvaita Ashrama. Mayavati, Pithoragarh, Himalayas.

[98] *The Vision and the Way of Vasistha.* 1993. Compiled by B.L. Atreya translated by Samvid, Indian Heritage Trust, Madras, India.

[99] Nagendra H R, Nagaratna R. 2001. *Yoga for Promotion of Positive Health.* Swami Vivekānanda Yoga Publications. Bangalore, India.

[100] *The Holy Gita* commentary by Swami Chinmayānanda Central Chinmaya Mission Trust, Sandeepany Sadhanalaya, Powai Park Drive, Mumbai, India.

[101] *Hath Yoga Pradipika: Light on hath yoga-* commentary by Swami Muktibodhānanda under the guidance of Swami Satyānanda Saraswati. Yoga Publication Trust, Ganga darshan, Munger, Bihar, India (Third edition).

[102] *The Gheranda Samhita*, translated by Rai Bahadur Srisa Chandra Vasu. Chaukhamba Sanskrit pratishthan, Jawaharnagar, Delhi, India. (First edition).

[103] *Hathratnavali of Śrinivasabhatta Mahayogindra.* Printed and published by Sri M Ramakrishna Reddy, Arthamaru. E.G. Dist. Andhra Pradesh, India.

[104] Antoni, MH., Baggett, L., Ironson, G., LaPerriere, A., August, S., Klimas, N., Schneiderman, N., and Fletcher, MA. 1991. Cognitive-behaviour stress management intervention buffers distress responses and immunological changes following notification of HIV-1 seropositivity. *Journal of Consulting and Clinical Psychology*, 59, 906-915.

[105] Antoni, MH., Cruess, DG., Klimas, N., Maher, K., Cruess, S., Kumar, M., et al. 2002. Stress management and immune system reconstitution in symptomatic HIV-infected gay men over time: Effects on transitional naïve T cells (CD4(+) CD45RA(+) CD29(+)). *American Journal of Psychiatry*, 159(1): 143-145.

[106] LaPerriere, A., Fletcher, M., Antoni, M., Klimas, N., Ironson, G., and Schneiderman, N. 1991. Aerobic exercise training in an AIDS risk group. *International Journal of Sports Medicine*, 12: 52-57.

[107] Gopal A, Mondal S, Gandhi A, Arora S, Bhattacharjee J. 2011. Effect of integrated yoga practices on immune responses in examination stress - A preliminary study. *Int J Yoga.* 4(1):26-32.

[108] Todd Cade, PT, Dominic N. Reeds, Kristin E. Mondy, Turner Overton et al. 2010. Yoga lifestyle intervention reduces blood pressure in HIV-infected adults with cardiovascular disease risk factors. *HIV Med.* 11(6): 379–388.

[109] Nagarathna R, Nagendra H R. 2011. *Efficacy Of Yoga Intervention In HIV Sero Positive Subjects –A Randomized Control Trial.* In Press.

[110] Kamei T, Toriumi Y, Kimura H, Ohno S, Kumano H, Kimura K. 2000. Decrease in serum cortisol during yoga exercise is correlated with alpha wave activation. *Percept Mot. Skills.* 90: 1027-32.

[111] Woolery, A., Myers, H., Sternlieb, B, Zeltzer L. 2004. A yoga intervention for young adults with elevated symptoms of depression. *Altern. Ther. Health Med.* 10(2):60-3.

[112] Schmidt T, Wijga A, Von Zur Mühlen A, Brabant G, Wagner TO. 1997. Changes in cardiovascular risk factors and hormones during a comprehensive residential three month kriya yoga training and vegetarian nutrition. *Acta Physiol Scand Suppl.*; 640:158-62.

[113] Yadav RK, Ray RB, Vempati R, Bijlani RL. 2005. Effect of a comprehensive yoga-based lifestyle modification program on lipid peroxidation. *Indian J. Physiol. Pharmacol.* 49: 358-62.

[114] Prasnopaniśad. *Commentary by swami chinmayānanda.* Central Chinmaya Mission Trust, Sandeepany Sadhanalaya, Powai Park Drive, Mumbai (Fourth Edition).

[115] Janakiramaiah, N., Gangadhar, B.N., Naga, Venkatesha Murthy, P.J., Harish, M.G., Subbakrishna, D.K., and Vedamurthachar, A. 2000. Antidepressant efficacy of Sudarshan Kriya Yoga (SKY) in melancholia: a randomized comparison with electroconvulsive therapy (ECT) and imipramine. *J. Affect Disord.* 57(1-3):255-9.

[116] Jerath R, Edry J.W, Barnes V.A, Jerath V. 2006. Physiology of long *prāna*yamic breathing: neural respiratory elements may provide a mechanism that explains how slow deep breathing shifts the autonomic nervous system. *Med. Hypotheses.* 67:566–571.

[117] Telles S, Nagarathna R, Nagendra HR. 1994 .Breathing through a particular nostril can alter metabolism and autonomic activities. *Indian J. Physiol Pharmacol.* 38: 133-137.

[118] Shannahoff-Khalsa DS. 2007. Selective Unilateral Autonomic Activation: Implications for Psychiatry *CNS Spectr.* 12(8):625-634.

[119] Shannahoff-Khalsa DS, Kennedy B. 1993. The effects of unilateral forced nostril breathing on heart. *Int. J. Neurosci.* 73: 47-60.

[120] Jain, R., Nagarathna, R., Nagendra, H.R., and Telles, S. 1999. Effect of '*prānic*' healing in chronic musculoskeletal pain – a single blind control study. *International Journal of Alternative and Complementary Medicine.* 17(8), 14-17.

[121] Nagendra H R. 2001. *Prānic Energisation Technique.* Swami Vivekānanda Yoga Prakashan. Bangalore.

[122] Nagendra H R, Nagarathna R. 2008. *New Perspectives in Stress Management.* Swami Vivekānanda Yoga Prakashan. Bangalore.

[123] *Mandukya Upanisad.* Commentary by swami chinmayānanda. Central ChinŚ Mission Trust, Sandeepany Sadhanalaya, Powai Park Drive, Mumbai (Fourth Edition).

[124] Pailoor Subramanya and Shirley Telles. 2009. A review of the scientific studies on cyclic meditation. *Int. J. Yoga*. 2(2): 46–48.

[125] Nagendra H R. 2005. *Mind Sound Resonance Technique*. Swami Vivekānanda Yoga Prakashan. Bangalore.

[126] Madanmohan. Effect of yogic practices on different systems of human body. icyer.com/documents/yogresearchMMT.pdf

[127] Maini S. 2000. The effect of Sahaja Yoga on Lipid Peroxidation. *MD Thesis*. Delhi University.

[128] Tooley GA, Armstrong SM, Norman TR, Sali A. 2000. Acute increases in night-time plasma melatonin levels following a period of meditation. *Biol Psychol*. 53: 69-78.

[129] Oswal P, Nagarathna R, Ebnezar J, Nagendra HR. 2011. The effect of add-on yogic *prāna* energization technique (YPET) on healing of fresh fractures: a randomized control study. *J. Altern .Complement Med.* 17(3):253-8.

[130] Sarang PS, Telles S. 2006. Oxygen consumption and respiration during and after two yoga relaxation techniques. *Appl. Psychophysiol Biofeedback*. 31(2):143-53.

[131] Sarang P, Telles S. 2006. Effects of two yoga based relaxation techniques on heart rate variability. *Int. J. Stress Manag*. 13: 460-75.

[132] Vempati RP, Telles S. 2000. Baseline occupational stress levels and physiological responses to a two day stress management program. *J. Indian Psychol.* 18:33–7.

[133] Patra S, Telles S. 2009. Positive impact of cyclic meditation on sleep. *Med SciMonit.* 15: CR375-81.

[134] Padmini T. 2009. Effect of yoga therapy on chronic low back pain - a randomized control study. *Ph.D Thesis*. SVYASA University, Bangalore.

[135] Malathi A, Damodaran A. 1999. Stress due to exams in medical students- a role of Yoga. *Indian J. Physiol Pharmacol* 43(2): 218-224.

[136] Satyapriya M, Nagendra HR, Nagarathna R, Padmalatha V. 2009. Effect of integrated yoga on stress and heart rate variability in pregnant women. *Int. J. Gynaecol Obstet.* 104:218-22.

[137] Chaya MS, Nagarathna R, Manjunath NK, Rao R et al. 2006. *The effects of laughter yoga on stress in the work place*. Laughter Yoga International commissioned scientific research project.

[138] Mora-Ripoll R. 2011. Potential health benefits of simulated laughter: A narrative review of the literature and recommendations for future research. *Complement Ther. Med.* 19(3):170-7.

[139] Berk LS, Tan SA, Fry WF, Napier BJ, Lee JW, Hubbard RW et al. 1989. Neuroendocrine and stress hormone changes during mirthful laughter. *Am. J. Med. Sci.* 298(6):390-6.

[140] Hayashi T, Tsujii S, Iburi T, Tamanaha T, Yamagami K, Ishibashi R. 2007. Laughter up-regulates the genes related to NK cell activity in diabetes. *Biomed. Res.* 28(6):281-5.

[141] Toda M, Kusakabe S, Nagasawa S, Kitamura K, Morimoto K. 2007. Effect of laughter on salivary endocrinological stress marker chromogranin A. *Biomed Res.* 2007. 28(2):115-8.

In: Stem Cells in Disease
Editor: Prasad S. Koka
ISBN: 978-1-62257-169-7
© 2012 Nova Science Publishers, Inc.

Chapter XII

Immunological Modulation of Neural Stem Cells in the Adult Brain

***Oscar Gonzalez-Perez*[1,2*], *Jose Manuel Garcia-Verdugo*[3] *and Alfredo Quiñones-Hinojosa*[4]**

[1]Laboratorio de Neurociencias,
Facultad de Psicologia Universidad de Colima, Colima, Mexico
[2] Department of Neuroscience, Centro Universitario de Ciencias de la Salud, Universidad de Guadalajara. Guadalajara, Jal. Mexico
[3]Laboratorio de Morfología Celular. Unidad Mixta CIPF-UVEG, Valencia, CIBERNED, Spain
[4] Department of Neurosurgery, Brain Tumors Surgery Program, the Johns Hopkins. University School of Medicine, Baltimore, MD, US

Abstract

Adult neurogenesis occurs only in discrete regions of adult central nervous system: the subventricular zone and the subgranular zone. These areas are populated by adult neural stem cells (aNSC) that are regulated by a number of molecules and signaling pathways, which control their cell fate choices, survival and proliferation rates. For a long time, it was believed that the immune system did not exert any control on neural proliferative niches. However, it has been observed that many pathological and inflammatory conditions significantly affect NSC niches. Even more, increasing evidence indicates that chemokines and cytokines play an important role in regulating proliferation, cell fate choices, migration and survival of NSCs under physiological conditions. Hence, the immune system is emerging is an important regulator of neurogenic niches in the adult brain, which may have clinical relevance in several brain diseases.

[*] Corresponding author: Facultad de Psicologia Universidad de Colima Av. Universidad 333 Colima, COL 28040 Mexico Tel/Fax:. +52 (312) 316-1091 E-mail: osglez@gmail.com.

Introduction

For most of last century, it was believed that cell proliferation in the brain was limited to glial cells, the supportive cells found around neurons. In the 1960s, newborn neurons were first described [1]. In the 1980's and 1990's, neurogenesis was demonstrated in the telencephalon of lizards, adult birds and in several mammalian species: mouse, rat, rabbit, cow, primate and humans [2-9]. In mammals, new neurons are continuously added to restricted brain regions, the olfactory bulb and the hippocampus. In these regions, new neurons are functional and appear to modulate olfaction and memory formation, respectively. New neurons in the adult nervous system derive from adult neural stem cells (aNSC), a group of cells that can self-renew and differentiate into all types of neural cells, including neurons, astrocytes and oligodendrocytes.

The brain is an immune-privileged organ because the selective permeability of the blood-brain barrier only allows certain substances and cells to enter and leave. Under normal physiological conditions, only macrophages, T cells and dendritic cells can access the brain [10-12]. After damage, an inflammatory process is initiated by the activation of astrocytes and microglia. This event is followed by parenchymal infiltration of macrophages and lymphocytes. The recruited immune cells release many anti- and pro-inflammatory mediators, chemokines, neurotransmitters and reactive oxygen species. This process generates the production and releasing of multiple inflammatory factors, which produces a positive feedback loop that results in both detrimental and positive consequences to neurogenesis [11, 13, 14]. Recently, it has been demonstrated that immune system regulates aNSC population through production of chemokines and cytokines [12, 13, 15]. aNSC have been proposed as an alternative for brain repair therapies but the molecular mechanisms that control survival, proliferation and cell fate are to be elucidated. In this chapter, we summarize emergent evidence indicating that immune mediators control aNSC population under physiological and pathological conditions.

1. The Brain Niches of Adult Neural Stem Cells

Active neurogenesis occurs only in discrete regions of the adult central nervous system. There are two regions were adult neurogenesis has been indisputably described: the subventricular zone (**SVZ**) and the subgranular zone within the hippocampus (**SGZ**). Some reports claim that neurogenesis may also occur in other brain areas, including amygdala [16], neocortex [17, 18], substantia nigra [19, 20], and striatum [21, 22]. However, neurogenesis in these areas appears to occur either at substantially lower levels or under non-physiological conditions.

1.1. The Subventricular Zone (SVZ)

The most important germinal region is the SVZ (Figure 1), which contains a subpopulation of astrocytes that function *in vivo* as aNSCs. SVZ astrocyte NSCs are also known as Type-B cells.

Currently Type-B cells are divided into two subtypes: B1 and B2. Type-B1 cells make contact with the ventricular cavity while B2 cells do not. Type-B1 cells show one short primary cilium towards the ventricular cavity (Figure 1), which is important to control cell proliferation and posse a long expansion that contact blood vessels [23].

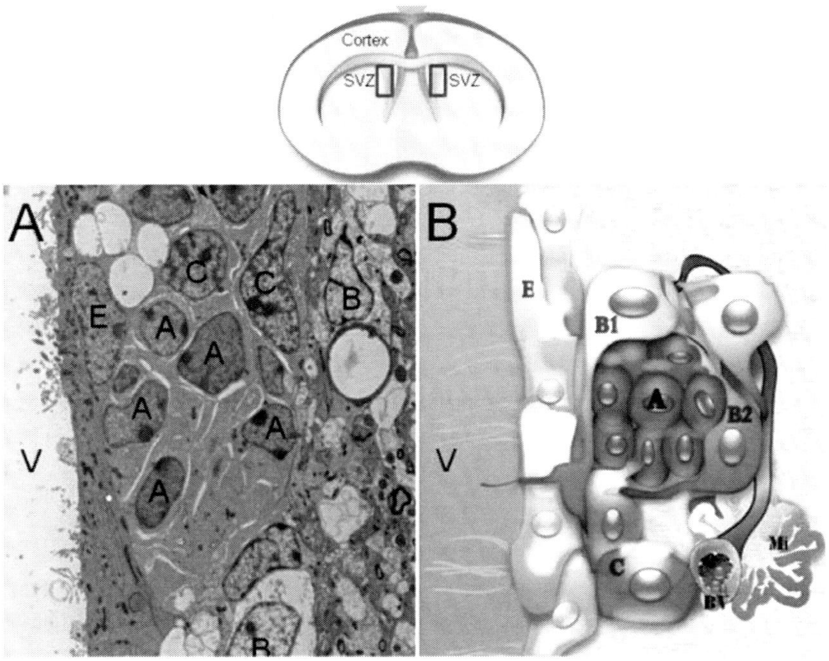

Figure 1. The adult subventricular zone in rodent. This neurogenic niche has been well-characterized by electron microscopy (A). Type-A cells (migrating neuroblasts) have an elongated cell body with one or two processes, profuse lax chromatin with small nucleoli (2 to 4), a scarce dark cytoplasm, abundant free ribosomes, microtubules oriented along the long axis of the cells, and nuclei occasionally invaginated. Their cytoplasmic membrane showed cell junctions intercalated with large intercellular spaces. Type-B cells have a light cytoplasm with a few ribosomes, extensive intermediate filaments and nuclei are typically invaginated. Their cell profiles are irregular that filled intercellular spaces between neighboring cells. Type-C cells are large and semi-spherical; their nuclei contain deep invaginations, lax chromatin occasionally clumped and large reticulated nucleoli. Type-C-cell cytoplasm is more electron-lucent than Type-A cells, but more electron-dense than Type-B cells, because it contains a few ribosomes and no intermediate filaments. Schematic drawing of the adult SVZ shows the cell organization of this region (B). Ependymal cells (Type-E cells) formed an epithelial monolayer that separates the SVZ from the lateral ventricles. These cells have spherical nuclei with lax chromatin, lateral cytoplasmic processes heavily interdigitated with apical junction complexes. The cell membrane contacting the ventricle contains microvilli and cilia, and their cytoplasm is electron-lucent with many mitochondria and basal bodies in the apical pole. A: Type- A cell; B: Type-B cell; C: Type-C cell cell; E: Ependymal cell; BV: Blood vessel; Mi: Microglia cell; V: Ventricle.

Type-B1 cells give rise to intermediate neural progenitors defined actively proliferating transit amplifying progenitors or Type-C cells. Type-C cells symmetrically divide to produce migrating neuroblasts (Type-A cells) that migrate ventrally through the RMS into the olfactory bulb to become interneurons [24-26], which appear to regulate the olfaction process [27]. Recently, it has been described that Type-B cells *in vivo* generate oligodendrocytes that migrate into the corpus callosum and fimbria fornix [28, 29]. Blood vessels play an important role in the SVZ and there is evidence that the activation of neurogenic niches is regulated by this vascular network [30].

1.2. The Subgranular Zone (SGZ)

The SGZ of the dentate gyrus in the hippocampus is a proliferative region that contains neuronal progenitors that give rise to granular neurons (Figure 2). The primary progenitors in this region are Type-B astrocytes, which have shown *in vitro,* via neurosphere and adherent monolayer cultures, multipotential properties.

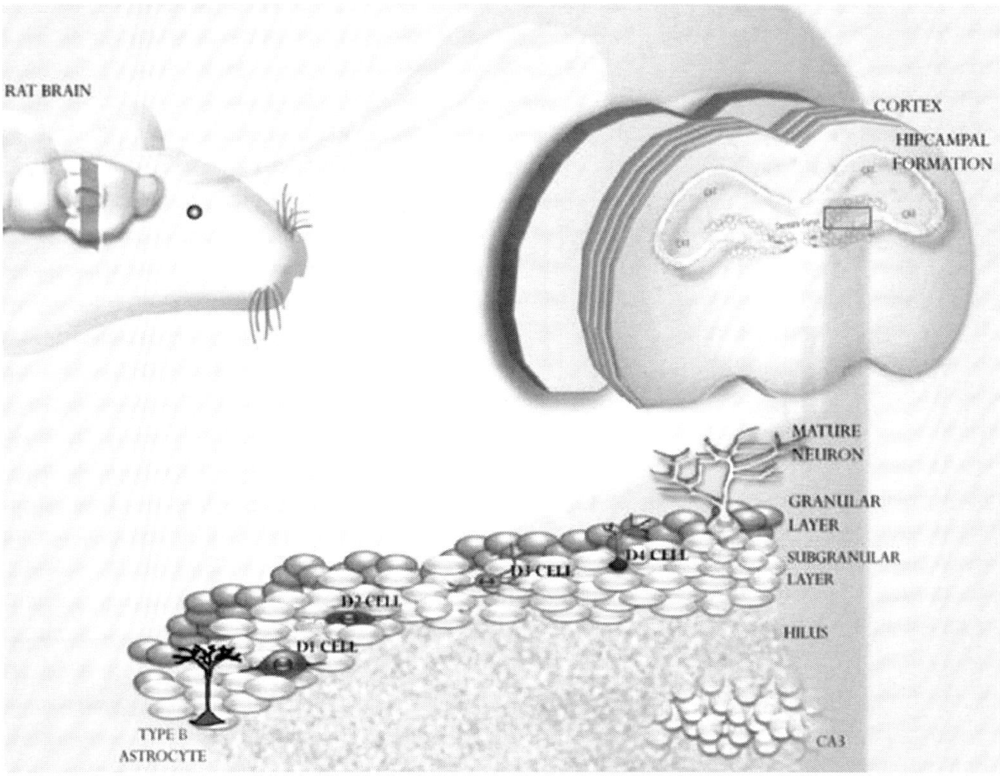

Figure 2. Schematic drawing of adult SGZ in rodent. Dentate gyrus of adult hippocampus continuously produces new neurons throughout life. Type-B cells are the primary progenitors that give rise to intermediate progenitors named Type-D cells, which give rise to granulate neurons.

In vivo, SGZ Type-B cells appear to have limited capacity for differentiation. Therefore, some authors consider SGZ precursors as neuronal progenitors instead of aNSCs. SGZ Type-B cells divide asymmetrically to give rise to type-D cells that differentiate locally into mature granular neurons. The function of these newly generated neurons appears to play a role in memory process, learning and depression [31].

1.3. Microglia in Neurogenic Niches

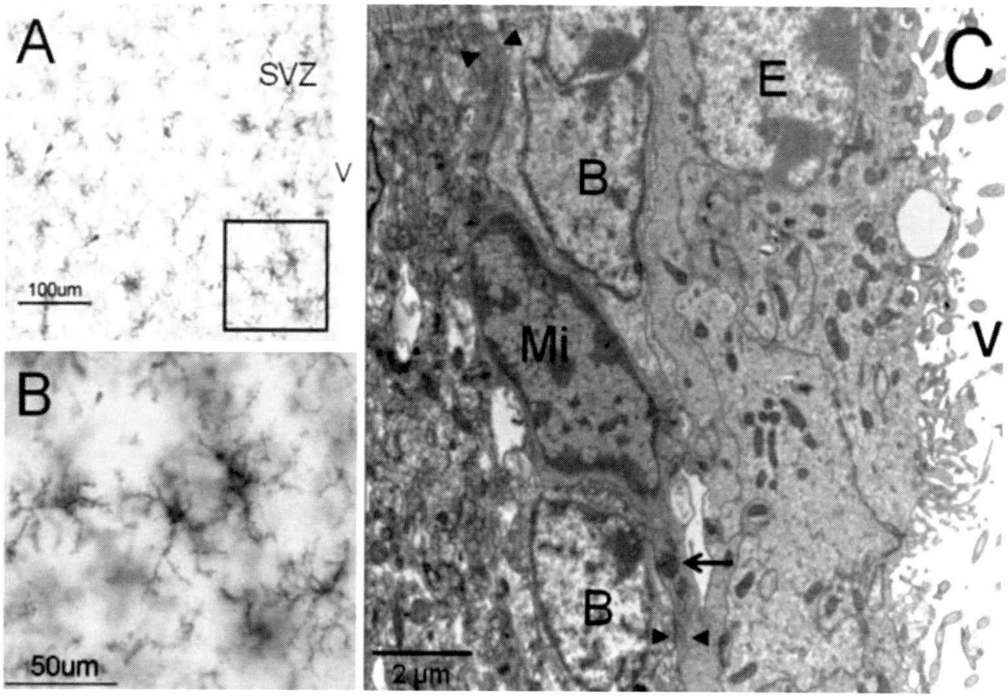

Figure 3. Microglia cells in the rodent SVZ. Iba-1 immunocytochemistry to detect microglia cells by light microscopy (A-B). In their "resting" stage microglia displays multiple thin branches, which confer a 'bushy' morphology to these cells. By electron microscopy (C), microglia (Mi) shows a typical dark nucleus and electrodense corpus in their cytoplasm (arrow). Frequently, microglial cytoplasmic expansions (arrow heads) are in close contact with Type-B cells. B: Type-B cell; E: Ependymal cell; V: Ventricle.

Microglia is the main immune effector cell in the nervous system, which have a hematopoietic origin [32] and populate the CNS throughout adulthood [33, 34]. Under physiological conditions microglia is a quiescent cell population, which constantly excavates the CNS for damaged neurons, plaques, and infectious agents [34, 35]. In both, the adult SVZ and SGZ, microglia is abundant and, remarkably, is in close contact to aNSC (Type-B cells), which suggest that local interactions are possible between immune cells and multipotential progenitors (figure 3). Attracted by endogenous and exogenous chemotactic factors, microglial cells constitute the "first line of defense" of the CNS against injury or infections [34]. During inflammation or brain injury, microglia is capable of secreting neurotrophic or neuron survival factors upon activation [35], some of these effects are summarized in the figure 4. Recent evidence indicate that microglia instructs aNSC by secreting factors essential for neurogenesis, but not NSC maintenance, self-renewal, or propagation [36]. These effects seem to be mediated a number of factors, such as: interleukin-1 (IL-1) and tumor necrosis factor alpha (TNF-α) that serve as autocrine activators [11, 37, 38]; interferon gamma (IFN-γ), which thrive the immune response toward a cytotoxic response mediated by Th1 cells [39-42]; insulin-like growth factor-1 (IGF-1) that promotes cell proliferation [43]; interleukin-4 (IL-4) that increases phagocytotic properties of microglia [44, 45]; leukemia inhibitory factor (LIF) that is usually related to growth promotion and cell differentiation [15, 46-48]. It has been suggested that microglia modulation of aNSC is mediated by activation of mitogen activated protein kinase and phosphatidylinositol-3-kinase/Akt signaling pathways [49]. However, other inflammatory cells produce chemokines and cytokines, which can also influence implicated proliferation, differentiation, survival, and migration of aNSC [50-55]. Their effects will be described in detail in the next section.

2. Immunological Control of Adult Neural Stem Cells

2.1. Cytokines and Chemokines

There are two types of immunological mediators: cytokines and chemokines. Cytokines are polypeptide regulators that have important roles in cellular communication [13]. Most, if not all, cells are regulated by cytokines. In the central nervous system, neuropoietic cytokines are a group of glycoproteins that control neuronal, glial and immune responses to injury or disease. They regulate neuronal growth, regeneration, survival, and differentiation by binding to high affinity receptors. The neuropoietic cytokine family includes interleukin-6 (IL-6), interleukin-18 (IL-18), IFN-γ, LIF, TNF-α, ciliary neurotrophic factor (CNTF) and others [13, 15]. Chemokines are small cytokines or proteins (8–14 kDa) that, according to the sequence motif of conserved N-terminal cysteine residues, are categorized into four groups: α-chemokines (CXC chemokines), which promote the migration of neutrophils and lymphocytes; β-chemokines (CC chemokines), which induce the migration of monocytes, NK cells and dendritic cells; γ-chemokines (C chemokines) that attract T cell precursors to the thymus; and δ-chemokines (CX3C chemokines), which serve as a chemoattractants and as an adhesion molecules [12]. Neurons express several receptors for immunological mediators, such as: CCR3, CXCR4, CXCR2, and CX3CR1, while astrocytes mainly express CXCR4, which make them responsive to chemokine gradients in the brain. CXCR4 is also highly expressed on the CD133+/nestin+ human neural precursors [56, 57]. Interestingly, CXCR4 expression is upregulated when embryonic precursors differentiate into neuronal precursors, whereas CXCL12 appears to drive astroglial differentiation [58]. Cytokines and chemokines alter self-renewal, progenitor cell division and differentiation of neural progenitors via JAK/STAT pathway and the Janus kinase-signal transducer [13, 15].

2.2. Effects of Cytokines and Chemokines on aNSC

After a brain injury, a number of inflammatory and immunological responses occur that modulate aNSC behavior (Table 1). Activated microglia produces IGF-1, which triggers the extracellular signal-regulated kinase (ERK) / mitogen-activated protein kinase (MAPK) pathway, increasing neurogenesis in the SGZ [43]. Interestingly, 'resting' microglia can also promote aNSC proliferation via the same signaling pathways [49]. Microglia-derived soluble factors such as IL-6 and LIF-1 induces astrocytic differentiation [59]. However, activated microglia appears to have a dual effect on aNSCs, for instance microglia activated by IL-4 drives the generation of oligodendrocytes (the axon supportive and myelin producer cells), whereas the IFN-γ-activated microglia induces a bias towards neurogenesis [44]. Acute LIF or CNTF exposure differentially affects development, growth, amplification and self-renewal of aNSCs [15, 46-48]. Chronic exposure to LIF or CNTF alters the formation of aNSC progenies and promotes aNSC self-renewal [15]. Phosphorylation of STAT3 induced by LIF is essential for maintaining NSC phenotype [60]. Conversely, leptin, which activates STAT3, inhibits differentiation of multipotent cells [15, 61]. aNSCs do not express a functional receptor for IL-6, thus they do not properly respond to IL-6. However, the stimulation of aNSCs with the active fusion protein of IL-6 and sIL-6R, designated as hyper-IL-6, induces aNSCs to differentiate into glutamate-responsive neurons and oligodendrocytes [62].

IFN- γ is pro-neurogenic, promotes neural differentiation and neurite outgrowth of murine aNSCs [39, 40]. However, IFN-γ has shown a dual effect on neurogenesis, because not only stimulate neuronal differentiation [40, 41] and NPC migration, but also inhibits aNSCs proliferation and reduces aNSCs survival [42]. However, the mechanism of this paradoxical effect is unknown. The IFN-γ-induced neuronal differentiation is probably mediated by c-Jun N-terminal kinase (JNK) pathway [63]. JNK pathway has been involved in neural differentiation of carcinoma cells, embryonic stem cells and PC12 cells [64-67]. Decreased neurogenesis has been observed by effect of TNF-α [11].

Table 1. Effects of chemokines and cytokines on adult NSCs

Cytokine / Chemokine	Effect on aNSCs	Reference
IFN- γ	Promotion of differentiation and neurite outgrowth. Reduction of proliferation and survival of multipotent progenitors.	[39, 40, 42]
IGF-1	Increasing of neurogenesis in SGZ	[43]
IL-4	Oligodendrogenesis	[44]
LIF	Neurogenesis promotions and NSC self-renewal (acute exposure)	[15, 46, 47]
CNTF	Neurogenesis promotions and NSC self-renewal (acute exposure)	[15, 79]
Leptin	Inhibition of differentiation of multipotent cells and glial progenitors	[15, 61]
TNF- α	Decreasing of neurogenesis	[11]
H-IL-6	Differentiation into glutamate-responsive neurons and oligodendrocytes	[62]
MCP-1	Migration of NSCs	[37, 38]
SDF-1	Promotion of migration, survival and proliferation of NSCs	[37, 70, 71, 73]
CCL2	Neuronal differentiation of SVZ progenitors	[74]

Other studies indicates that TNF-α is a positive regulator of neurogenesis and promotes neurosphere grown by reducing aNSC apoptosis [68]. However, TNF-α increases the expression of MCP-1, a chemokine that induces migration of aNSCs thorough the MCP-1 receptor CCR2 [37, 38]. MCP-1 has protective effects on neurons against excitotoxicity mediated by NMDA receptors [69]. SDF-1 chemokyne promotes migration of neural progenitors and increases survival of aNSCs [37, 70, 71], but contrasting reports demonstrated that SDF-1 has a dual effect on neural progenitors producing quiescence [72] or inducing cell proliferation [73]. Other chemokine as CCL2 has no effects on proliferation and cell survival, but promotes neuronal differentiation of SVZ progenitors [74]. Hematopoietic growth factors have also been involved in the regulation of adult NSCs (Figure 4).

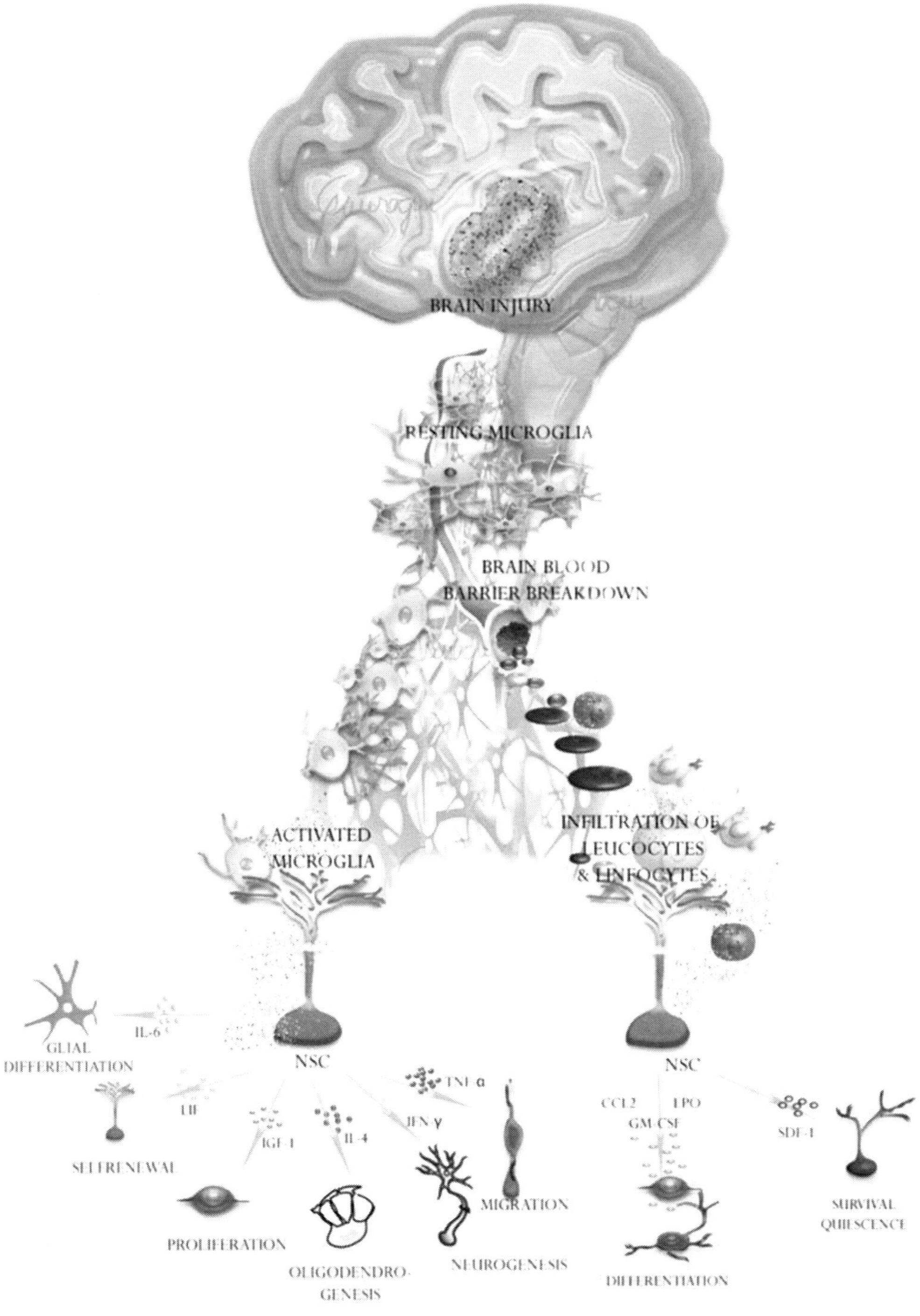

Figure 4. Effects of immune cells on adult neural stem cells. Cell effectors such as microglia, lymphocytes and leucocytes can induce a wide variety of effects on aNSC upon brain injury.

Granulocyte-macrophage colony stimulating factor (GM-CSF) stimulates neuronal differentiation of aNSCs [75]. Granulocyte-colony stimulating factor (G-CSF) drives neuronal differentiation of aNSCs *in vitro* [76] and enhances neurogenesis and functional recovery. Erythropoietin (EPO) drives neuronal differentiation of aNSCs *in vitro* [77, 78]. Interestingly, EPO-receptor deficient mice display reduced neurogenesis [77, 78]. Yet, as findings in this field are relatively recent, there exist a number of cytokines and chemokines to be investigated as possible regulators of neurogenesis and neuroprotection.

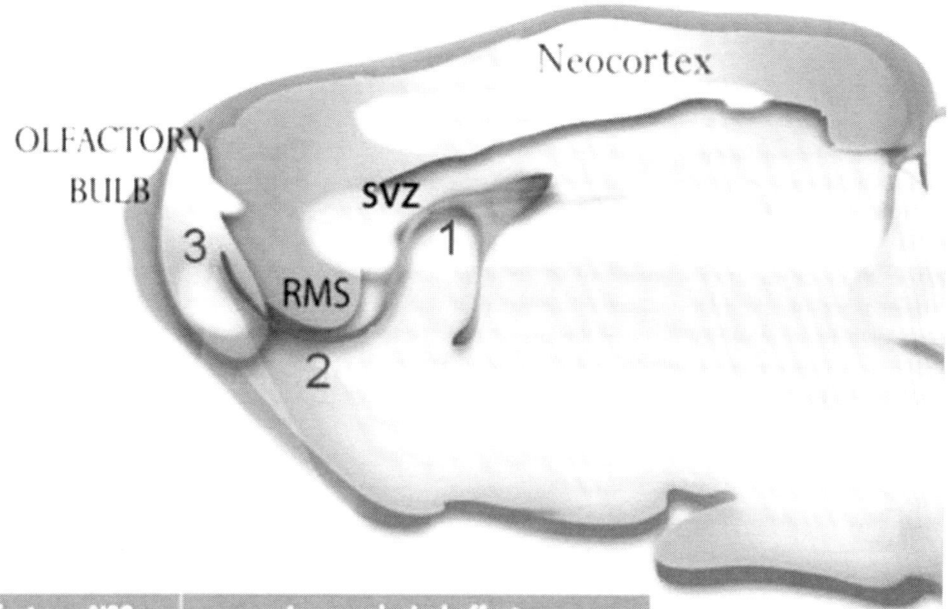

Effect on aNSC	Immunological affector
Proliferation (1)	TNF-α, LIF, CNTF, SDF-1, IGF-1 and IFN-γ
Survival and Migration (1,2)	TNF-α a, MCP-1, SDF-1, and IFN-γ
Differentiation (3)	IL-6, LIF-1, IL-4, IFN-γ, CCL2, EPO, G-CSF and GM-CSF

\

Figure 5. Immunological mediators have multiple effects on aNSC. There are some crucial steps in the neurogenic processs: Proliferation, survival, migration, differentiation. Immune effectors that affect proliferation mainly target the SVZ (1). Effectors that modulate survival and migration aim both SVZ and RMS (2), whereas immunological effects on differentiation are reflected in the olfactory bulb (3).

Conclusion

The immunological mediators affect proliferation, survival, migration and differentiation of aNSC (Figure 5). TNF-α, LIF, CNTF, SDF-1 and IGF-1 are considered important regulators of aNSC proliferation. Cell differentiation is driven mainly by IL-6, LIF-1, IL-4, IFN-γ, CCL2, EPO, G-CSF and GM-CSF. Migration of neural progenitors is promoted by MCP-1 and SDF-1, whereas cell survival is positively regulated by TNF-α and SDF-1, but negatively regulated by IFN-γ. In summary, further studies are necessary to elucidate some paradoxical effects on aNSC of immunological factors and signaling pathways involved in these processes.

Acknowledgments

OGP was supported by CONACyT's grant (CB-2008-101476). AQH supported by The National Institute of Health and the National Institute of Neurological Disorders and Stroke (NIH/NINDS; grant R01 NS070024). JMGV Instituto de Salud Carlos III (Ciberned, Centro de Investigacion Principe Felipe y Red de Terapia Celular, Ministerio de Ciencia e Innovación (SAF2008-01274), Alicia Koplowitz's Foundation. We also thank Fernando Jáuregui for his assistance in the design and preparation of figures.

References

[1] Altman, J. Postnatal neurogenesis and the problem of neural plasticity., in *Developmental neurobiology.*, W.A. Himwich, Editor. 1970, C.C.Thomas: Springfield. 197-237.

[2] Goldman, SA; Nottebohm, F. Neuronal production, migration, and differentiation in a vocal control nucleus of the adult female canary brain. *Proc.Natl.Acad.Sci. USA*, 1983, 80, 2390-2394.

[3] Alvarez-Buylla, A; Nottebohm, F. Seasonal and species differences in the production of long projection neurons in adult birds. *Neuroscience*, 1989, 15, 962.

[4] Galileo, DS; et al., Neurons and glia arise from a common progenitor in chicken optic tectum: Demonstration with two retroviruses and cell type-specific antibodies. *Proc.Natl.Acad.Sci. USA*, 1990, 87, 458-462.

[5] Alvarez-Buylla, A; Garcia-Verdugo, JM; Tramontin, AD. A unified hypothesis on the lineage of neural stem cells. *Nat. Rev. Neurosci*, 2001, 2, 2(4. 4), 287-93.

[6] Temple, S. The development of neural stem cells. *Nature*, 2001, 414(6859), 112-7.

[7] Gage, FH. Neurogenesis in the adult brain. *J. Neurosci.*, 2002, 22(3), 612-3.

[8] Sanai, N; et al., Unique astrocyte ribbon in adult human brain contains neural stem cells but lacks chain migration. *Nature,* 2004, 427(6976), 740-4.

[9] Garcia-Verdugo, JM; et al., The proliferative ventricular zone in adult vertebrates: a comparative study using reptiles, birds, and mammals. *Brain Res. Bull.*, 2002, 57(6), 765-75.

[10] Hickey, WF. Leukocyte traffic in the central nervous system: the participants and their roles. *Semin. Immunol.*, 1999, 11(2), 125-37.

[11] Whitney, NP; et al., Inflammation mediates varying effects in neurogenesis: relevance to the pathogenesis of brain injury and neurodegenerative disorders. *J Neurochem,*, 2009, 108(6), 1343-59.

[12] Bonecchi, R; et al., Chemokines and chemokine receptors: an overview. *Front Biosci,* 2009, 14, 540-51.

[13] Miller, RJ; et al., *Chemokine action in the nervous system. J. Neurosci.*, 2008, 28(46), 11792-5.

[14] Das, S; Basu, A. Inflammation: a new candidate in modulating adult neurogenesis. *J. Neurosci. Res.*, 2008, 86(6), 1199-208.

[15] Bauer, S. Cytokine control of adult neural stem cells. *Ann N Y Acad. Sci.,* 2009, 1153, 48-56.

[16] Bernier, PJ; et al., Newly generated neurons in the amygdala and adjoining cortex of adult primates. *Proc. Natl. Acad. Sci, USA*, 2002, 99(17), 11464-9.
[17] Gould, E; et al., Neurogenesis in the neocortex of adult primates. *Science*, 1999, 286(5439), 548-52.
[18] Takemura, NU. Evidence for neurogenesis within the white matter beneath the temporal neocortex of the adult rat brain. *Neuroscience*, 2005, 134(1), 121-32.
[19] Zhao, M; et al., Evidence for neurogenesis in the adult mammalian substantia nigra. *Proc. Natl. Acad. Sci., USA*, 2003, 100(13), 7925-30.
[20] Yoshimi, K; et al., Possibility for neurogenesis in substantia nigra of parkinsonian brain. *Ann. Neurol,* 2005, 58(1), 31-40.
[21] Van Kampen, JM; Robertson, HA. A possible role for dopamine D3 receptor stimulation in the induction of neurogenesis in the adult rat substantia nigra. *Neuroscience,* 2005, 136(2), 381-6.
[22] Bedard, A; Gravel, C; Parent, A. Chemical characterization of newly generated neurons in the striatum of adult primates. *Exp. Brain Res*, 2006, 170(4), 501-12.
[23] Han, YG; et al., Hedgehog signaling and primary cilia are required for the formation of adult neural stem cells. *Nat. Neurosci.,* 2008, 11(3), 277-84.
[24] Lois, C; Alvarez-Buylla, A. Proliferating subventricular zone cells in the adult mammalian forebrain can differentiate into neurons and glia. *Proc.Natl.Acad.Sci.USA,* 1993, 90, 2074-2077.
[25] Lois, C; Alvarez-Buylla, A. Long-distance neuronal migration in the adult mammalian brain. *Science*, 1994, 264, 1145-1148.
[26] Alvarez-Buylla, A; Garcia-Verdugo, JM. Neurogenesis in adult subventricular zone. *J. Neurosci*, 2002, 22(3), 629-34.
[27] So, K; et al., The olfactory conditioning in the early postnatal period stimulated neural stem/progenitor cells in the subventricular zone and increased neurogenesis in the olfactory bulb of rats. *Neuroscience,* 2008, 151(1), 120-8.
[28] Menn, B; et al., Origin of oligodendrocytes in the subventricular zone of the adult brain. *J Neurosci*, 2006, 26(30), 7907-18.
[29] Gonzalez-Perez, O; et al., Epidermal Growth Factor Induces the Progeny of Subventricular Zone Type B Cells to Migrate and Differentiate into Oligodendrocytes. *Stem Cells,* 2009, 27(8), 2032-2043.
[30] Shen, Q; et al., Adult SVZ stem cells lie in a vascular niche: a quantitative analysis of niche cell-cell interactions. *Cell Stem Cell*, 2008, 3(3), 289-300.
[31] Aimone, JB; Wiles, J; Gage, FH. Potential role for adult neurogenesis in the encoding of time in new memories. *Nat Neurosci,* 2006, 9(6), 723-7.
[32] Eglitis, MA; Mezey, E. Hematopoietic cells differentiate into both microglia and macroglia in the brains of adult mice. *Proc. Natl. Acad. Sci. USA*, 1997, 94(8), 4080-5.
[33] Cuadros, MA; Navascues, J. Early origin and colonization of the developing central nervous system by microglial precursors. *Prog. Brain Res.*, 2001, 132, 51-9.
[34] Tambuyzer, BR; Ponsaerts, P; Nouwen, EJ. Microglia: gatekeepers of central nervous system immunology. *J. Leukoc Biol.*, 2009, 85(3), 352-70.
[35] Pivneva, TA. *Microglia in normal condition and pathology.* Fiziol Zh, 2008, 54(5), 81-9.
[36] Walton, NM; et al., Microglia instruct subventricular zone neurogenesis. *Glia,* 2006, 54(8), 815-25.

[37] Widera, D; et al., MCP-1 induces migration of adult neural stem cells. *Eur. J. Cell Biol.,* 2004, 83(8), 381-7.

[38] Schwamborn, J; et al., Microarray analysis of tumor necrosis factor alpha induced gene expression in U373 human glioblastoma cells. *BMC Genomics*, 2003, 4(1), 46.

[39] Johansson, S; Price, J; Modo, M. Effect of inflammatory cytokines on major histocompatibility complex expression and differentiation of human neural stem/progenitor cells. *Stem Cells*, 2008, 26(9), 2444-54.

[40] Wong, G; Goldshmit, Y; Turnley, AM. Interferon-gamma but not TNF alpha promotes neuronal differentiation and neurite outgrowth of murine adult neural stem cells. *Exp. Neurol.,* 2004, 187(1), 171-7.

[41] Song, JH; et al., Interferon gamma induces neurite outgrowth by up-regulation of p35 neuron-specific cyclin-dependent kinase 5 activator via activation of ERK1/2 pathway. *J. Biol. Chem.*, 2005, 280(13), 12896-901.

[42] Ben-Hur, T; et al., Effects of proinflammatory cytokines on the growth, fate, and motility of multipotential neural precursor cells. *Mol. Cell Neurosci.,* 2003, 24(3), 623-31.

[43] Choi, YS; et al., IGF-1 receptor-mediated ERK/MAPK signaling couples status epilepticus to progenitor cell proliferation in the subgranular layer of the dentate gyrus. *Glia*, 2008, 56(7), 791-800.

[44] Butovsky, O; et al., Microglia activated by IL-4 or IFN-gamma differentially induce neurogenesis and oligodendrogenesis from adult stem/progenitor cells. *Mol. Cell Neurosci*, 2006, 31(1), 149-60.

[45] von Zahn, J; et al., Microglial phagocytosis is modulated by pro- and anti-inflammatory cytokines. *Neuroreport,* 1997, 8(18), 3851-6.

[46] Bauer, S; Patterson, PH. Leukemia inhibitory factor promotes neural stem cell self-renewal in the adult brain. *J. Neurosci.,* 2006, 26(46), 12089-99.

[47] Oshima, K; et al., LIF promotes neurogenesis and maintains neural precursors in cell populations derived from spiral ganglion stem cells. *BMC Dev. Biol.,* 2007, 7, 112.

[48] Covey, MV; Levison, SW. Leukemia inhibitory factor participates in the expansion of neural stem/progenitors after perinatal hypoxia/ischemia. *Neuroscience,* 2007, 148(2), 501-9.

[49] Morgan, SC; Taylor, DL; JM. Pocock, Microglia release activators of neuronal proliferation mediated by activation of mitogen-activated protein kinase, phosphatidylinositol-3-kinase/Akt and delta-Notch signalling cascades. *J. Neurochem.,* 2004, 90(1), 89-101.

[50] Faiz, M; et al., Substantial migration of SVZ cells to the cortex results in the generation of new neurons in the excitotoxically damaged immature rat brain. *Mol. Cell Neurosci.,* 2008, 38(2), 170-82.

[51] Liu, XS; et al., Functional response to SDF1 alpha through over-expression of CXCR4 on adult subventricular zone progenitor cells. *Brain Res*, 2008, 1226, 18-26.

[52] Robin, AM; et al., Stromal cell-derived factor 1alpha mediates neural progenitor cell motility after focal cerebral ischemia. *J. Cereb. Blood Flow Metab*, 2006, 26(1), 125-34.

[53] Tiveron, MC; et al., Molecular interaction between projection neuron precursors and invading interneurons via stromal-derived factor 1 (CXCL12)/CXCR4 signaling in the cortical subventricular zone/intermediate zone. *J. Neurosci*, 2006, 26(51), 13273-8.

[54] Yan, YP; et al., Monocyte chemoattractant protein-1 plays a critical role in neuroblast migration after focal cerebral ischemia. *J. Cereb Blood Flow Metab.*, 2007, 27(6), 1213-24.
[55] Bhattacharyya, BJ; et al., The chemokine stromal cell-derived factor-1 regulates GABAergic inputs to neural progenitors in the postnatal dentate gyrus. *J. Neurosci.*, 2008, 28(26), 6720-30.
[56] Ni, HT; et al., High-level expression of functional chemokine receptor CXCR4 on human neural precursor cells. *Brain Res. Dev. Brain Res.*, 2004, 152(2), 159-69.
[57] Tran, PB; et al., Chemokine receptors are expressed widely by embryonic and adult neural progenitor cells. *J. Neurosci. Res.*, 2004, 76(1), 20-34.
[58] Peng, H; et al., Differential expression of CXCL12 and CXCR4 during human fetal neural progenitor cell differentiation. *J. Neuroimmune Pharmacol.*, 2007, 2(3), 251-8.
[59] Nakanishi, M; et al., Microglia-derived interleukin-6 and leukaemia inhibitory factor promote astrocytic differentiation of neural stem/progenitor cells. *Eur. J. Neurosci*, 2007, 25(3), 649-58.
[60] Burdon, T; Smith, A; Savatier, P. Signalling, cell cycle and pluripotency in embryonic stem cells. *Trends Cell Biol*, 2002, 12(9), 432-8.
[61] Udagawa, J; Nimura, M; Otani, H. Leptin affects oligodendroglial development in the mouse embryonic cerebral cortex. *Neuro Endocrinol. Lett*, 2006, 27(1-2), 177-82.
[62] Islam, O; et al., Interleukin-6 and neural stem cells: more than gliogenesis. *Mol. Biol Cell*, 2009, 20(1), 188-99.
[63] Kim, SJ; et al., Interferon-gamma promotes differentiation of neural progenitor cells via the JNK pathway. *Neurochem Res.*, 2007, 32(8), 1399-406.
[64] Zentrich, E; et al., Collaboration of JNKs and ERKs in nerve growth factor regulation of the neurofilament light chain promoter in PC12 cells. *J. Biol. Chem.*, 2002, 277(6), 4110-8.
[65] Akiyama, S; et al., Activation mechanism of c-Jun amino-terminal kinase in the course of neural differentiation of P19 embryonic carcinoma cells. *J. Biol Chem.*, 2004. 279(35), 36616-20.
[66] Wang, H; et al., Activation of c-Jun amino-terminal kinase is required for retinoic acid-induced neural differentiation of P19 embryonal carcinoma cells. *FEBS Lett*, 2001. 503(1), 91-6.
[67] Amura, CR; et al., Inhibited neurogenesis in JNK1-deficient embryonic stem cells. *Mol. Cell Bio*l, 2005, 25(24), 10791-802.
[68] Widera, D; et al., Tumor necrosis factor alpha triggers proliferation of adult neural stem cells via IKK/NF-kappaB signaling. *BMC Neurosci*, 2006, 7, 64.
[69] Eugenin, EA; et al., MCP-1 (CCL2) protects human neurons and astrocytes from NMDA or HIV-tat-induced apoptosis. *J. Neurochem.*, 2003, 85(5), 1299-311.
[70] Peng, H; et al., Stromal cell-derived factor 1-mediated CXCR4 signaling in rat and human cortical neural progenitor cells. *J. Neurosci Res.*, 2004, 76(1), 35-50.
[71] Molyneaux, KA; et al., The chemokine SDF1/CXCL12 and its receptor CXCR4 regulate mouse germ cell migration and survival. *Development*, 2003, 130(18), 4279-86.
[72] Krathwohl, MD; Kaiser, JL. HIV-1 promotes quiescence in human neural progenitor cells. *J. Infect Dis.*, 2004, 190(2), 216-26.

[73] Gong, X; et al., Stromal cell derived factor-1 acutely promotes neural progenitor cell proliferation in vitro by a mechanism involving the ERK1/2 and PI-3K signal pathways. *Cell Biol. Int,* 2006, 30(5), 466-71.

[74] Liu, XS; et al., Chemokine ligand 2 (CCL2) induces migration and differentiation of subventricular zone cells after stroke. *J. Neurosci Res.,* 2007, 85(10), 2120-5.

[75] Kruger, C; et al., The hematopoietic factor GM-CSF (granulocyte-macrophage colony-stimulating factor) promotes neuronal differentiation of adult neural stem cells in vitro. *BMC Neurosci*, 2007, 8, 88.

[76] Schneider, A; et al., The hematopoietic factor G-CSF is a neuronal ligand that counteracts programmed cell death and drives neurogenesis. *J. Clin. Invest*, 2005, 115(8), 2083-98.

[77] Chen, ZY; et al., Endogenous erythropoietin signaling is required for normal neural progenitor cell proliferation. *J. Biol. Chem.*, 2007, 282(35), 25875-83.

[78] Shingo, T; et al., Erythropoietin regulates the in vitro and in vivo production of neuronal progenitors by mammalian forebrain neural stem cells. *J. Neurosci.*, 2001, 21(24), 9733-43.

[79] Shimazaki, T; Shingo, T; Weiss, S. The ciliary neurotrophic factor/leukemia inhibitory factor/gp130 receptor complex operates in the maintenance of mammalian forebrain neural stem cells. *J. Neurosci.,* 2001, 21(19), 7642-53.

In: Stem Cells in Disease
Editor: Prasad S. Koka

ISBN: 978-1-62257-169-7
© 2012 Nova Science Publishers, Inc.

Chapter XIII

Establishment of a Brain Tumor Tissue Repository in India: Maintaining Quality Standards

Aparna Khanna[1], Samba Siva Reddy[1], Majahar Jan[1], Swapnil Totey[1], T. Vasudev Rao[2], Shailesh A.V. Rao[2], Arun L. Naik[2], Satish Totey[1] and Neelam K. Venkataramana[1*]

[1]ANSA Research Foundation (ARF), Indiranagar, Bangalore, Karnataka, India
[2]BGS Global Hospitals, Bangalore, Karnataka, India

Abstract

Tumor tissue repositories (TTRs) play a pivotal role in both basic and translational research by acting as a conduit to facilitate innovative research, thereby providing solutions to treat the incurable disease – 'Cancer'. One of the fundamental requirements to achieve this goal would be the acquisition of high quality tumor tissue specimens that are stored in such a manner that its integrity is preserved. Further, a quality system should be in place that assures the compliance of procedures that are the key to a smooth functioning of inter-related departments that play a key role in the entire operations

To address this, we have initiated an effort to build a tumor tissue repository of brain tumor tissues in the Southern part of the Indian sub-continent. One of the cardinal features of brain tumors is the heterogeneity, both phenotypically and genotypically. Moreover, significant gaps exist in current understanding of the molecular pathways involved in the genesis, progression, and biological and clinical behavior of brain tumors. We hope that our initiative will provide researchers accessibility to a reserve of high quality tissues in this part of the globe. We have created and validated a complete histology service including tissue processing, embedding, sectioning and H&E staining for fixed tissues, in addition to creating and staining frozen sections. To our knowledge, such a structured initiative to store brain tumor samples is the first of its kind in the India.

Keywords: Tumor tissue repository, RNA, DNA, histology, quality standards, data management, ethics

* Corresponding author: Dr. Neelam K Venkataramana, ANSA Research Foundation #560, 1st Floor, "A" Main, Indiranagar, Bangalore, Karnataka -560 038, INDIA. E.mail: drnkvr@gmail.com.

1. Introduction

Tumor tissue banks/repositories are organized services for the purpose of collection, storage and distribution of tumor samples for further use in basic and translational cancer research. Commonly in a hospital set-up, the functional divisions of a tumor tissue repository are the surgery, pathology, molecular biology and the bioinformatics departments (Qualman et al., 2004). More recently with the advent of the 'omics' platform, there is an absolute necessity of high quality cancer tissues or peripheral blood for research on genome, transcriptome, proteome and metabolome. Thus, the establishment of high quality banks of biological resources at large medical centers or institutes is a fundamental pre-requisite to state-of the art translational cancer research (Mager et al., 2007).

Currently there are a few tumor tissue repositories worldwide and most of them primarily focus on one type of tumor. Some of the prominent tumor tissue banks globally are; MD Anderson Cancer Centre in United State of America and deals with head and neck tumors and was established approximately fifteen years ago (Mishra et al., 2009). In Canada, the Ontario Tumor Bank stores tumor related human biospecimens, which consists of all tumors. The Canadian Breast Cancer Foundation (CBCF), currently funds the CBCF Tumor Bank (CBCF TB, formerly ARTB) and is created by a merger of components of two existing tumor-banking initiatives, the CLS repository in Calgary and the tumor bank of the PolyomX Program in Edmonton. As the name suggests, the bank specializes in the collection of breast cancer tissues. The European tumor frozen tissue bank (TuBA frost) is a virtual tumour tissue bank developed in close collaboration with the European Organization for Research and Treatment of Cancer (EORTC) and 10 other participants from seven European countries. The uniqueness of the bank is that it is searchable through a query system on the internet, which is provided with rules for access and use of the tissues complete with a European code of conduct to comply with the various legal and ethical regulations in European countries (Riegman et al., 2006).

In India, barring a few research institutions, there is no concerted effort to store bio-specimens for translational cancer research, more so with tumor tissue samples. Presumably, one of the major reasons for this is the huge investment as well as the manpower that is required from the hospitals or organizations, interested to kick off this ambitious project (Mishra., et al. 2009). However, given the huge disease burden as well as the diversity in the Indian population, such a dedicated endeavor would definitely help in providing a valuable resource to researchers and scientists working towards finding solutions to treat cancers. Currently, in India, there are three existing banks; the human brain bank at National Institute of Mental Health and neurosciences (NIMHANS) at, Bangalore, Tata Memorial Hospital (TMH) Tumor tissue bank, Mumbai (Gajiwala, 2003) and the Advanced Center for Treatment Research and Education in Cancer (ACTREC), Navi-Mumbai. The Human Brain Bank at NIMHANS collects and store brain and brain tissues from infective conditions as well as fresh samples, for research purposes. The ACTREC bank currently stores samples only from oral cancer patients. However, most of them are at very primitive stage and unable to cater research institutes or drug companies if large volumes are needed.

The aim of this initiative is to collect and store tumor tissue samples and blood from cancer patients with relevant clinical records, thereby facilitating cancer research. These activities are expected to encourage basic, developmental, and translational studies in many areas of cancer research including molecular biology, immunology, genetics and proteomic research as well as biomarker discovery. Due to diversity seen in the Indian population and with research moving towards personalized medicine, the approach of this initiative intends to act as a bridge for cancer researchers by providing them with a diverse selection of high quality tumor-related specimens in large volumes. To begin with, we are focusing on building a brain tumor tissue repository. To our knowledge, this is one of the Country's first initiative to establish a brain tumor tissue bank.

One of the prime concerns regarding collection and storage of tissues has been the preservation of tissue integrity and to define quality parameters to ensure that certain standards are met.

Our article describes in detail the quality criteria that we have established during the entire procedure.

2. Experimental Procedures

2.1. Organizational Structure

Organizational issues in providing high-quality human tissues stored in bio-banks and clinical information for the support of biomedical research has been well documented (Reigman et al., 2006); Bell WC, 2009, 2010). Establishing an Organizational structure for collection and quick storage of samples is of prime importance in banking tumor tissues. Thus it becomes mandatory to integrate the tumor tissue banking activities with the pathology activities so that human tissues for research should minimize the likelihood that surgical specimens are compromised diagnostically. From the tissue bank perspective, the main goal of establishing an organizational structure is to minimize warm ischaemia time and tissue degradation, which is essential in ensuring that the tissue is fit to be used for a variety of research purposes. The entire logistics from tissue retrieval, sending to the hospital's pathology department, and sending to the ARF's Central laboratory for processing will be followed with extreme caution to avoid delay in time from excision of tissue to storage.

2.2. Ethics and Regulatory Framework

A consent form was prepared and after obtaining permission from the Institutional Ethics Committee (IEC), the study was initiated. The International Society for Biological and Environmental Repositories (ISBER) guidelines were taken into consideration when preparing the Informed consent form (ICF) (www.isber.org). Important points that were included in the consent form were the right to withdraw, maintaining confidentiality, no specified use of tissues and potential commercial use. After obtaining the duly signed informed consent form (ICF), the tumor tissue samples were collected from the hospitals from patients who underwent brain tumor resections. Immediately after surgery, the samples are collected and divided appropriately depending on the tumor size The samples are then transported to the Central laboratory for further processing and mirror image of the sample were sent to the hospital's pathological laboratory for further diagnosis, gross morphological characterization and grading. The flow chart of the details is given in Figure 1. Blood was also drawn from the patients prior to surgery and stored. Clinical details in the form of case record forms (CRFs) are collected from patients. The case record is comprehensive and covers detailed information so as to maximize the data available to the researchers interested in a particular research. Alternatively, we will also modify the procedures for collection and storage depending on the researcher's requirements for a specific study.

2.3. Collection and Transport of Tissues

After surgery, the tumor tissue is divided into two parts. One part is preserved for processing and its mirror image is sent to the Hospital's pathological department for further diagnosis. Sites with tumor and normal tissue are selected by gross examination of the surgical specimen. Each margin of the research sample is fixed in formalin as a critically important quality assurance step to document the histology of the research sample. Preservation techniques for DNA, RNA, protein, and tissue architecture need to be considered when storing samples. It has been reported that RNA and DNA can be isolated from FFPE specimen using commercially available kits but fresh freezing is still considered best for RNA and DNA isolation (Van Maldegem F., 2008). Irrespective of the exact preservation solution, the time that elapses between the procurement of the specimen until fixation or immersion into preservative and freezing is the most important factor. The temperature at which the sample is kept, transported, and processed also needs to be considered and standardized. The tissue that is to be processed for cryotome sections were transported in the sterile tube at $4^{o}C$. The tissue that was to be processed for DNA and RNA was transported in the stabilization reagent RNA *later*® (Ambion,Texas,US). For paraffin embedding the tissue was transported in 10% neutral buffered formalin. Average total time of collection and transportation to the Central laboratory is 2.5 hours.

2.4. Formalin Fixed Paraffin (FFP) and Optimum Cutting Temperature (OCT) Embedded Tissue Processing

For paraffin embedding, the tissues after transporting in neutral buffered formalin (NBF) are processed in an automated tissue processor (Leica TP1020, Germany) according to standard protocols.

Briefly, in step 1 and 2, after placing the tissues (2-3 mm), in cassettes, the tissue is fixed in NBF for 3 hrs. Next, in subsequent steps, tissue is placed in jars containing isopropyl alcohol for 3-4 hrs to remove water and formalin. Finally, the tissues are cleared with chloroform for 3-3.5 hrs. The entire processing takes about 10-12 hrs. Next, the processed tissues are transferred to the paraffin embedding station (Leica EG1150H; Leica EG1150C) for paraffin embedding. Serial sections of paraffin block were cut at 5-8 um thickness on a microtome. This procedure is routinely used for hematoxylin staining (H&E) and immunohistochemical (IHC) staining of tissue sections cut from paraffin blocks.

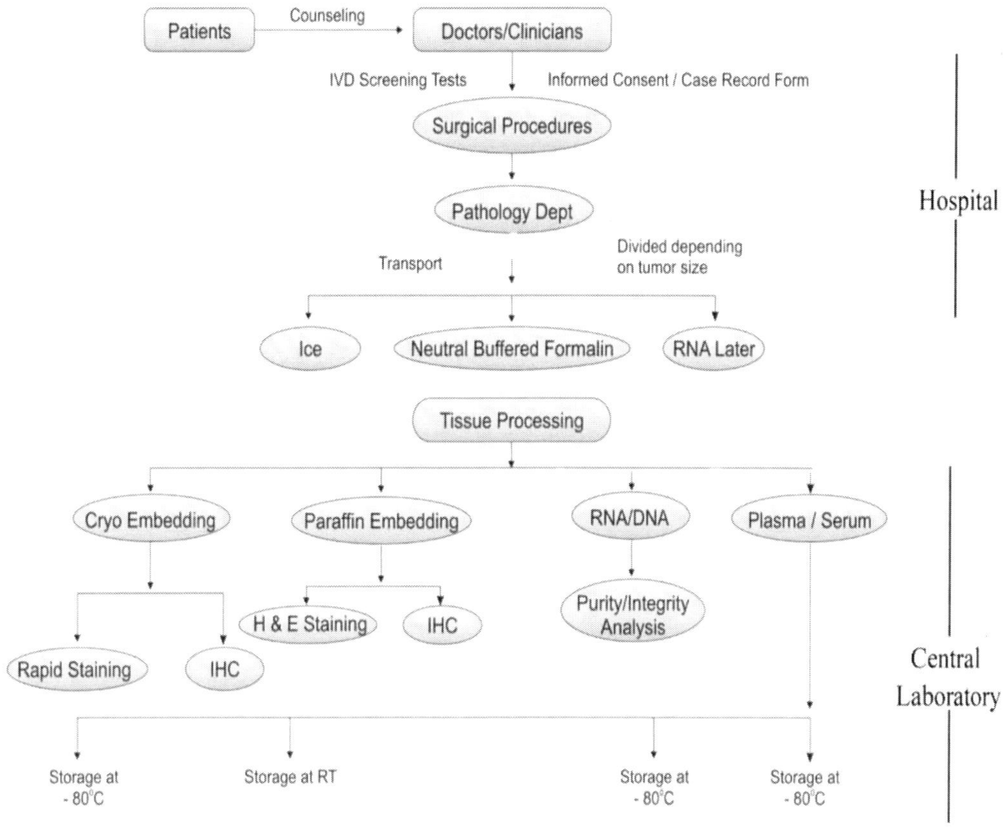

Figure 1. Work flow for collection, transport, processing and storage of tumor tissues.

The most frequently used methods of freezing tissues for biobanking purposes are liquid nitrogen or isopentane cooled with liquid nitrogen (Steu et al., 2007). For OCT embedding the samples are directly placed onto a metal chuck provided with the OCT compound (Tissue Freezing Medium®, Leica, Germany) and frozen using the cooling chamber of the cryostat (Silva EG., 1987). To avoid artifacts due to ice crystal formation, the samples are rapidly frozen in the OCT (Vonsatell et al., 1995). The cryomolds are then transferred to -80°C for long term storage. To generate frozen sections, the OCT tissue block is fixed on the chuck in the cryostat and sections are cut. (4-5 um) This procedure has been used for both rapid section and tissue banking (Steu et al., 2008).

2.5. Immunohistochemistry

Sections (4-5um) were mounted on glass slides and placed in a water bath for 45-50°C. After fixing the slides, deparaffinization in xylene, to unmask the antigenic epitopes, antigen retrieval was performed. This was done by immersing the slide in pre-heated retrieval solution (Tris-EDTA) at 95-100°C, and using the microwave method of antigen retrieval. The microwave oven has been effectively used for tissue fixation and for rapid histochemical and immunohistochemical staining (Leong et al., 1988; Hopwood et al., 1984; Shi et al., 1991). Immunostaining was performed using the two step protocol as per the manufacturer's instructions (Novolink Mini Polymer Detection System, Leica). Before staining, the slides are treated with peroxidase block to neutralize endogenous peroxidase and were then pre-incubated with protein block and then incubated for 45-60 min at room temperature with primary antibodies (Ki 67 (RTU-Ki-67-MM1, Leica) and Vimentin (RTU-VIM-V9, Leica). Subsequently, after washing the slides with TBS, standard immunohistochemical detection of the bound antibody was done using the secondary antibody for 30 min, followed and treated with horseradish peroxidase–conjugated streptavidin. Reaction products were developed with 3,3 9-di After neutralization of endogenous peroxidase and microwave antigen retrieval, slides were preincubated with blocking serum and then incubated overnight with primary antibodies. Subsequently, the sections were serially rinsed, incubated with secondary antibodies, and treated with horseradish peroxidase–conjugated streptavidin. Reaction products were developed with 3, 3 -diaminobenzidine solution and counterstained with hematoxylin. Positive control tissue sections were used to test if the protocol works. Negative control slides, in which incubation with the primary antibody was omitted, were also included in all staining procedures, to test the specificity of the antibodies used for immunohistochemical analysis.

2.6. RNA and DNA Extraction from Brain Tumor Samples

After transporting the specimen in RNA later, it is incubated overnight in RNAlater solution at 4°C so that the solution penetrates the tissue, the fluid drained, and then frozen at −80°C. For RNA extraction, the TRIzol® (GIBCO-BRL) method was used. Briefly, the tissues were minced properly by vigorous pipetting) in the reagent (15-25 mg of tissues in 1ml). Proper care was taken to see that the tissue is minced properly. Next, 0.2 ml of chloroform was added and mixed vigorously. After centrifugation at 1200 rpm for 15 min, the upper aqueous phase was transferred to another tube and precipitated with isopropanol (0.5 ml) at -200C overnight. After centrifugation, the pellet was washed with 70% ethanol. The pellet was left to air dry and dissolved in DEPC treated water. For quality check, the samples were outsourced to Genotypic Technology [P] Ltd, Bangalore, India.. RNA yield and purity was analyzed using a NanoDrop 1000 spectrophotometer. RNA integrity was assessed using the 2100 bioanalyzer (Agilent).

DNA isolation was done by using QIAamp DNA mini kit (Qiagen,CA, USA) using the manufacturer's protocol. The entire procedure is carried out a room temperature. 15 to 30 mg tissue was taken for DNA isolation. Tissue was minced properly and transferred to a 1.5 ml tube. Buffer ATL and Proteinase K was added and tissue was kept for digestion at 56ºC over night. After the digestion with lysis buffer AL was added to the tube and incubated at 70ºC for 10mins.Absolute ethanol was added to the tube and mixed thoroughly to yield a homogeneous solution. Mixture was collected into the QIAamp spin column and centrifuged for 1 min. QIAamp spin column was placed in a clean collection tube, washed with buffer AW1 and AW2 by centrifugation. DNA elution was done in buffer AL. The yield as well as purity was checked by A260/280 ratio using a spectrophotometer (Biophotometer, Eppendorf). DNA extraction was also carried out from paraffin sections in order to compare both the methods (tissue stored in RNA later and as paraffin blocks).

2.7. Serum/Plasma Processing

Each tumor sample has a matched peripheral blood sample which can be used to isolate germline DNA, if required. Blood samples were transported on ice and then centrifuged to separate the serum or plasma at 2500 rpm for 15 min within 3-5 hrs of collection. The serum or plasma are then stored at -80°C.

2.8. Data and Inventory Management

The entire database is managed by an integrated Hospital Management System (HMS), software, (designed by Insta health Solutions Pvt Ltd, Bangalore) that gives flexible choices to meet evolving needs and enhance the overall value by providing complete sample management along with inventory control. Once the tissues are received by the central laboratory, transport temperature is recorded. Tissues are then registered in the database with the tissue type and the unique identification number generated by the HMS.

Table 1. Summary sheet of the brain tumor samples stored in the repository

ARF ID	Age yrs	Gender M/F	Histopathological Diagnosis	ARF ID	Age yrs	Gender M/F	Histopatholological Diagnosis
ARF/BT/0001	65	F	Astrocytoma	ARF/BT/0026	22	M	Glioblastoma
ARF/BT/0002	42	M	Glioblastoma	ARF/BT/0027	50	M	Meningioma
ARF/BT/0003	38	M	Meningioma	ARF/BT/0028	54	M	Adenocarcinoma
ARF/BT/0004	44	F	Meningioma	ARF/BT/0029	46	M	Oligodendroglioma
ARF/BT/0005	53	M	Meningioma	ARF/BT/0030	30	M	Lymphoma
ARF/BT/0006	35	F	Meningioma	ARF/BT/0031	65	F	Glioblastoma
ARF/BT/0007	42	M	Nerve Sheath	ARF/BT/0032	55	F	Oligodendroglioma
ARF/BT/0008	58	F	Meningioma	ARF/BT/0033	25	M	Meningioma
ARF/BT/0009	59	M	Nerve Sheath	ARF/BT/0034	64	M	Pituitary tumor
ARF/BT/0010	28	F	Chordoma	ARF/BT/0035	45	F	Mixed Glioma
ARF/BT/0011	37	F	Oligodendroglioma	ARF/BT/0036	28	M	Pituitary tumor
ARF/BT/0012	25	M	Neurocytoma	ARF/BT/0037	35	M	Oligodendroglioma
ARF/BT/0013	63	F	Meningioma	ARF/BT/0038	32	F	Nerve Sheath
ARF/BT/0014	52	F	Meningioma	ARF/BT/0039	65	M	Meningioma
ARF/BT/0015	40	M	Malignant Mesenchymal tumor	ARF/BT/0040	35	M	Nerve Sheath
ARF/BT/0016	52	M	Glioblastoma	ARF/BT/0041	86	F	Meningioma
ARF/BT/0017	57	F	Glioblastoma	ARF/BT/0042	52	F	Pituitary tumor
ARF/BT/0018	47	M	Oligodendroglioma	ARF/BT/0043	59	M	Pituitary tumor
ARF/BT/0019	30	M	Nerve Sheath	ARF/BT/0044	39	F	Meningioma
ARF/BT/0020	30	M	Mixed Glioma	ARF/BT/0045	40	F	Astrocytoma
ARF/BT/0021	65	M	Oligodendroglioma	ARF/BT/0046	72	F	Meningioma
ARF/BT/0022	55	F	Glioblastoma	ARF/BT/0047	21	F	Nerve Sheath
ARF/BT/0023	56	F	Meningioma	ARF/BT/0048	29	M	Pituitary tumor
ARF/BT/0024	11	F	Medulloblastoma	ARF/BT/0049	27	M	Astrocytoma
ARF/BT/0025	47	M	Glioblastoma	ARF/BT/0050	44	M	Pituitary tumor

The HMS allows for sample registration, collects sample details based on forms, inventory control, Cost/Price management and generates MIS Reports. Further, it allows easy retrieval of sample based on diagnosis and sample types. It also incorporates a full fledged user and access control management. The registry is organized as different sections, namely – TTR summary sheet, RNA later, Paraffin embedding, Cryomolds, RNA extraction, DNA Extraction and finally plasma/serum. Each section has a sub-section, which works like an inventory and storage system giving details regarding the availability and location of a particular sample. As an example, Table 1 shows the data captured in the TTR summary sheet of the brain tumor samples stored in the repository.

2.9. Quality Systems

For defining the quality criteria while developing our tumor tissue repository, the following parameters have been included:

- Tumor diagnosis, percent cellularity of tumor and stroma and percent of necrosis, which is properly documented based on the histopathology report.
- Morphological reviews of tissue sections to ensure consistency for intended use
- Assessment of Nucleic acid (DNA and RNA) quality before storage of samples. The extracted RNA and DNA samples are outsourced to Genotypic Technology [P] Ltd, Bangalore, India for obtaining the integrity and purity of the extracted samples. The yield and purity of the RNA and DNA is analyzed by using a NanoDrop 1000 spectrophotometer. RNA integrity was measured using the 2100 Agilent bioanalyzer (Agilent).
- Documentation in the form of Standard Operating procedures (SOPs) for all operations beginning with the requisition forms, transport conditions, storage, ready traceability of tissues, methodologies followed, and lastly inventory management. After the surgery, the samples are immediately sent to the Central laboratory with the filled in tissue transport form.
- Effective and secure long-term storage of tissue samples is essential. Blocks and slides produced for routine diagnostic purposes or slides produced from frozen sections are of great value as a complement to the frozen repository. They will be stored under appropriate conditions to prevent degradation and coupled with a secure (lockable and controlled) access, accurate and up-to-date inventory system. Paraffin embedded tissues and slides are stored under climate controlled conditions (temperature, humidity and sunlight).
- Proper back-up and a non-stop electrical supply in order to maintain the quality of the biospecimens in case of a power shut-down.
- Audits will be conducted to check the equipment maintenance e.g. the temperature and alarm of the freezers, electricity backup, the adequate training of the staff, correct documentation of patient data, adherence to safety standards and ethical, legal and patient consent practices.

3. Results and Discussion

3.1. Distribution of Samples Stored in the Repository and Their Characteristics

According to the report by the Central Brain Tumor Registry in the United States, (CBTRUS), for 2004-2006 (CBTRUS Statistical Report., 2010), the distribution of primary brain and CNS tumors showed that the most frequently reported histology is the predominately non–malignant meningioma, which accounts for almost 34% of all tumors, followed by glioblastoma (17%). Gliomas account for 32% of all tumors and 80% of malignant tumors. Glioblastoma accounts for the majority of gliomas, while astrocytoma and glioblastoma combined account for about. three quarters of all gliomas. The predominately non–malignant pituitary and nerve sheath tumors account for 13% and 9% of all tumors, respectively. Acoustic neuromas account for 62% of all nerve sheath tumors.

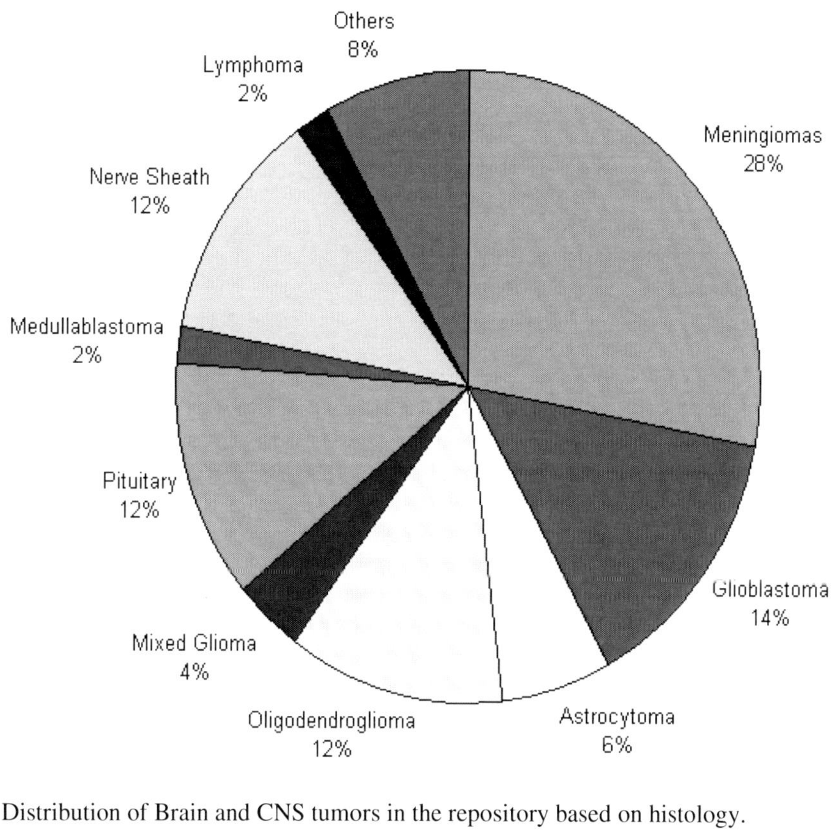

Figure 2. Distribution of Brain and CNS tumors in the repository based on histology.

Our data of 50 brain tumor tissue samples collected from May 2010 till 30th August, 2010 are depicted in Table 1. Although the samples size is small, we wanted to determine the distribution of the brain tumor samples stored in the repository, from patients undergoing brain resection, collected primarily from the Southern part of India. Figure 2 shows the distribution of all the samples stored in the TTR, based on histology. It was observed that out of 50 samples, 28% were classified as meningiomas, 36% were gliomas. The percentage of pituitary and nerve sheath tumors accounted for 12% each. Some of the rare tumors found were the medullablastoma and lymphoma sample. Out of the gliomas, gliobastoma was the highest (14%), followed by oligodendrogliomas (12%). Males accounted for 56% of the cases and females for 44% of all the cases.

Table 2. Assessment of RNA and DNA samples stored in the repository

	DNA		RNA				
ARF ID	OD 260/280	Conc ug/ul	OD 260/280	Conc ug/ul	QC Purity	QC Integrity	RIN
ARF/BT/0001	1.83	0.10	2.05	0.20	Optimal	Optimal	6.3
ARF/BT/0003	1.94	0.25	1.80	0.03	Sub-optimal	Good	7.7
ARF/BT/0004	1.96	0.13	1.77	0.03	Optimal	Optimal	6.8
ARF/BT/0005	1.71	0.20	2.03	1.70	Optimal	Degraded	2.9
ARF/BT/0006	2.05	0.18	2.01	0.50	Optimal	Good	8.8
ARF/BT/0008	1.89	0.10	1.75	0.09	Optimal	Optimal	7.3
ARF/BT/0009	1.87	0.02	1.96	1.16	Optimal	Admissible	5.9
ARF/BT/0011	1.50	0.10	1.76	0.04	Optimal	Admissible	6.0
ARF/BT/0013	1.80	0.30	2.08	0.70	Optimal	Good	7.4
ARF/BT/0014	1.80	0.35	1.97	1.70	Optimal	Optimal	7.0
ARF/BT/0015	1.80	0.25	1.97	2.00	Optimal	Degraded	2.4
ARF/BT/0016	1.60	1.30	2.05	1.00	Optimal	Admissible	6.1
ARF/BT/0021	2.06	0.32	2.05	0.60	Optimal	Admissible	6.5
ARF/BT/0022	1.82	0.03	2.06	1.74	Optimal	Good	6.9
ARF/BT/0023	1.83	0.15	1.70	1.10	Sub-optimal	Admissible	5.0

Vol: 50 ul.

The age-specific incidence for all primary brain and CNS tumors was found to highest amongst the 20-44 age group. (Table 1). Most of the meningiomas were of benign nature, as they belonged to the Grade I in nature since there were fibrous, meningothelial, transitional or transitional psammamotous types. Only one atypical meningioma (Grade II) was observed and tissue was collected (Table 2).

Knowing the histological composition and the quality of stored tissue is the first step toward keeping good quality standards in any tumor tissue banking. To address the same, all tissues sections were confirmed by pathological diagnosis, based on their gross, microscopic, immunohistochemical, and ultrastructural features, and an assessment of their clinical behavior (grade classification).

3.2. Histopathological and Immunohistochemical Analysis of the Brain Tumor Samples

As we are aware, brain tumors are given a histopathological grade of malignancy based on the features in H & E stained slides, and Immunohistochemical (IHC) analysis. Apart from the histopathological report generated by the hospital, to determine whether our paraffin embedded and cryosections are processed appropriately, we stained some random samples from the repository. Some examples of the H& E staining of the samples stored in the repository are given in Figure 3a is a micrograph of H & E stained section of glioma tissues.

As is seen with GBM, cells were highly pleomorphic and microvascular proliferation was seen. Figure 3b shows the typical herringbone pattern of spindle cells seen in fibrous meningiomas. Next, the cryosections were also subject to H & E and IHC staining to find out whether OCT embedded tissues had any adverse effect on tissue morphology or any artifacts due to lyophilization effect.

Figure 3 e and f are H& E stained sections of meningiomas after cryoembedding. We did not observe any ice crystals after staining. Further, IHC analysis of cryosections with vimentin showed scattered areas of vimentin positive cells, and uniform staining pattern was seen.(Figure 5 a).

Immunohistochemistry (IHC) has provided major insights about the classification of brain tumors by identifying cellular markers of phenotype and about tumor growth potential with nuclear markers of proliferation (Mc Keever., 1998). In essence, the grade of malignancy is an attempt to estimate the proliferative and invasive capacity and this helps in a definitive diagnosis of the particular tissue type. For the same, we performed IHC staining with Ki-67 antibody, which has since long been used as a cellular proliferative marker (Gerdes etal., 1983).

Similarly, the fibroblast intermediate filament 'vimentin', commonly found in fibroblast and other mesenchymal cells, has also been found present in glial cells.

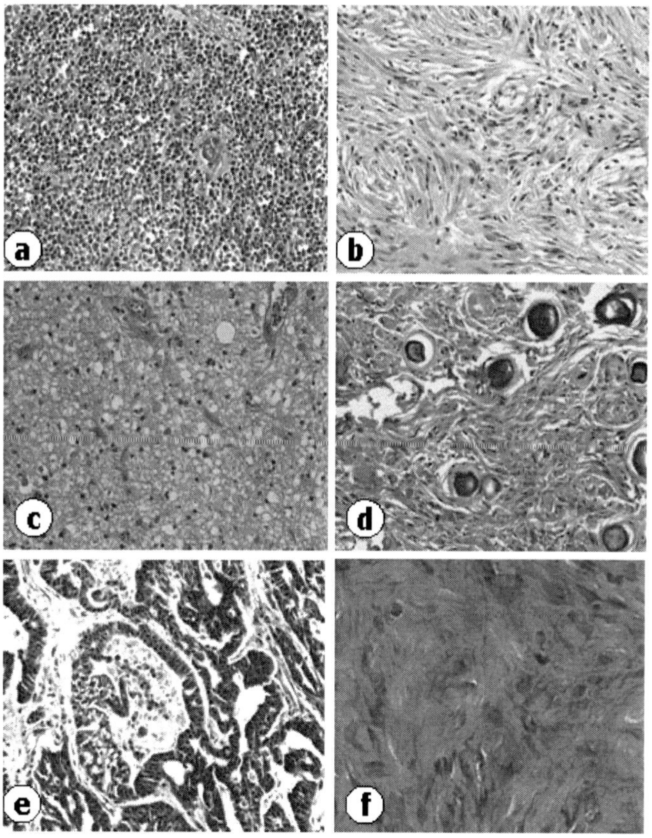

Figure 3. H & E staining of FFPE and Cryosections.

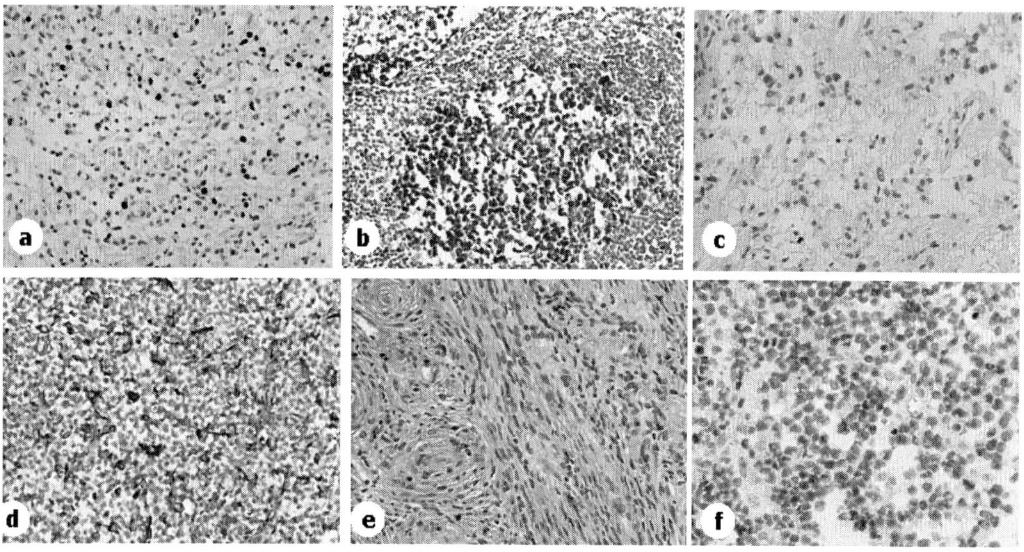

Figure 4. IHC Stain of glioma (Ki-67) and a lymphoma (Vimentin).

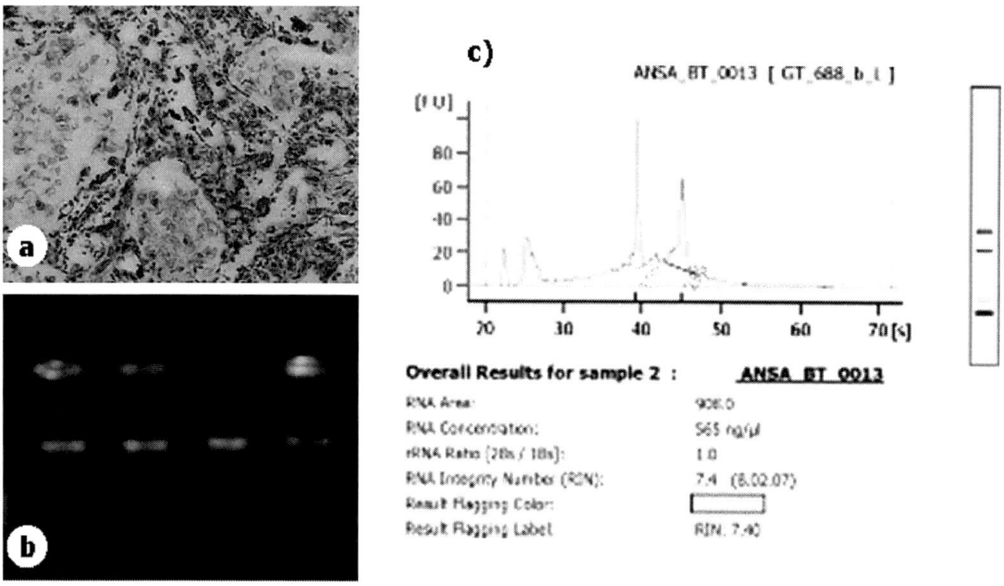

Figure 5. Examples of Quality analyses of OCT embedded Cryosections, DNA and RNA extracted from tumor tissues.

Reports suggest that vimentin can potentially be a useful marker for distinguishing undifferentiated GFAP-negative glial tumors and mesenchymal tumors from primitive neuroectodermal tumors (Yung et al., 1985). Figure 4a denotes IHC staining of two tumor types of a glioma stained with Ki-67 and Figure 4b is the IHC stain of a lymphoma with vimentin. Results showed Ki-67 (Figure 4a) showed nuclear staining (brown) in the glioma sections.

The positive control section (Figure 4b) showed a mixture of Ki-67 positive and negative cells darkly stained positive nuclei, whereas the negative control (without primary antibody) did not show any staining. Similarly, IHC analysis showed that the tumor cells contained scattered areas of vimentin-positive cells (Figure 4b). The positive control slide also stained positive, whereas no staining pattern was observed in the negative control slide, with the same section. Hence, we conclude that standardization of procedures for paraffin embedding, sectioning, H & E staining and immunostaining of brain tumor samples have been established in the laboratory.

3.3. Standardization of Procedures for Isolation of Nucleic Acid from the Tumor Tissue Samples

It has been reported (Spruessel A et al., 2004) that control of variables such as tissue ischaemia time is mandatory to obtain reliable data in screening programs for molecular targets and diagnostic molecular patterns. Their study focused upon the impact of ischaemia on gene and protein expression profiles of healthy and malignant colon tissue and revealed that initial changes in gene and protein expression profiles were already observed 5– 8 min after colon resection. Fifteen minutes after surgery, 10–15% of all detectable genes and proteins differed significantly from baseline values and 30 min after surgery this had increased to 20%. Similar reports by Huang et al., 2006, on human colon cancer specimens, quantified the effects of warm ischaemia – aliquots of tissue were frozen at 5, 10, 15, 20, 40 and 60 min after excision and the microarray data analysed. They concluded that ischaemic times of less than 20 min provide relatively stable gene expression profiles and that an ischaemic time of more than 40 min results in significant deviations from baseline. Thus, we would attempt to store all tissue specimens at the earliest to ensure that the molecular analysis would accurately reflect the state of the cells.

3.3.1. Measurement of the Yield/Purity of the Brain Tumor Tissues

Confirming the purity and integrity of the DNA/RNA extracted was important and hence we analyzed 15 random samples. As mentioned in the "Materials & Methods" section of the article, DNA was isolated using the column method (Qiagen, CA, USA). Table 2 shows the quantity and purity of the DNA isolated from various brain tumor types. The yield of DNA from 10-15 mg of the tumor tissues varied from 0.3-1.3 ug/ul. According to the manufacturer's protocol, typically 25 mg of brain tissues should yield 15-30 ug of DNA. A common observation was that irrespective of the nucleic acid extracted, the texture of the tumor played a vital role in deciding the yield. Hard tissue yielded low nucleic acid as compared to the softer tissues, probably due to improper digestion of the tissue. The majority of the samples showed the A260/280 ration between 1.8-2.0. The agarose gel electrophoresis of the samples showed that the DNA was intact (Figure 5b). Although, the purity of the samples was admissible/ optimal, the yield was still low. We are now in the process of improvisation of methods to increase the yield of the DNA isolated from the different tissue types. We have also carried out DNA extraction from FFPE sections, and have obtained the same yield with a high degree of purity (data not shown).

3.3.2. Assessment of the RNA Quality of the Samples Using Trizol Method

Compared to the more robust nature of DNA, RNA being more fragile is always the more problematic. Preservation of RNA for molecular analysis is of prime importance in genomic studies. We used the Trizol method of RNA extraction from tumor samples. Avoiding RNA degradation is a major challenge in the process. We took precautions right from the time of tumor resection, by immediately placing the tissue in RNA*later*® (Ambion, Texas, US). Reports have shown that tissue integrity has been preserved using RNA*later*® (Florell et al., 2001). There were no discernable differences between H&E frozen or paraffin embedded sections stored in RNA later. Further, immunohistochemical analysis as well as microarray experiments revealed that RNA later did not further experiments. Few samples that had been collected earlier and not transported in RNA*later*® got degraded (unpublished observations). One of the reasons probably could be due to the fact that they were not transported in RNA*later*®. Table 2 and Figure 5c denotes the results of the quality of the RNA extracted from the samples. Two of the samples in spite of being collected in RNA*later*® were found to have degraded RNA. To find out whether this was because of the handling process, we repeated the procedure again and found the same result. Hence, we conclude that this was not due to a procedural fault rather the sample was already degraded before the extraction procedure, probably due to trauma before transport. We observed that the yield of RNA also varied. The purity of the samples was between 1.7- 2.0 and almost all was qualified as ‘optimal’ according to the QC report generated by Genotypic Technology [P] Ltd. The quality control of RNA is based on the analysis of the ratio of 28S and 18S. The RIN values which is an indicator of the integrity of the isolated RNA, was comparable among samples and was between 5.0-8.8, (Table 2), except for two samples wherein degradation was observed. RIN, ribosomal RNA ratios, optical density, RNA yields, showed that intact RNA was obtained from 80% of the samples (Table 2). After completing six months of storage in RNA*later*®, samples will be assessed for their integrity as part of our QC process.

Conclusion

In this article, we have discussed the various aspects needed to be considered while setting up a tumor tissue repository in India. Given the heterogeneity in brain tumor samples, we feel that this repository would definitely serve as a gold-mine for researchers interested in looking at diverse tissue types from different geographic origins. The repertoire of samples is intended to provide academicians/researchers a diverse ethnic group of tissues for intensive research in various areas, given that such an initiative is not presently available in the Indian sub-continent. Our main objective has been to collect, store and preserve the tissues to the quality as intended by researchers for their use. We intend to carry out molecular characterization in order to find more definitive diagnostic markers for brain tumor tissues, especially gliomas and also plan to carry out research in the area of glioma stem cells. We are in the process of moving into tissue microarrays for high-throughput storage of samples. One of our long-term goals is to extend the TTR to other tissues as well. We are also working towards becoming a part of the existing global repositories.

Acknowledgments

The authors would like to thank Prof S.K.Shankar, Dr Anita Mahadevan (NIMHANS, Bangalore, India), Dr Rajiv Sarin and Dr Kishore Amin, (ACTREC, Navi-Mumbai, India) for permitting them to visit the brain bank at NIMHANS and the biobank at ACTREC respectively, before initiating the project. The authors would also like to thank Dr Mahendra Rao, Life Technologies, US for critical reviewing of the manuscript. The authors would also like to gratefully acknowledge all the patients who have donated their tissues for furthering cancer research. The work carried out was supported by Advanced Neuro-Science Institute, Bangalore and BGS Global Hospitals, Bangalore.

References

[1] Bell, WC., Sexton, KC., Grizzle WE., 2009a. How to efficiently obtain human tissues to support specific biomedical research projects. *Cancer Epidemiol Biomarkers* 18, 1676-9.

[2] Bell ,WC., Sexton, KC., Grizzle WE., 2010b.Organizational issues in providing high-quality human tissues and clinical information for the support of biomedical research. *Methods Mol. Bio* l576, 1-30.

[3] CBTRUS Statistical Report *Primary brain and central nervous system tumors diagnosed in the united states in 2004-2006,* February 2010.

[4] Florell, SR., Layfield, LJ., Gerwels, JW., 2001.A comparison of touch imprint cytology and Mohs frozen-section histology in the evaluation of Mohs micrographic surgical margins. *J. Am. Acad. Dermatol.* 44, 660-4.

[5] Gajiwala AL., 2003. Setting up a Tissue Bank in India: The Tata Memorial Hospital Experience. *Cell Tissue Bank.* 20, 193-201.

[6] Gerdes J, Schwab U, Lemke H, Stein H.1983. Production of a mouse monoclonal antibody reactive with a human nuclear antigen associated with cell proliferation. *Int. J. Cancer.* 31, 13-20.

[7] Hopwood, D., Coghill, G., Ramsay, J., Milne, G., Kerr M., 1984 . Microwave fixation: its potential for routine techniques, histochemistry, immunocytochemistry and electron microscopy. *Histochem J.* 16, 1171-91.

[8] Huang, Y., Jiang, X., Wang, W., Duan, J., Chen, G., 2006. Separation and determination of l-tyrosine and its metabolites by capillary zone electrophoresis with a wall-jet amperometric detection. *Talanta* 70, 1157-63.

[9] Leong, AS., Raymond, WA., 1988.Demonstration of AgNOR-related proteins in microwave-fixed tissues. *J. Pathol.* 156, 352.

[10] Mager, MD., Melosh, NA., 2007. Lipid bilayer deposition and patterning via air bubble collapse. *Langmuir* 23, 9369-77.

[11] McKeever P., 1998. Insights about brain tumors gained through Immunohistochemistry and in Situ hybridization of nuclear and phenotypic markers. J. Histochemistry and Cytochemistry 46, 585-594.

[12] Mishra, L., Rajkumar, N., Singh, S., Dubey, R., Yadav, G., 2009. A Comparative Study of Propofol and Isoflurane Anaesthesia using Butorphanol in Neurosurgery. *Indian J Anaesth* 53, 324-9.

[13] Qualman, SJ., France, M., Grizzle, WE., LiVolsi, VA., Moskaluk, CA., Ramirez , NC., Washington MK.,2004. Establishing a tumour bank: banking, informatics and ethics. *Br. J. Cancer* 90, 1115-9.

[14] Riegman, PH., Oomen, MH., Dinjens, WN., Oosterhuis, JW., Lam, KH., Spatz, A., Ratcliffe, C., Knox, K., Mager, R., Kerr, D., Pezzella, F., Van Damme, B., Van De Vijver, M., Van Boven, H., Morente, MM., Alonso, S., Kerjaschki, D., Pammer, J., López-Guerrero, JA., Llombart-Bosch, A., Carbone, A., Gloghini, A., Teodorovic, I., Isabelle, M., Passioukov, A., Lejeune, S., Therasse, P., Van Veen, EB., 2006. TuBaFrost: European virtual tumor tissue banking. *Adv. Exp. Med. Biol.* 587, 65-74.

[15] Shi S, Key M, Kalra K., 1991. Antigen Retrieval in Formalin-fixed, Paraffin-embedded Tissues: An Enhancement Method for Immunohistochemical Staining Based on Microwave Oven Heating of Tissue Sections. *J. Histochemistry and Cytochemistry* 39, 741-748.

[16] Silva, EG., 1987.Chorionic villous-like structures in metastatic testicular choriocarcinoma. *Cancer* 60, 207-10.

[17] Spruessel, A., Steimann, G., Jung, M., Lee, SA., Carr, T., Fentz, AK., Spangenberg, J., Zornig, C., Juhl, HH., David, KA.,2004. Tissue ischemia time affects gene and protein expression patterns within minutes following surgical tumor excision. *Biotechniques* 36, 1030-7.

[18] Steu, S., Baucamp, M., von Dach, G., Bawohl, M., Dettwiler, S., Storz, M., Moch ,H., Schraml, P., 2008. A procedure for tissue freezing and processing applicable to both intra-operative frozen section diagnosis and tissue banking in surgical pathology. *Virchows Arch* 452, 305-12.

[19] Troyer, D., 2008. Biorepository standards and protocols for collecting, processing, and storing human tissues. *Methods Mol. Biol.* 441,193-220.

[20] Van Maldegem, F., de Wit, M., Morsink, F., Musler ,A., Weegenaar, J., van Noesel, CJ., 2008. Effects of processing delay, formalin fixation, and immunohistochemistry on RNA Recovery From Formalin-fixed Paraffin-embedded Tissue Sections. *Diagn Mol. Pathol.* 17, 51-8.

[21] Vonsattel, JP., Aizawa, H., Ge, P., DiFiglia, M., McKee, AC., MacDonald, M., Gusella, JF., Landwehrmeyer ,GB., Bird, ED., Richardson, EP, Jr., et al.1995 An improved approach to prepare human brains for research. *J. Neuropathol. Exp. Neurol.* 54, 42-56.

In: Stem Cells in Disease
Editor: Prasad S. Koka
ISBN: 978-1-62257-169-7
© 2012 Nova Science Publishers, Inc.

Chapter XIV

Sca-1 Expression Pattern in the Mouse Limbal Epithelium and its Association with Cell Cycle

Prosun Das, Sumanta Chatterjee, Pratima Basak, Madhurima Das, Jacintha Archana Pereira, Ranjan Dutta, Malay Chaklader, Ketaki Bagchi, Gautam Bhaduri, Samaresh Chaudhuri, and Sujata Law *

Stem Cell Research and Application Unit, Department of Biochemistry and Medical Biotechnology, Calcutta School of Tropical Medicine, Kolkata, India

Abstract

Stem Cell Antigen-1 or Sca-1 is a cell surface receptor protein commonly used to detect adult murine haematopoietic stem cell population. Outside the haematopoietic system Sca-1 is similarly expressed in stem and progenitor cells in a wide variety of tissues and organs such as skeletal muscle, mammary gland, prostate, heart, liver and dermis. Thus Sca-1 has become a candidate marker in the search of tissue specific stem cells. The maintenance of a healthy corneal epithelium is achieved by a unique population of stem cell located in the limbal epithelial region. This limbal epithelium mainly contains limbal epithelial stem cells and its immediate progenitor early transient amplifying cells (e-TAC) which have self renewal capacity. As stem cells in other organs have been identified by their expression of Sca-1, in our study we wanted to determine whether this antigen could be present in the limbal epithelial region which contains stem cell population by using immunofluorescence through flow cytometric analysis of Sca-1 and its association with the cell cycle.

* Corresponding Author: Dr. Sujata Law, Assistant Professor. Stem Cell Research and Application Unit, Department of Biochemistry and Medical Biotechnology, Calcutta School of Tropical Medicine, C.R Avenue, Kolkata-700073, India. E-mail: msuj2002@yahoo.co.in, Cell Phone: 9051259521.

Introduction

Stem cell antigen-1 or Sca-1 is a common marker used to detect adult murine hematopoietic stem cell population is an 18 KDa mouse glycosyl phosphatidylinositol anchored cell surface protein of the Ly6 gene family, expressed mainly on cells which have self renewal potential [1]. Recent studies suggests that stem cells are present in all self renewing tissues and have tremendous potential for cell division, but are normally slow cycling presumably to preserve their proliferative potential and thus play a crucial role in tissue homeostasis [2,3]. Some of the organ/tissue exhibit stem cell population with particular characteristics and functional properties which is common to haematopoietic stem cells. Recent research work identified that presence of Sca-1 not only present in haematopoietic system but also in other tissue specific stem cells. The murine mammary epithelial cells [4,5] and cells having sphere forming ability of mouse skin [6], skeletal system [7], heart [8], liver [9], and proximal part of prostatic duct [10,11]express such a population of Sca-1 positive cells.

The ocular system is designed in a highly specialized manner where the system bears several integral parts with distinct functional properties. The anterior part of the eye represent cornea and covered by corneal epithelium. The maintenance of corneal epithelium is dependent on stem cells located in the limbal region is a well accepted phenomenon [12-14]. The mouse limbal epithelium is two to four cell layers thick and contains stem cell population [2, 15]. These limbal epithelial stem cell share some features common to other adult somatic stem cells like smaller cell size [16], self renewal capacity [17], long life span [18], slow cycling and also act as a "reporter cell" that function in cross talk [2]. These stem cells have low granularity and high nucleus-to-cytoplasm (N/C) ratio [14,19]. Limbal epithelial stem cells give rise to their immediate progenitor early-Transient Amplifying cells (e-TAC) which are relatively undifferentiated under normal steady state and rapidly proliferate on appropriate stimulation [20]. Like stem cells, these cells too have the self renewable potential and play a major role in amplifying the cells to maintain the total number of epithelial cells [3, 18, 20].

The compartmentalization of the limbal epithelial stem cell within the limbus gives us a valuable opportunity to study the behavior of adult stem cells [21]. In the present study we wanted to evaluate whether there is any expression of membrane bound Sca-1 receptor in the limbal epithelial region which denotes the stem/progenitor cell population and its association with the cell cycle status.

Materials and Methods

Inbred Swiss albino mice of both sexes aged about 2-4 months were taken for the experimental purpose. Ten such mice weighed approximately 18-20 gm were selected and maintained with standard diet and clean water *ad libitum* and the use of animals was approved by Institutional Animal Ethical Committee.

Isolation of Mouse Limbal Epithelial Sheets

After cervical dislocation 10 pairs of eye globes were taken out from mice with forceps and washed three times in chilled Phosphate Buffer Saline (PBS). The anterior half of the eye globes were separated from the posterior part using fine scissor and then enzymatically digested at 37° C for 3 hours in RPMI-1640 (Gibco, BRL -USA) containing 1.2 U/ml Dispase II (Roche, Germany). After 3 hours of Dispase digestion the peripheral epithelium of the cornea loosened from the underlying stroma whereas the central corneal epithelium still remained attached with the stroma. Under dissecting microscope the peripheral part of the corneal epithelial sheet- the "limbus" was carefully removed using fine scissor.

Single Cell Preparation

After removing the peripheral or limbal epithelial sheets, they were suspended in calcium free HBSS containing 0.25% Trypsin (Sigma-Aldrich) and 0.01% EDTA (HiMedia, India) and incubated at 37°C for 10 minutes with intermittent gentle shaking and brief pipetting. After trypsinization step the supernatant was collected into excess of RPMI-1640 medium with 10% FBS (Lonza Verviers SPRL) in ice-tray to stop the trypsin digestion. The second step of trypsinization procedure was done with the residual limbal epithelium. The single cell suspension was then filtered through a nylon mesh and centrifuged for 10 minutes (250 g) at 4° C. The cell pellet was then resuspended into fresh RPMI-1640 media. Cells were counted in haemocytometer chamber.

Cell Culture and Colony Forming Assay

Isolated limbal epithelial single cells were cultured in RPMI-1640 media supplemented with and without 20% FBS (Fetal Bovine Serum) in 1% gelatin coated 35mm tissue culture dish (Corning, USA) at a density of 2×10^4 cells/ml [22]. The cells attached to the plastic dish within 24 hours after seeding. The media was changed after 24 hours and thereafter every 3rd day. The non-adherent cells were pulled out as the media was changed. Mean percentage of cell was calculated by counting the cells in the haemocytometer chamber. In culture the proliferating capacity of the limbal epithelial cells was observed at 24 hours and on the 7th day.

The colony forming assay was done by seeding a low density of limbal epithelial cells (100 cells/well) in 6-well plate for 2 weeks and the colony growth visualized by crystal violet staining. The numbers of colonies were scored using an inverted microscope (CK Olympus, Tokio). Colony forming efficiency (CFE) was determined by the following formula Colony Forming Efficiency (CFE %) =

$$\frac{\text{Counted colony number} \times 100}{\text{Initial seeding cell number}}.$$

Immunofluorescent Staining

Limbal epithelial cells were incubated for 30 minutes at 37° C in dark with 2 μl of phycoerythrin (PE) labeled anti mouse Sca-1-PE monoclonal antibody (BD-Bioscience, USA). After 30 minutes of incubation cells were washed 3 times in PBS to wash off the excess fluorescence. A small amount of cell suspension was then mounted on dewaxed slide and allowed to dry in dark. Sample slide was then observed under fluorescence microscope.

Flow Cytometry Analysis

Isolated epithelial cells from limbus were resuspended in ice cold RPMI-1640 media and kept on ice for flow cytometric analysis.

a) *Light Scattering Analysis*: Trypsin digested limbal epithelial cells were resuspended into phosphate buffer saline containing 5% FBS and the light scattering property of the cells were measured in flow cytometer BD FACS Calibur (Becton Dickenson ,USA) using CellQuest Pro Software.
b) For the identification of membrane bound Sca-1 expression, limbal epithelial cells were subjected to flow cytometric analysis following staining with anti-Sca-1-PE monoclonal antibody. Briefly, $1x10^6$ cells/ml were fixed with 3% paraformaldehyde, washed and incubated with 2 μl of anti Sca-1-PE (BD- Bioscience, USA) conjugated antibody in dark at 37°C for 30 minutes. Finally the cells were washed thrice in PBS and flow cytometric analysis was done by BD-FACS Calibur using CellQuest Pro Software.

7 AAD Assay

Prior to analysis, to distinguish between the viable and non-viable cells of the isolated limbal epithelium, 7-Amino-actinomycin D (7'AAD) (BD Biosciences) flowcytometry assay was performed. Briefly, 1×10^6 cells/ml were fixed with 3% paraformaldehyde, then washed and incubated with 5 μl of dye for 15 minutes before analysis. Finally the cells were washed thrice in PBS and analysis was done by BD-FACS Calibur using CellQuest Pro Software.

Cell Cycle Analysis by Flow Cytometry

The cell cycle pattern of isolated limbal epithelial cells were analyzed by the DNA QC particle kit (BD Biosciences, USA) containing Propidium Iodide (PI). Briefly, the cells were washed two times with PBS by centrifugation for 3 minutes at 4° C and then fixed with 50% ethanol for 30 minutes at room temperature.

The cells were then suspended in PBS containing RNAse (1 mg/ml, 20 μl) (sigma), PI (10 mg/ml, 2.5 μl) and 0.2% Nonidet P-40 (Sigma-Aldrich) and incubated for 30 minutes at room temperature.

The cell cycle status was analyzed with BD-FACS Calibur using CellQuest Pro and Mod Fit LT (Variety Sales House, USA) software.

Results

Isolation of Limbal Epithelial Cell

The number of epithelial cells collected after Dispase digestion and Trypsin treatment from one mouse was 0.5-1 $\times 10^5$ cells/ml on average (Figure 1) and we used 10 mice at a time.

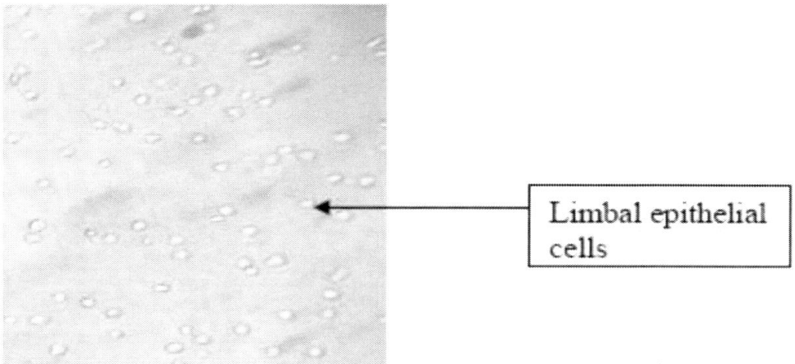

Figure 1. Single cells from limbal epithelium after trypsin–EDTA digestion in a petri-dish at seeding density.

Cell Culture and Colony Forming Assay

The proliferative potential (7th day *ex-vivo* culture) of limbal epithelial single cells was higher in RPMI-1640 media with 20 % FBS in comparison to non-FBS media (Figure 2A, 2B).

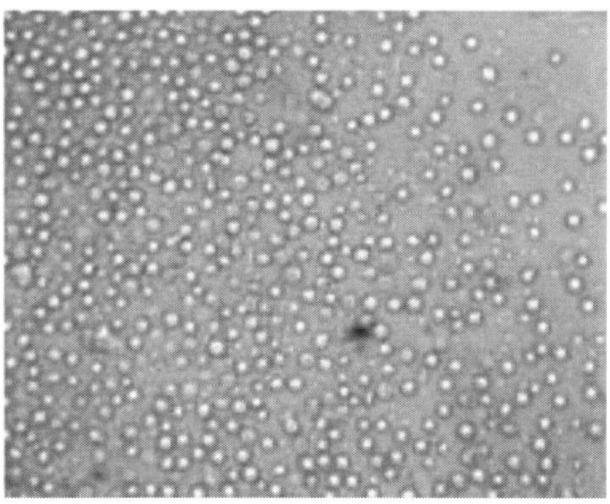

Figure 2A. Single cell culture of isolated limbal epithelial cells at 7th day in non FBS RPMI-1640 media.

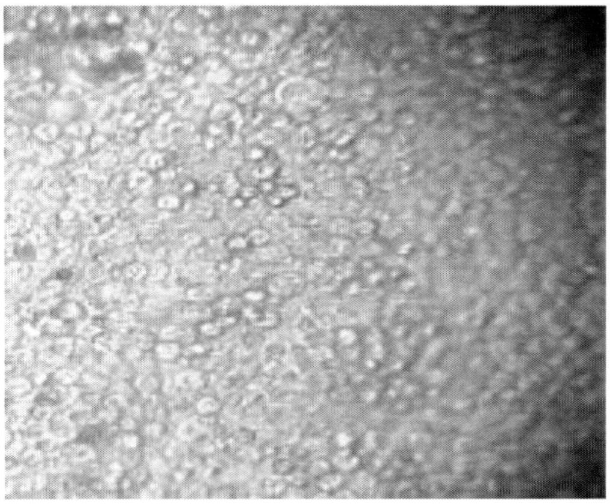

Figure 2B. Limbal epithelial cells became confluent in serum (20%) supplemented media on 7th day of culture. Cells exhibited uniformity of shape, compactness and large nucleus-to-cytoplasm (N/C) ratio.

The Colony Forming Efficiency (CFE) of limbal epithelial cells was 12.2 ±1.1 % (Figure 3) after 14 days of *ex-vivo* culture where the colonies showed uniformity of shape and size.

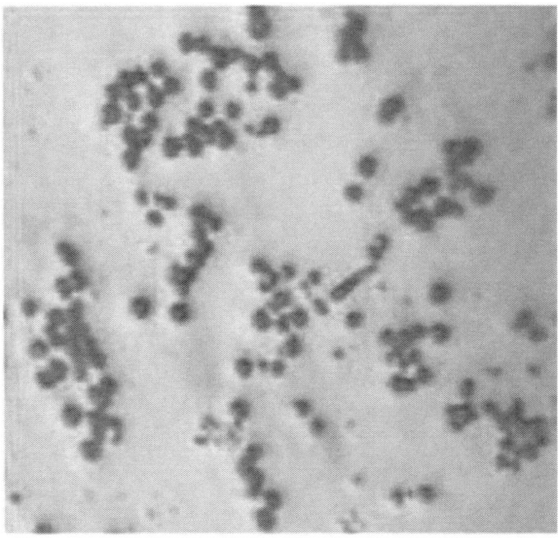

Figure 3. Limbal epithelial cells formed colonies in RPMI-1640 media supplemented with 20% FBS. 100 cells/well were seeded in 6 well plates and after 2 weeks colonies were visualized by crystal violet staining and scored using an inverted microscope. Cells within the colony were uniform in shape and size.

Immunofluroscence Study

The monoclonal antibody staining of membrane receptor showed the presence of Sca-1 expression on a significant number of cells of isolated limbal epithelium (Figure 4).

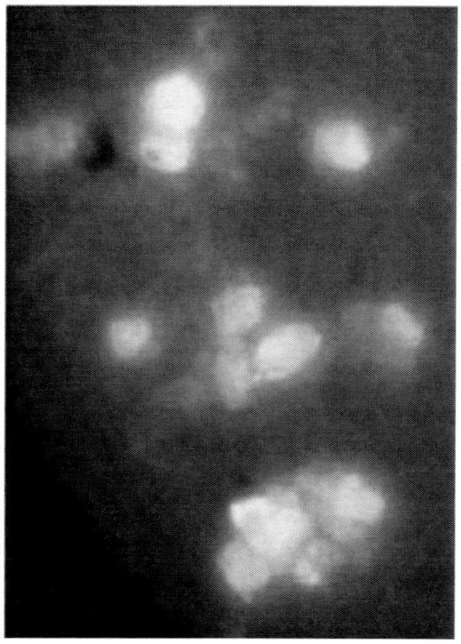

Figure 4. Fluorescence microscopy by immunofluorescent staining represents Sca-1 expression on a significantly large number of cells of isolated limbal epithelium.

Flow Cytometric Analysis

The light scattering property of the isolated limbal epithelial cells showed distinct populations of cells which are in FSC^{low}/SSC^{low} zone (Figure 5A). Phenotypic characterization of Sca-1 receptor expression by limbal epithelial cells from the gated zone indicated presence of a significantly higher percentage of Sca-1 positivity i.e. approximately 92.76% of isolated cells were Sca-1 positive (Figure 5B).

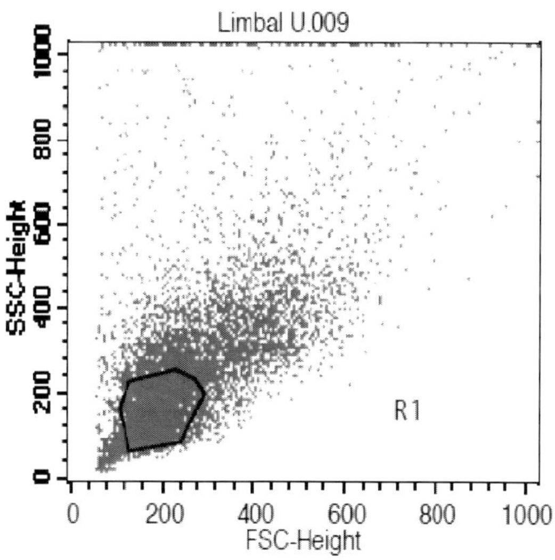

Figure 5A. Light scattering phenomenon of the isolated limbal epithelial cells showed, distinct population of cells are in FSC low/SSC low zone in fluorescence activated cell sorter (FACS) analysis.

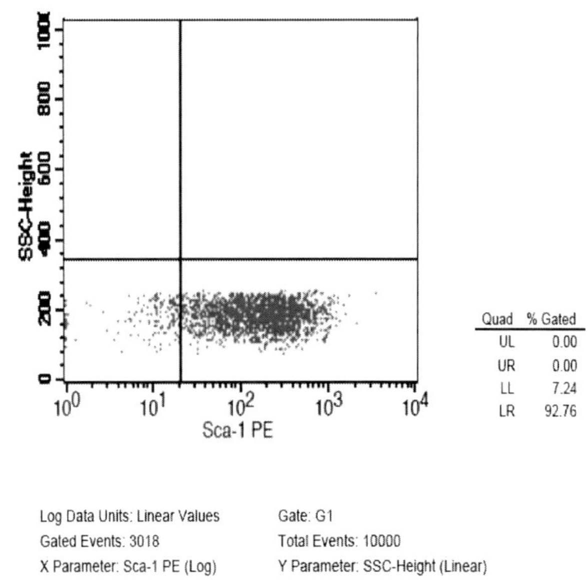

Figure 5B. Fluorescence analysis of FSC ^{low}/SSC ^{low} gated zone indicated presence of high population of Sca-1 positive cells. Approximately 92.76 % of isolated cells were Sca-1 positive.

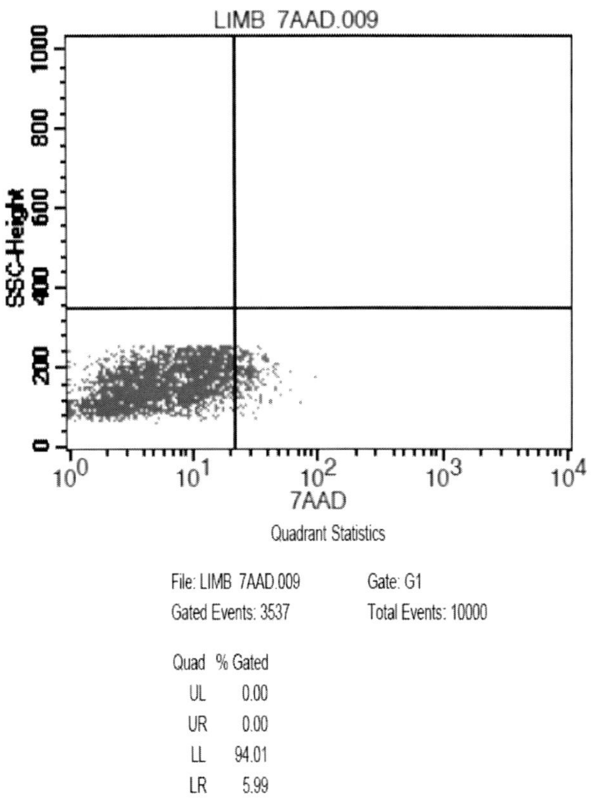

Figure 6. 7AAD assay by flow cytometric analysis indicated that almost all the isolated limbal epithelial cells were viable (94.01%).A very insignificant population of cells (5.99%) showed 7AAD positivity.

7AAD Assay

The cell viability was determined by 7AAD assay which depicted viable cell population (94.01%) (Figure 6) by flow cytometric analysis and only 5.99 % of cells were 7AAD positive i.e. non-viable.

Cell Cycle Analysis

The cell cycle analysis (Figure 7A, 7B) of limbal epithelial cells showed 97.14 % (M1 region) positivity through G0/G1 phase and 2.87% (M2 region) positivity in S-G2-M phase by Mod Fit LT software of flow cytometric analysis.

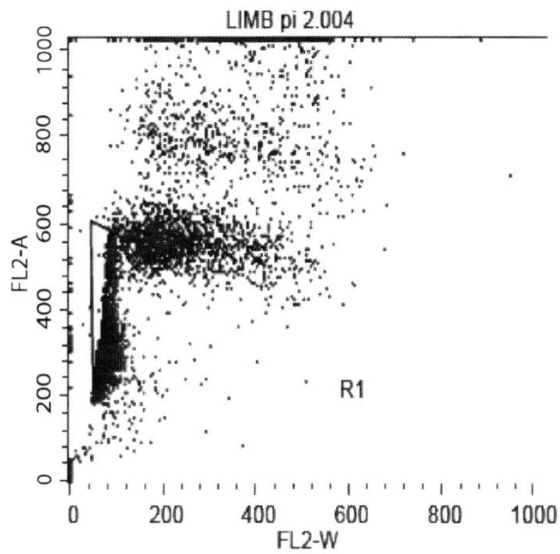

Figure 7A. The gated population of isolated limbal epithelial cells were plotted with dot plot of FL2W/FL2A for cell cycle and DNA content analysis in flow cytometry.

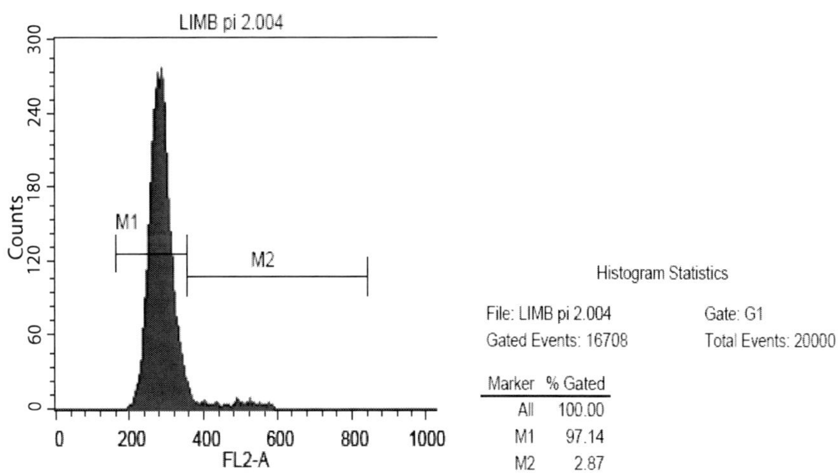

Figure 7B. 97.14 % population of isolated limbal epithelial cells were in the G0/G1 phase of the cell cycle. A very small fraction of cells were in the mitotic phase (2.87%).

Discussion

Limbus is an anatomical and functional location of limbal stem cells as well as immediate progenitor early-Transient Amplifying cells which have the capacity of self renewal to maintain the transparency and function of corneal epithelial cells [23].

In our experiment we successfully isolated single epithelial cells from the limbus which reflected a dense population of low SSC / FSC zone in flow cytometric analysis with 94.01 % viability (Figure 6). The low FSC/SSC zone represents stem cell rich population in all self renewing tissues consisting predominantly with nucleus within a small amount of less granular cytoplasm [16, 19, 24]. In our study the gated population in the low FSC v/s SSC zone in the flow cytometric analysis (Figure 5A) denoted the limbal stem and progenitor e-TAC rich population as the limbal epithelial immature cells have high nucleus-to-cytoplasmic ratio with smaller cell size and low granularity.

Using radiolabelled thymidine, Cotsarelis and his co-workers demonstrated that the cells of limbal epithelium of mice are normally slow cycling in nature, but can be made to cycle much more rapidly in response to wounding and growth promoter [2].In our present study the *in-vitro* culture of limbal epithelium which is an enriched source of stem/progenitor cells showed that limbal cells have a higher *in-vitro* proliferative potential which is stimulus (20% FBS) (Figure 2A,2B) dependent [25,26] and different from *in-vivo* condition where these cells usually remain in slow cycling status [2]. The particular compact zone of cell population which we have isolated from the limbus showed uniformity in their shape and size and also depicted significant colony forming ability at the 14th day of culture(Figure 3) ensured presence of a rich primitive stem, progenitor cell population.

Expression of Sca-1 is not limited only to HSCs but also observed in other tissue specific stem cells and cancer cells which have the self renewal capacity [27]. The flow cytometric analysis showed that, a large population of cells in the limbal epithelium is Sca-1 positive (Figure 5B). As the Sca-1 population is too large (92.76%), so we can state that not only the stem cell population but also the e-TAC population expresses Sca-1 in *in-vivo* condition which is the background base of our experimental cell source. The parallel study carried out with fluorescence microscopy of the fluorescinated antibody labeled cells also confirmed that the isolated population is enriched with Sca-1 positive cells (Figure 4). Previous experiments revealed that hematopoietic stem cells from Sca-$1^{-/-}$ mice showed decreased repopulation potential, resulted from a primary defect in the self renewal capacity of stem cells [28, 29]. So, as the limbal stem and e-TACs have the self renewing potential [2] we can suggest that Sca-1 is directly or collectively involved in the self renewal capacity of the limbal stem/progenitor cells which explains the appearance of a large population of Sca-1 positive cells in the flow cytometry analysis of limbal zone.

Flow cytometry technique is unique to study the cell cycle of an accessible cell population such as the limbal epithelium. The distribution of DNA content in cell populations can be accurately and rapidly determined by flowcytometry, offering advantages over radiolabelling and scintillation counting. In contrast to other methods, flowcytometry provides more precise information about the cell cycle of isolated limbal epithelium. Nancy *et al* reported that limbal epithelial cell population are arrested in early G1 phase and under homeostatic condition does not go through other cell cycle phases [20]. In our experiment we observed that, high population of limbal epithelial cells are in the G0/G1 phase of cell cycle

(Figure 7A, 7B). As the rate of proliferation and centripetal movement of mouse limbal e-TAC is very slow in normal *in-vivo* condition [30-33] so it further proves the increased appearance of G0/G1 phase of the cell cycle in our experiment. All these findings support our data that limbal epithelial cells are slow cycling and retain G0/G1 phase of the cell cycle under normal condition.

Recent data showed that Sca-1 plays an important role in cellular differentiation, proliferation and cell cycle exit [29].It has been reported earlier that, Sca-1 positive mouse hematopoietic stem cells have low DNA content which indicated that they were in the G0/G1 phase of cell cycle [27,34] In our present study we found, high population of limbal Sca-1 positive cells are in the G0/G1 phase which significantly correlates with others data on other tissue specific stem cells where expression of Sca-1 was necessary for cell cycle withdrawal [11, 35, 36].

As Sca-1 is expressed both on limbal stem cells and its immediate progenitor cells i.e. e-TACs we can state that expression of Sca-1 is not only limited on undifferentiated immature quiescent G0 cell population but also gets expressed on the cells which are in the early G1 phase of cell cycle and have long cell cycle time. So we can suggest that Sca-1 has a definite role on cell cycle withdrawal and negatively regulate cell proliferation.

In conclusion we propose that Sca-1 expression serves as a protective mechanism to maintain an adequate pool of limbal stem/progenitor cell population throughout the life. Normally they remain at G0/G1 phase of the cell cycle and expression of Sca-1 negatively regulates the cell cycle to maintain quiescence. As Sca-1 is highly expressed on the limbal epithelial cells so we can say that, like other stem/ progenitor cell population, here Sca-1 too has a role to maintain the level of signaling receptor in such a manner that self renewal and the G0/G1 cell cycle status of limbal epithelial cells are regulated and balanced for the maintenance of corneal epithelium in normal physiological condition.

Acknowledgment

We are thankful to the Indian Council of Medical Research for their sponsorship and The Director, Calcutta School of Tropical Medicine for the facilities provided.

References

[1] Yutoku M, Grossberg AL, Pressman D. A cell surface antigenic determinant present on mouse plasmacytes and only about half of mouse thymocytes. *J. Immunol*, 1974, 112(5), 1774-1781.

[2] Costaralis G, Cheng S-Z, Dong G, Sun T-T, Lavker RM. Existence of slow- cycling limbal epithelial basal cells that can be preferentially stimulated to proliferate: Implications on epithelial stem cells. *Cell*, 1989, 57, 201-209.

[3] Lajtha LJ. *Stem cell concepts in stem cells: their identification and characterization,* C.S. Potten, ed. (New York: L Churchill Livingston). 1983, 1-11.

[4] Woodward WA, Chen MS, Behbod F and Rosen JM. On mammary stem cells. *J. Cell Sci,* 2005, 118 (16), 3585-3594.

[5] Welm BE, Tepera SB, Venezia T, Graubert TA, Rosen JM, Goodell MA. Sca-1 (pos) cells in the mouse mammary gland represent an enriched progenitor cell population. *Dev. Biol,* 2002, 245 (1), 42-56.

[6] Toma JC, Akhavan M, Fernandes KJ *et al.* Isolation of multipotent adult stem cells from the dermis of mammalian skin. *Nat. Cell Biol,* 2001, 3(9), 778-784.

[7] Lee JY, Qu-Petersen Z, Cao B *et al.* Clonal isolation of muscle-derived cells capable of enhancing muscle regeneration and bone healing. *J Cell Biol,* 2000, 150(5), 1085-1100

[8] Matsuura K, Nagai T, Nishigaki N, Oyama T, Nishi J *et al.* Adult cardiac Sca-1 positive cells differentiate into beating cardiomyocytes. *J. Biol. Chem,* 2004, 279(12), 11384-11391.

[9] Petersen BE, Grossbard B, Hatch H, Pi L, Deng J, Scott EW. Mouse A6-positive hepatic oval cells also express several hematopoietic stem cell markers. *Hepatology,* 2003, 37(3), 632-640.

[10] Burger PE, Xiong X, Coetzee S Salm SN, Moscatelli D,Goto K, Wilson EL. Sca-1 expression identifies stem cells in the proximal region of prostatic ducts with high capacity to reconstitute prostatic tissue. *Proc Natl Acad Sci,* 2005, 102(20), 7180-7185.

[11] Xin L, Lawson DA, Witte ON. The Sca-1 cell surface marker enriches for a prostate-regenerating cell subpopulation that can initiate prostate tumorigenesis. *Proc. Natl. Acad. Sci,* 2005, 102(19), 6942-6947.

[12] Buck RC. Measurement of centripetal migration of normal corneal epithelial cells in the mouse. *Invest Ophthal. and Vis. Sci,* 1985, 26(9), 1296-1299.

[13] Schermer A, Galvin S, Sun TT. Differentiated-related expression of a major 64K corneal keratin *in vivo* and in culture suggests limbal location of corneal epithelial stem cells. *J. Cell Biol.,* 1986, 103, 49-62.

[14] Chen Z, De Paiva CS, Luo L, Kretzer FL, Pflugfelder SC, Li DQ. Characterization of putative stem cell phenotype in human limbal epithelia. *Stem cells,* 2004, 22, 355-366.

[15] Krulova M, Pokorna K, Lencova A, Fric J, Zajicova A, Filipec M, Forrester JV, Holan V. A rapid separation of two distinct populations of mouse corneal epithelial cells with limbal stem cell characteristics by centrifugation on percoll gradient. *Invest Ophthalmol Vis. Sci,* 2008, 49(9), 3903-3908.

[16] Romano AC, Espana EM, Yoo SH, Budak MT, Wolosin JM, Tseng SC. Different cell sizes in human limbal and central corneal basal epithelia measured by confocal microscopy and flow cytomerty. *Invest Ophthalmol. Vis. Sci,* 2003, 44(12), 5125-5129.

[17] Majo F, Rochat A , Nicolas M, Jaoude GA and Yann BY. Oligopotent stem cells are distributed throughout the mammalian ocular surface. *Nature,* 2008, 456, 250-254.

[18] Ebrahimi M, Taghi-Abadi E, Baharvand H. Limbal stem cells in review. *J. of Ophthalmol and Vis. Res,* 2009; 4 (1), 40-58.

[19] Arpitha P, Prajna NV, Srinivasan M and Muthukkaruppan V. High expression of p63 combined with a large N/C ratio defines a subset of human limbal epithelial cells: implications on epithelial stem cells. *Invest Ophthalmol Vis. Sci, 2005,* 46(10), 3631-3636.

[20] Joyce NC, Meklir B, Joyce SJ and Zieske JD. Cell cycle protein expression and proliferative status in human corneal cells. *Invest Ophthalmol. Vis. Sci,* 1996, 37(4), 645-655.

[21] Shortt AJ, Secker GA, Munro PM, Khaw PT, Tuft SJ, Daniels JT. Characterization of the limbal epithelial stem cell niche: novel imaging techniques permit in vivo

observation and targeted biopsy of limbal epithelial stem cells. *Stem Cells*, 2007, 25 (6), 1402-1409.

[22] Qu L, Yang X, Wang X, Zhao M, Mi S, Duo Z, Wang H. Reconstitution of corneal epithelium with cryopreserved corneal limbal stem cells in a rabbit model. *The Vet. J.*, 2009, 179 (3), 392-400.

[23] Dua HS, Shanmuganathan VA, Powell-Richards AO, Tighe PJ, Joseph Br J A. Limbal epithelial crypts: a novel anatomical structure and a putative limbal stem cell niche. *Ophthalmol* 2005; 89: 529-532.

[24] Majore I, Moretti P, Hass R, Kasper C. Identification of subpopulations in mesenchymal stem cell-like cultures from human umbilical cord. *Cell Communication and Signaling,* 2009, **7**:6.

[25] Pelligrini G, Golisano O, Paterna P, Lambiase A, Bonini S, Rama P, and De Luca M. Location and clonal analysis of stem cells and their differentiated progeny in the human ocular surface. *The J. of Cell Biol*, 1999, 145(4), 769-782.

[26] Cruse EF, Tseng SCG. A serum-free clonal growth assay for limbal, peripheral, and central cornel epithelium. *Invest Ophthalmol Vis. Sci,* 1991, 32(7), 2086-2095.

[27] Holmes C, Stanford WL. Concise Review: Stem Cell Antigen-1: Expression, Function, and Enigma. *Stem Cells*, 2007, 25, 1339–1347.

[28] Ito CY, Li CYJ, Bernstein A, Dick JE, Stanford WL. Hematopoietic stem cell and progenitor defects in Sca-1/Ly-6A–null mice. *Blood*, 2003, 101(2), 517-523.

[29] Bonyadi M, Waldman SD, Liu D, Aubin JE, Grynpas MD and Stanford WL. Mesenchymal progenitor self-renewal deficiency leads to age-dependent osteoporosis in Sca-1_Ly-6A null mice. *Proc. Natl. Acad. Sci.*, 2003, 100(10), 5840–5845.

[30] Pokroy R,Tendler Y,Pollack A,Zinder O,Weisinger G.p53 expression in the normal murine eye. *Invest Ophthalmol. Vis. Sci,* 2002, 43(6), 1736-1741.

[31] Potten CS, Wichmann HE, Loeffler M, Dobek K, Major D. Evidence for discrete cell kinetic subpopulations in mouse epidermis based on mathematical analysis. *Cell Tissue Kinet,* 1982, 15(3), 305-329.

[32] Nagasaki T and Zhao J. Centripetal movement of corneal epithelial cells in the normal adult mouse. *Invest Ophthalmol. Vis. Sci,*, 2003, 44(2), 558-566.

[33] Kaufmann B, Bay H and Hollaender A. Distribution of mitoses in the corneal epithelium of the rabbit and the rat. *Anat. Res*, 1944, 90,161 178.

[34] Chatterjee S, Basak P, Das P, Das M, Pereira JA, Dutta RK, Chakladar M, Law S, Chaudhuri S. Primitive Sca-1 positive bone marrow HSC in mouse model of aplastic anemia: A comparative study through flowcytometric analysis and scanning electron microscopy. *Stem Cell Int, 2010,* doi:10.4061/2010/614395 1-7.

[35] Epting CL, Lopez JE, Shen X, Liu L, Bristow J and Bernstein HS. Stem cell antigen-1 is necessary for cell-cycle withdrawal and myoblast differentiation in C2C12 cells._*J. of Cell Sci*, 2004,117, 6185-6195.

[36] Shen H, Boyer M and Cheng T. Flow Cytometry-Based Cell Cycle Measurement of Mouse Hematopoietic Stem and Progenitor Cells. *Hematopoietic Stem Cell Protocols,* 2008, 430, 77-86.

In: Stem Cells in Disease
Editor: Prasad S. Koka

ISBN: 978-1-62257-169-7
© 2012 Nova Science Publishers, Inc.

Chapter XV

Foreword: Stem Cell Applications and Tissue Engineering Approaches in Sports Medicine - From Bench to Bedside

Wasim S. Khan
University College London Institute of Orthopaedic and Musculoskeletal Sciences, Royal National Orthopaedic Hospital, Stanmore, Middlesex, United Kingdom

Abstract

Musculoskeletal tissue is frequently damaged or lost in sports injuries. Although surgery has been successful in repairing, realigning and replacing damaged musculoskeletal structures, the challenge of the coming years is to establish whether a paradigm shift from fixation towards regeneration of tissue is possible, clinically feasible and financially viable. There has been an increasing interest in stem cell applications and tissue engineering approaches in surgical practice to deal with damaged or lost tissue caused by sports injuries [1-3]. Tissue engineering is the science of generating tissue using molecular and cellular techniques, combined with material engineering principles, to replace tissue. Although there have been developments in almost all surgical disciplines [1], the greatest advances are being made in orthopaedics, especially in sports medicine [3]. This is due to many factors including the familiarity with bone marrow derived mesenchymal stem cells.

Stem Cells

Stem cells are a self-renewing cell population that can be isolated from tissues of individuals of various ages and maintain capacity for multilineage differentiation. Protocols for the culture and, chondrogenic, osteogenic and adipogenic differentiation of bone marrow derived mesenchymal stem cells have been described [4-6]. By the end of last century, there was considerable interest in the use of mesenchymal stem cells for clinical tissue engineering applications. Unlike embryonic stem cells, the use of autologous postnatal mesenchymal stem cells is generally well accepted by society. Mesenchymal stem cells are less tumourogenic than their embryonic counterparts [7] and provide an autologous source of cells eliminating concerns regarding rejection and disease transmission. Cells with mesenchymal stem cell characteristics have been isolated from many different adult tissues including bone marrow, adipose tissue, skeletal muscle, synovial tissue, the infrapatellar fat pad, and more recently, cartilage [8-14].

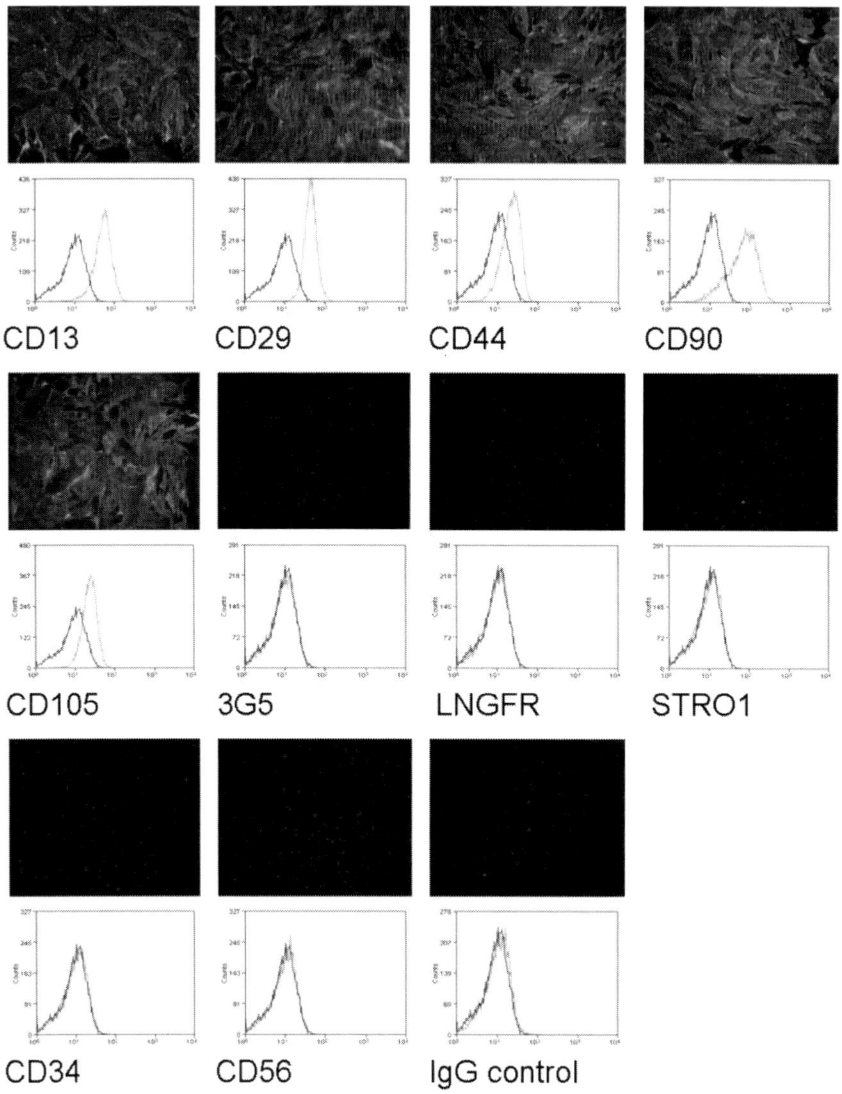

Figure 1. Cell surface staining on passage 2 synovial fat pad derived MSCs from a patient performed using a panel of antibodies and FITC-conjugated secondary antibody (green), and DAPI (blue). Results showed strong staining for CD13, CD29, CD44, CD90 and CD105, and negative staining for 3G5, LNGFR, STRO1, CD34 and CD56. No staining was observed for the IgG control. The staining pattern was confirmed by flow cytometry characterisation and showed the increase in fluorescence (green) compared with the autofluorescence (black) [9].

Although bone marrow-derived mesenchymal stem cells are multipotent with good differentiation potential, their use does have limitations that are becoming more relevant with greater clinical applicability. Bone marrow-derived mesenchymal stem cells are scarce and form only 0.001-0.01% of the total nucleated cells in bone marrow aspirates [15]. Human bone marrow-derived mesenchymal stem cells from older donors have been shown to be fewer in number, and have a reduced lifespan, proliferation and differentiation potential [16-20]. Compared to cells harvested from the bone marrow, other sources e.g. synovial fat pad derived mesenchymal stem cells are easier to obtain and may be associated with a higher yield of mesenchymal stem cells and better differentiation potential [21-24]. These cells are identified using cell surface markers as shown in Figure 1 [25], and the most commonly reported positive markers are CD105, CD90, CD44, CD73, CD29, CD13, CD146, CD106, and CD166, and the most frequently reported negative markers are CD34, CD14, CD45, CD56, CD11b and CD10 [26]. A list of antibodies and their primary role and function is outlined in Table 1. Irrespective of the merits of the various tissue sources, a large amount of work has been done on bone marrow derived cells. The therapeutic use of bone marrow-derived mesenchymal stem cells has been applied to many different tissue types that are vulnerable to sports injuries. Avenues of treatment include direct injection mesenchymal stem cells into the defect, however although minimally invasive, research has highlighted flaws which have been improved upon with the use of scaffolds.

Table 1. A list of some commonly used stem cell antibodies and their primary role and function

Antibody	Primary role and function
SH2	Monoclonal antibody that identifies CD105
SH3	Antibody that identifies CD73
SB-10	Monoclonal antibody that recognises CD166
CD10	Receptor for common acute lymphocytic leukaemia antigen
CD11b	Receptor for integrin αM
CD13	Receptor for aminopeptidase N
CD14	Lipopolysaccharide receptor for haematopoietic lineage
CD29	Receptor for integrin β1
CD34	Receptor for haematopoietic lineage
CD44	Receptor for hyaluronate
CD45	Receptor for leucocyte common antigen
CD56	Receptor for neural cell adhesion molecule (NCAM)
CD73	Receptor for a molecule involved in B cell activation
CD90	Receptor for thy-1
CD105	Receptor for endoglin; the TGF β receptor type III
CD106	Receptor for vascular cell adhesion molecule 1 (VCAM-1)
CD146	Receptor for Muc-18
CD166	Receptor for a type I membrane glycoprotein, activated leucocyte cell adhesion molecule (ALCAM)

One of the features of sports injury is the varying tissue distribution that can be affected ranging from cartilage to ligaments and tendons. This issue sets out to discuss these challenges and specifically the role of stem cells in these injuries.

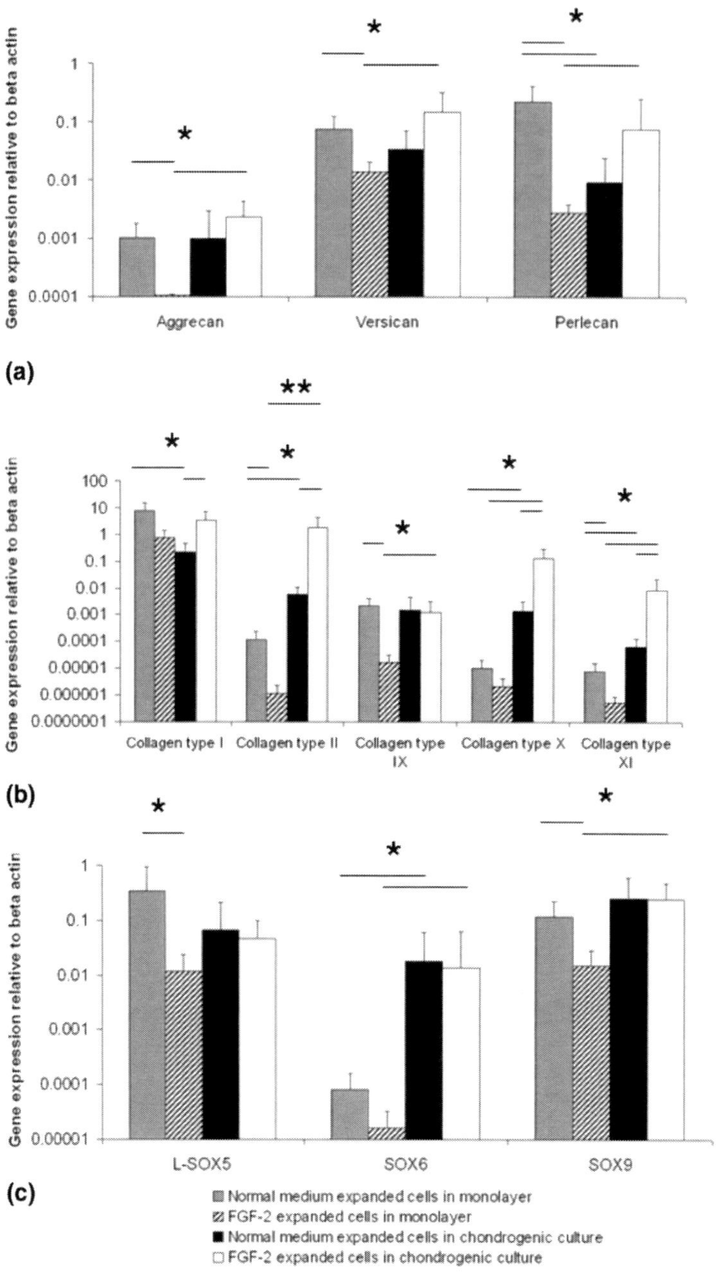

Figure 2. Gene expression in chondrogenic cultures of synovial fat pad derived MSCs. Relative gene expression for proteoglycans (a), collagens (b), and SOX genes (c) in monolayer with and without FGF-2-supplemented medium to determine basal levels and following subsequent chondrogenesis for 14 days is shown. Data are mean ± standard error of the mean (n = 6). *P <0.05, **P <0.001 (analysis of variance with Bonferroni correction). The results show that in monolayer culture, the expression of genes characteristic of chondrocytes, such as aggrecan, collagen types II, IX and XI, SOX5 and SOX9 were significantly lower in cells expanded with FGF-2 compared to those without. On subsequent chondrogenic culture, cells expanded with or without FGF-2 showed a chondrogenic response with increased levels of the chondrogenic genes. However, the cells expanded with FGF-2 showed greater increases in gene expression for collagen types I, II, X and XI compared to cells expanded without FGF-2 [22].

Cartilage

Articular cartilage is frequently damaged in sports injuries but shows only a limited capacity for repair. Focal cartilage lesions left untreated or treated inadequately, progress to more extensive secondary osteoarthritic lesions [27]. The frequent outcome for arthritis in large joints such as the knee is surgical intervention for joint replacement that although tends to be successful in older sedentary patients, the limited lifetime of prostheses makes it much less desirable for younger and more active patients [28, 29].

Non-cell based treatment options for the repair of focal cartilage lesions include abrasive chondroplasty, subchondral drilling and microfracture, but these result in the formation of fibrocartilage rather than the desired hyaline cartilage and are more appropriate for smaller lesions [30]. Autologous Chondrocyte Implantation (ACI) and Matrix-carried Autologous Chondrocyte Implantation (MACI) are currently used in clinical practice to treat larger full thickness chondral defects in the knee [31], but they involve injury to non-weight bearing cartilage. With prolonged expansion in culture chondrocytes lose their ability to proliferate and to express cartilage specific proteins [32]. Although short-term clinical results have been good, evidence suggests formation of fibrocartilage and progression of degenerative changes in the joint [32]. There are a small number of studies using mesenchymal stem cells and further in vitro and in vivo studies are needed before this treatment is optimised. There are many strategies being explored to optimize the use of mesenchymal stem cells for potential clinical applications including the use of mesenchymal stem cell sources other than bone marrow, and the use of growth factors as shown in Figure 2 [22].

Tendons and Ligaments

Tendons and ligaments are also frequently injured in sports. Due to their relatively avascular nature, repair is slow and often incomplete. Stem cells offer a new approach to augment healing of native tissues, as well as providing materials to surgically replace injured structures that are beyond repair. In this issue we discuss the various roles of stem cells in natural repair processes compared to engineered tissues to assist healing or replace tissues. Rotator cuff disease is particularly becoming more prevalent and is a significant source of pain and disability. Current methods of treating rotator cuff dysfunction have inconsistent results and there is a high rate of recurrent tear and failure. This has prompted the search for novel solutions and the use of tissue engineered strategies and approaches. In this issue, we also specifically look at the current state of tissue engineering methods for rotator cuff regeneration.

References

[1] Khan WS, Malik AA, Hardingham TE. Stem Cell Applications and Tissue Engineering Approaches in Surgical Practice. *J. Perioper Pract.* 2009;19(4):130-5.

[2] Khan WS, Johnson DS, Hardingham DS. The Potential Use of Stem Cells for Knee Articular Cartilage Repair. *Knee* 2010;17(6):369-74.

[3] Malik AA, Khan WS. Stem Cell Applications and Tissue Engineering Approaches in Orthopaedic Surgery and Musculoskeletal Medicine. *Curr. Stem Cell Res.* Ther. (in press).

[4] Freidenstein AJ, Chailakhjan RK, Lalykina KS. The development of fibroblast colonies in monolayer cultures of guinea pig bone marrow and spleen cells. *Cell Tissue Kinet.* 1970;4:393-403.

[5] Johnstone B, Hering TM, Caplan AI, Goldberg VM, Yoo JU. In vitro chondrogenesis of bone marrow-derived mesenchymal progenitor cells. *Exp. Cell Res.* 1998;238:265-72.

[6] Pittenger MF, Mackay AM, Beck SC, et al. Multilineage potential of adult human mesenchymal stem cells. *Science.* 1999;284:143-7.

[7] Raghunath J, Salacinski HJ, Sales KM, Butler PE, Seifalian M. Advancing cartilage tissue engineering: the application of stem cell technology. *Curr. Opin. Biotech.* 2005;16:503-9.

[8] Erices A, Conget P, Minguell JJ. Mesenchymal progenitor cells in human umbilical cord blood. *Br. J. Haematol.* 2000;109:235-42.

[9] De Bari C, Dell'Accio F, Tylzanowski P, Luyten FP. Multipotent mesenchymal stem cells from adult human synovial membrane. *Arthritis Rheum.* 2001;44:1928-42.

[10] Zuk PA, Zhu M, Mizino H, et al. Multilineage cells from human adipose tissue: implications for cell-based therapies. *Tissue Eng.* 2001;7:211-28.

[11] Dragoo JL, Samimi B, Zhu M, et al. Tissue-engineered cartilage and bone using stem cells from human infrapatellar fat pads. *J. Bone Joint Surg. Br.* 2003;85:740-7.

[12] Peng H, Huard J. Stem cells in the treatment of muscle and connective tissue diseases. *Curr. Opin. Pharmacol.* 2003;3:329-33.

[13] Wickham MQ, Erickson GR, Gimble JM, Vail TP, Guilak F. Multipotent stromal cells derived from the infrapatellar fat pad of the knee. *Clin. Orthop.* 2003;412:196-212.

[14] Dowthwaite GP, Bishop JC, Redman SN, et al. The surface of articular cartilage contains a progenitor cell population. *J. Cell Sci.* 2004;117:889-97.

[15] Jones EA, Kinsey SE, English A, et al. Isolation and characterisation of bone marrow multipotential mesenchymal progenitor cells. *Arthritis Rheum.* 2002;46:3349-60.

[16] Nishida S, Endo N, Yamagiwa H, Tanizawa T, Takahashi HE. Number of osteoprogenitor cells in human bone marrow markedly decreases after skeletal maturation. *J. Bone Miner Metab.* 1999;17:171-7.

[17] Muschler GF, Nitto H, Boehm CA, Easley KA. Age and gender related changes in the cellularity of human bone marrow and the prevelance of osteoblastic progenitors. *J. Orthop Res.* 2001;19:117-25.

[18] Mendes SC, Tibbe JM, Veenhof M, et al. Bone tissue-engineered implants using human bone marrow stromal cells: Effect of culture conditions and donor age. *Tissue Eng.* 2002;8:911-20.

[19] Stenderup K, Justesen J, Clausen C, Kassem M. Aging is associated with decreased maximal life span and accelerated senescence of bone marrow stromal cells. *Bone.* 2003;33:919-26.

[20] Khan WS, Marsh DR. A Literature Review on the Effects of Ageing on Mesenchymal Stem Cells. *Curr. Res. J. Biol. Sci.* 2009;1(1):1-6.

[21] Khan WS, Adesida AB, Hardingham TE. Hypoxic Conditions Increase HIF2a and Enhance Chondrogenesis in Stem Cells from the Infrapatellar Fat Pad of Osteoarthritic Patients. *Arthritis Res. Ther.* 2007;9(3): R55.

[22] Khan WS, Tew SR, Adesida AB, Hardingham TE. Human Infrapatellar Fat Pad Derived Stem Cells Express the Pericyte Marker 3G5 and Show Enhanced Chondrogenesis After Expansion in Fibroblast Growth Factor-2. *Arthritis Res. Ther.* 2008;10(4):R74.

[23] Zuk PA, Zhu M, Ashjian P, et al. Human adipose tissue is a source of multipotent stem cells. *Mol. Biol. Cell.* 2002;13:4279-95.

[24] Sakaguchi Y, Sekiya I, Yagishita K, Muneta T. Comparison of human stem cells derived from various mesenchymal tissues- Superiority of synovium as a cell source. *Arthritis Rheum.* 2005;52:2521-9.

[25] Khan WS, Adesida AB, Tew SR, Andrew JG, Hardingham TE. The epitope characterisation and the osteogenic differentiation potential of human fat pad-derived stem cells is maintained with ageing in later life. *Injury.* 2009;40(2):150-7.

[26] Mafi P, Hindocha S, Mafi R, Griffin M, Khan WS. Sources of Adult Mesenchymal Stem Cells Applicable for Musculoskeletal Applications- A Systematic Review of the Literature. *Open Orthop. J.* (in press).

[27] Parsons IM, Sonnabend DH. What is the role of joint replacement surgery? *Best Pract. Res. Clin. Rheumatol.* 2004;18:557-72.

[28] Kurtz S, Ong K, Lau E, Mowat F, Halpern M. Projections of primary and revision hip and knee arthroplasty in the United States from 2005 to 2030. *J. Bone Joint Surg.* 2007;89A:780-5.

[29] Hunziker EB. Articular cartilage repair: basic science and clinical progress; a review of the current status and prospects. *Osteoarthritis Cartilage.* 2001;10:432-63.

[30] Brittberg M, Peterson L, Sjogren-Jansson E, Tallheden T, Lindahl A. Articular cartilage engineering with autologous chondrocyte transplantation. *J. Bone Joint Surg.* 2003;85A:109-15.

[31] Cancedda R, Dozin B, Giannoni P, Quarto R. Tissue engineering and cell therapy of cartilage and bone. *Matrix Biol.* 2003;22:81-91.

[32] Clar C, Cummins E, McIntyre L, et al. Clinical and cost-effectiveness of autologous chondrocyte implantation for cartilage defects in knee joints: systematic review and economic evaluation. *Health Technol Assess.* 2005;9:1-82.

In: Stem Cells in Disease
Editor: Prasad S. Koka
ISBN: 978-1-62257-169-7
© 2012 Nova Science Publishers, Inc.

Chapter XVI

The Role of Bone Marrow Derived Mesenchymal Stem Cells in Sports Injuries

***B. A. Tucker*[1], *S. S. Karamsadkar*[2], *Wasim S. Khan*[3*] *and P. Pastides*[4]**

[1]University College London Medical School, London, UK
[2]University College London Medical School, London, UK
[3]University College London Institute of Orthopaedics and Musculoskeletal Sciences, Royal National Orthopaedic Hospital, Stanmore, Middlesex, UK
[4]University College London Institute of Orthopaedics and Musculoskeletal Sciences, Royal National Orthopaedic Hospital, Stanmore, Middlesex, UK

Abstract

The therapeutic use of bone marrow-derived mesenchymal stem cells (BM-MSCs) has been applied to many different tissue types that are vulnerable to sports injuries. Avenues of treatment include direct injection of BM-MSCs into the defect, however although minimally invasive, research has highlighted flaws which have been improved upon with the use of scaffolds. BM-MSCs have been applied via many different scaffold types, for example PLGA, collagen gel and coral each with advantages and disadvantages of which can be improved through further research. As a cell source for tissue engineering, BM-MSCs are ideal due to the minimal invasion of aspiration, high *in vitro* proliferation rate and the ability to maintain their differentiating capacity. The vast majority of these studies are at the small animal stage and therefore further work using larger animal models, and ideally humans is required.

Keywords*:* Scaffold, injection, cell culture, differentiation, integration

* Corresponding Author: Mr Wasim S Khan, Clinical Lecturer, University College London Institute of Orthopaedics and Musculoskeletal Science, Royal National Orthopaedic Hospital, Stanmore, Middlesex, London, HA7 4LP, UK. Telephone number: +44 (0) 7791 025554. Fax number: +44 (0) 20 8570 3864. E-mail address: wasimkhan@doctors.org.uk.

Introduction

Bone marrow-derived mesenchymal stem cells (BM-MSCs) have been implicated in the repair and regeneration of musculoskeletal injury. The multi-potential nature gives BM-MSCs adipogenic, chondrogenic and osteogenic properties (Pittenger et al. 1999, Charbord et al. 2010, Kagami et al. 2011).

Musculoskeletal injury is a common consequence occurrence in sport. 3% of all acute Scandinavian hospital visits are sport related with 22.5 per 1000 inhabitants acquiring a sport injury in a 12 month period (de Loes 1990;Lindqvist et al. 1996). This highlights the magnitude of sports injuries; it is essential therefore that novel, more effective treatments are continually explored. Potentially BM-MSCs are one such option. Currently a lot of research is being carried out into this area to determine this and thus a review is essential to critique and clarify their findings.

Sports injuries are commonly involved with muscle, tendon, ligament, bone, meniscus and cartilage. This review will look at the role of BM-MSCs in the treatment of these tissues.

Muscle

Sporting activity can exert abnormal biomechanics onto muscle which can lead to injury. Such injuries include muscle strain and tears which can sufficiently hinder the patient's mobility. Over three Australian football seasons the incidence of hamstring strains was 86.4 per 10,000 player hours (Orchard et al. 1998).

Muscle repair and regeneration is primarily mediated by resident multipotent stem cells. BM-MSCs have been shown to aid this process by migrating into the regenerating muscle, acting as a reserve for muscle precursors. In cases of extended damage, BM-MSCs maintain the population of more differentiated, muscle-forming precursors. However, when BM-MSCs were administered systemically they had minimal effect ,thus disproving their potential as therapy in muscle for sports injuries (Ferrari et al. 1998). Conversely, a recent study from three human donors compared the myogenic properties of MSCs from adipose tissue (AT), bone marrow (BM) and synovial membrane (SM). They concluded that AT-MSCs appear to be the best choice in view of their efficient contribution to myoregeneration and because their harvesting is less demanding than that of BM- or SM-MSCs (de la Garza-Rodea et al. 2011).

LaBarge and Blau (2002) presented evidence which clearly demonstrates that adult BM-MSCs contribute to muscle tissue in a biological stepwise progression. They noted that BM-MSCs respond to two biological stimuli; firstly they were capable of occupying the muscle stem cell niche after irradiation-induced damage, which resulted in the ablation of endogenous cells. Secondly, as a result of exercise induced damage, they participated in the regeneration of multi-nucleated muscle fibres at a frequency significantly greater than any previous reports for any bone marrow to muscle conversion. This is suggestive that BM-MSC could potentially be a reservoir of reparative cells for damages muscles.

Tendon

In addition to transmitting muscular force some tendons serve as a store of elastic energy (Fukashiro et al. 1995). This is particularly exhibited in the Achilles tendon which is essential in endurance running which therefore undergoes repetitive cyclical loading resulting in overuse injury (Kvist 1994), a consequence of which is tendon rupture. Of the total number of partial tendon ruptures, 75% were related to sporting activities many of which involved repetitive jumping and sprinting (Kvist 1994) with an odds ratio of 14.9 compared to controls. Conversely, longer distance runners are at higher risk of Achilles tendinopathy with an odds ratio of 31.2 compared to controls (Kujala et al. 2005). Other injuries include patellar tendinopathy which can give significant functional deficit and be a career ending injury (Koen et al. 2005).

One study (Chong et al. 2007) looking at rabbit Achilles tendon using a fibrin gel into which BM-MSCs were seeded, demonstrated an increased modulus of elasticity by 32% and an increased proportion of collagen type I compared to the fibrin gel alone group at 3 weeks. However, after 6 and 12 weeks no difference was observed between groups.

Also looking at rabbit Achilles tendon, Ouyang et al used 3 groups: group 1 received BM-MSCs seeded onto a poly-lactide-co-glycolide (PLGA) scaffold; group 2, a PLGA scaffold alone and group 3 received no laceration to act as a control. Group 1 exhibited greater tissue formation and remodelling compared to group 2. Both groups 1 and 2 had similar histological appearance to native tendon by 12 weeks. The tensile stiffness and modulus in group 1 was 87% and 62.6% respectively of a normal tendon whereas in group 2 they were more modest (56.4% and 52.9%). Therefore a prolonged effect is indicated. (Ouyang et al. 2003).

A collagen gel-BM-MSC composite was studied using incised rabbit patellar tendons. The results showed improved biomechanics for example stiffness increased by 15% when compared to the cell-free controls. 40% of the treatment group expressed more physiological, well integrated collagen. However the remaining 60% of specimens showed no differences in appearance to rabbits receiving collagen gel alone. This study therefore indicates BM-MSCs have an advantageous biomechanical effect which is not translated histologically (Awad et al. 1999).

Damage at the tendon bone interface was also explored (Ouyang et al. 2004) using fibrin glue seeded with BM-MSCs and just fibrin glue in the control leg. In the control group a fibrovascular interface tissue was visible, which by 6 weeks showed some perpendicular collagen type I and III fibres similar to Sharpeys fibres. The treatment group in comparison had more perpendicular collagen fibres illustrating accelerated tendon healing and consisted of collagen type I, II and III thus demonstrating their ability to promote fibrocartilage-like tissue formation which aids in the healing process.

Further to the above findings, Gulotta et al (2010) showed that MSCs can be modified further to better tendon repair. Using sixty rats that underwent unilateral detachment and repair of the supraspinatus tendon, thirty animals received MSCs in a fibrin glue carrier and 30 received adenoviral MT1-MMP (Ad-MT1-MMP)-transduced MSCs. At four weeks, the Ad-MT1-MMP group had more statistically significant more fibrocartilage, higher ultimate load to failure, higher ultimate stress to failure and higher stiffness values as compared with the other group.

Cyclic loading of tendons treated with MSCs may also increase the mechanical properties. Using acellurised rabbit paw flexor tendons, three different groups of were compared; fresh tendons and tendons reseeded with either MSCs or fibroblasts (Angelidis et al. 2010). Half of them underwent either cyclical loading or were left in stationary incubation for 5 days. The ultimate tensile stress and elastic modulus of loaded tendons were significantly higher than all the tendon groups in the incubation group and comparable to the cyclically loaded fresh tendons.

The results from these studies show improved biomechanical properties of the tendon when BM-MSCs are inserted. This may simply be due to an increased cross sectional area provided by the cells. However, these results were not always seen histologically. In relation to a normal tendon, these results are not very significant, for example, Awad et al (1999) found the modulus, maximum stress and strain energy for the treated repairs were only 7%, 16% and 32% respectively of normal patellar tendons. The studies indicate BM-MSCs can be used to increase the rate of tendon healing but have varying effects on the final outcome of the tendon.

Ligament

Ligaments are essential where movement is exaggerated and forceful, as seen in sports, as they stabilise joints and guide them through their normal range of motion. Additionally, they act as a proprioceptive input into the nervous system. This allows for the coordination of complex movement required in sport (Frank 2004).

Injuries to ligaments are very common in athletes, particularly those in the knee, namely the medial collateral and anterior cruciate ligaments (ACL). ACL tears can be caused by direct blows to the outside of the knee as occurring in contact sports or by torsional forces created at the knee whilst the foot is firmly planted on the ground or upon landing. The annual incidence of ACL injury in Denmark is 3 per 10,000 inhabitants with a greater frequency in athletes (Nielsen et al. 1991). ACL injuries dominate some sports, making up 43% of all soccer related injuries in Sweden. These can be career ending with only 30% of soccer players active in the sport three years after injury (Roos et al. 1995). Ligament injuries do not only threaten immediate sporting careers but can have future implications such as increased risk of osteoarthritis (OA) (Gillquist et al. 1999).

Effective treatment is essential for the successful recovery of athletes and their return back to sport. In cases of severe tears or complete rupture, surgery is a viable option. This involves either primary repair by suturing the ligament (Gobbi et al. 2009) or reconstruction using extra- or intra-articular tendon grafts therefore causing donor site morbidity. BM-MSCs potentially enhance the efficacy of some of the current treatments (Lim et al. 2004) or may act as a treatment in their own right (Kanaya et al. 2007). When comparing BM-MSCs to ACL fibroblasts and skin fibroblasts, BM-MSCs showed the greatest proliferation and collagen production. However, these results have been yielded from just one animal (Van Eijk et al. 2004).

One study(Kanaya et al. 2007) used partially torn ACLs of 98 rats to explore the role of intra-articularly injected BM-MSCs. The right ACLs were partially transected and a sham operation carried out on the left. One group then received autologous BM-MSCs suspended in phosphate buffered solution (PBS) and the control group an equal amount of pure PBS. The ultimate failure load of the femur-ACL-tibia complex of the BM-MSC group (70.5%) was significantly higher than the PBS group (58.2%). The transected area of the ACLs in the PBS group retracted, with no reperative tissue at any time points after surgery. Conversely, in the BM-MSC group no retraction was observed, with reparative tissue containing BM-MSCs spanning the transection as early as 2 weeks post surgery. A histological grading score for the BM-MSC group was significantly better than for the PBS group. The BM-MSCs survived the intra-articular environment and enhanced the healing of partial tears resulting in more biomechanically and histologically viable results.

Ligament reconstruction has several drawbacks including early tendon autograft pull-out andBM-MSCs have been investigated in enhancing this fixation. Bilateral ACL reconstructions using hamstring tendon autografts were carried out on rabbits. The treatment limb autograft was coated with autologous BM-MSCs using a fibrin glue carrier. The control limb autograft received only fibrin glue. At 8 weeks post surgery the control had a distinct fibrous interface with the bone, containing collagen type I and III with occasional fibres resembling Sharpey's fibres bridging the gap. Conversely the treatment group had matured zones of cartilage rich in collagen type II resembling normal entheses. The overall mean failure load (66%) and overall mean stiffness (51%) were significantly higher in the BM-MSC reconstructions compared with the controls. Nevertheless, as many as 44% of BM-MSC limbs failed by pullout, leaving this issue unresolved. Regardless, their use has resulted in more physiologic and biomechanically stronger ACL reconstructions (Lim et al. 2004).

BM-MSCs have clearly been defined as optimum cell sources for ligament repair, enhancing the end result biomechanically, histologically and physiologically. Their methods of application have greatly varied yet their role is synonymous thus illustrating their potential for future therapy.

Bone

Demanding sports such as running, places multiple, high impact loading cycles on bone. This leads to the accumulation of micro-fractures which propagate to form bigger cracks. The annual incidence of stress fracture in athletes is 21.1%, making up 20% of all musculoskeletal injuries obtained. Sprints, hurdles and jumps are commonly associated with foot fractures; as is middle and long distance running with long bone and pelvic fractures (Bennell et al. 1996).

Closed tibial fractures take on average 28 weeks to heal (Wiss et al. 1995), inhibiting the athlete from training during this time, making rapid effective treatment essential. Scaffolds seeded with BM-MSCs have been assessed for their potential as a treatment which would increase the rate and quality of fracture healing.

The results of using a coral scaffold with and without BM-MSCs were compared to fresh bone marrow (FBM) seeded scaffolds and to untreated bone defects in sheep. The BM-MSC seeded scaffold allowed bone deposition at the same rate as scaffold degradation; it was the only composite to allow bony union to occur after 16 weeks which resembled physiological bone. Conversely, scaffold degradation outweighed bone deposition in coral and FBM scaffolds. Nevertheless the coral scaffold was osseoconductive resulting in bone deposition in the medullary centre (Petite et al. 2000).

In a different study evaluating the effect of BM-MSCs in healing rates of femoral fractures in rats, a porous hydroxyapatite-tricalcium phosphate ceramic cylinder was used. In one leg the rat received the cylinder alone and in the contralateral leg received the cylinder embedded with BM-MSCs and in some rats the defects were left empty to act as controls. In all control rats non-union occurred. By 12 weeks union was complete in the BM-MSC group with bony ingrowth into the pores of the scaffold displaying increased strength (215%), stiffness (245%) and torsional energy absorbed (212%) compared to the scaffold side. On the scaffold side the pores of the implant were predominantly filled with fibrous tissue(Bruder et al. 1998b).

In a similarly designed study, a ceramic cylinder (65% hydroxyapatite, 35% β-tricalcium phosphate) was again used but to investigate fracture healing in a dog model. The dogs either received a cylinder alone, a ceramic cylinder with BM-MSCs or no treatment. The untreated group all displayed atrophic non-union with little or no bone formation and no visible callus. In the dogs with cell-free cylinders union occurred between the implant and the bone cortex in ten of twelve dogs by 16 weeks however no callus was visible and most of the pores were filled with fibrous tissue. In the BM-MSC group, bone was distributed evenly throughout the implant and integrated well with the host bone. By 8 weeks solid union had occurred in all 12 bone implant interfaces with a continuous bridge of mineralized bone surrounding the defect. An osseous callus formed around the implant and the adjacent host bone in 84% of specimens. The implant pores were filled with woven or lamellar bone in direct contact with the ceramic (Bruder et al. 1998a).

In mice tibial fractures inserted BM-MSCs were shown to improve fracture callus strength, ultimate displacement and reduced callus stiffness compared to cell-free controls. These combined decrease the structural rigidity thereby decreasing the brittleness of the tissue. The BM-MSCs also caused an increased amount of bone, callus volume and mineralisation. Thus a more organised bridge is formed between the bone ends, improving the healing process and the final properties of the bone (Granero-Molto et al. 2009).

Ben-David et al (2011) proved the efficacy of a gelatin-based hydrogel scaffold to support osteogenic differentiation of rat bone marrow-derived mesenchymal stem cells. MSCs which were cultured on hydrogel under osteogenic conditions demonstrated typical osteogenic differentiation which included cluster formation with positive Alizarin Red staining, sedimentation of calcium phosphate confirmed by scanning electron microscopy and spectroscopy and expression of mRNA osteogenic markers.

The preferred treatment for large bone defects is currently autologous bone grafts. However, the supply of suitable bone is limited and its collection is painful, with a risk of infection, nerve damage, and a loss of function. BM-MSC embedded scaffolds offer a safer, less destructive alternative, and as illustrated, produce good results in terms of bone deposition, callus biomechanics and time to union.

Meniscus

The menisci function to dissipate stress over a larger area, decreasing the force felt by the articular cartilage; reducing the risk of osteoarthritis. They also function to absorb shock during dynamic loading and assist in joint lubrication. These functions are served by the ability of the menisci to withstand rotational, translational and compressive forces(Walsh et al. 1999). Additionally the menisci provide stability to the injured knee when the cruciate ligaments are deficient (Fithian et al. 1990).

Meniscal tears often occur in conjunction with ACL injuries with an incidence of 62% (Noyes et al. 1980). Medial meniscal tears, ACL injuries and medial collateral ligament tears form the O'Donoghue triad (O'Donaghue 1950)-a common injury in high contact sports. Lesions in the vascular region of the meniscus heal well but lesions in the avascular area are unable to repair. A treatment option for large tears is allograft but the results of this are variable. A further option is isolating meniscal cells from the resected region however the quantity and quality of these cells is often poor. Prosthetic replacement has received promising results from early animal studies but further studies are needed. Another approach currently being researched is the use of BM-MSCs seeded scaffolds.

In one study a fibrin glue scaffold was inserted into rats with and without BM-MSCs, with a further group receiving no treatment. The control group showed many polyglonal cells by 12 weeks in the defect, however no extracellular matrix (ECM) was synthesised. The cell-free scaffold group by 12 weeks had many small round cells within the fibrin glue which were synthesising ECM in 25% of specimens. The BM-MSC group by 12 weeks contained an abundance of round cells within the scaffold which were surrounded completely by ECM in 75% specimens and cartilage-like tissue could be seen (Izuta et al. 2001).

In another study, circular meniscal punch defects of up to 2 mm were created in the avascular zone of rabbit menisci and left empty or filled with hyaluronan-collagen composite matrices without cells, loaded with platelet-rich plasma, autologous bone marrow, or autologous mesenchymal stem cells (Zellner et al. 2010). In some experiments, matrices with stem cells were precultured in chondrogenic medium for 14 days before implantation. Rabbits were then allowed free cage movement after surgery for up to 12 weeks. Untreated defects and defects treated with cell-free implants had muted fibrous healing responses. Neither bone marrow nor platelet-rich plasma loaded in matrices produced improvement in healing compared with cell-free implants. However, mesenchymal stem cells in hyaluronan-collagen composite matrices stimulated the development of completely integrated meniscus-like repair tissue within the avascular zones.

Alternatively, the effect of cell-seeded collagen type I scaffolds have been investigated in rabbits (Walsh et al. 1999). The rabbits all underwent bilateral partial menisectomy and then either received no treatment, autogenous periosteal graft, type I collagen sponge or a type I collagen sponge with BM-MSCs. Osteoarthritic changes developed in all groups, particularly at the later time points. These were increased by the autogenous periosteal graft and decreased with the collagen scaffold, especially when used with BM-MSCs. The addition of BM-MSCs to the collagen sponge enhanced fibrocartilage regeneration with mature bundles of collagen and proteoglycan. The transition from regenerated to normal meniscus was smooth and well-healed.

Rabbits with meniscal resection of the pars intermedia received either a hyaluronon/gelatine scaffold alone, or with BM-MSCs or received no treatment. The BM-MSC knees had high cellularity of chondrocyte-like morphology and extensive ECM resembling that of normal meniscus however the degree of order and collagen fibril diameter was lower. There was nearly complete filling of the defects with good integration of the scaffold. The amount of fibrocartilage seen was significantly more than seen in the empty scaffold. The cell-free scaffold group had a partially filled defect with good integration with the repair tissue; however the ECM laid down by the cells did not contain any type II collagen. The control group receiving no form of treatment had a limited healing response, leaving the majority of the defect unfilled (Angele et al. 2008).

The effect of BM-MSCs when applied within a blood clot by sutures to a defected middle third of meniscus in goats was investigated. Group 1 of this study received just sutures, group 2 sutures and a blood clot, group 3 sutures, a blood clot and BM-MSCs and the final group received nothing. Group 1 had 4 healed and 4 partially healed knees (3 at 75% and 1 at 50%) with no failed repairs. The repair tissue was unorganized with hypercellular focal areas composed largely of macrophages, giant cells and leukocytes. In group 2 5 were healed and 2 patially healed (by 50%) and 1 failed repair. The repaired section was more organised with less cellularity than in group 1. Group 3 had 3 healed, 1 partially healed (25%) and 4 failed repairs. The repair site had reduced cellularity, increased matrix and increased orientation of the matrix. Group 4 had 7 knees with no healing and 1 partial healing (25%). This study found BM-MSCs were detrimental to meniscal healing. (Port et al. 1996)

These studies, except study 4, demonstrate the positive effects BM-MSCs can have on meniscal healing by producing ECM. Their ability to withstand the avascular conditions makes them an ideal treatment for this area. The differing results shown by Port et al may be due to different study design for example inserting the cells into the fibrin clot *in vivo* rather than preculturing them within the scaffold which causes greater cell retention.

Cartilage

Articular cartilage provides low friction, wear resistant joint surfaces. Their high load bearing and shock absorbing capacity are essential to withstand the excessive mechanical force experienced across joints during sporting activity (Williams et al. 2007). Cartilage lesions are common in sport analysis showed 49% were caused by athletic activity (Aroen et al. 2004). Once damaged cartilage is vulnerable due to its poor ability to heal, even small defects may degenerate over time, ultimately causing osteoarthritis (Redman et al. 2005). Thus, treatment to enhance healing is essential to maintain the short and long term function of the joint.

Current treatments such as arthroscopic management, autologous osteochondral transfer and autologous chondrocyte implantation (ACI) have shown positive results but have several drawbacks. For example, Nejadnik et al compared the use of BM-MSCs to ACI. This showed significant clinical improvement for both treatments with no significant difference between them. Therefore clinically, BM-MSCs are as effective as ACI in cartilage repair with the benefit of BM-MSCs requiring less invasive surgery, minimised donor site morbidity, 1 less anaesthesia application and reduced costs (Nejadnik et al. 2010). Abrasion arthroplasty or microfracture treatment causes formation of reparative tissue. However it is fibrous in nature and thus very different from normal articular cartilage both functionally and morphologically (Hunt et al. 2002). Similarly, osteochondral transfer is limited by the cartilage defect size (Hangody et al. 2003;Jakob et al. 2002) and causes donor site morbidity (Redman et al. 2005). Thus, to avoid these limitations, BM-MSCs have been investigated as possible alternative treatment.

Im et al. suspended BM-MSCs in Ham F-12 medium before injecting into full thickness cartilage defects in the patellar groove of rabbits. The control defects received cell free medium. At 14 weeks the BM-MSC group contained reparative tissue resembling articular cartilage with a fully repaired subchondral bone layer. However, the reparative tissue of the control defects was thin, irregular and undifferentiated with less matrix collagen type II. Histological grading scores indicated the treatment group (14.8) performed significantly better than the control (8.9). Nevertheless, junctions between the reparative tissue and the surrounding cartilage were identifiable and could become a starting point for degeneration beyond the 14 week period. Furthermore, leakage of cells from the defect occurred- a consequence of the repair technique. Thus, the findings suggest the use of BM-MSCs in this way enhances cartilage repair but does not guarantee cartilaginous healing (Im et al. 2001).

Using a rabbit model Wakitani et al. (1994), BM-MSCs or periosteum derived mesenchymal stem cells (PD-MSCs) were seeded into a type 1 collagen gel and implanted into large (3x6mm), full thickness osteochondral defects located in the weight bearing surface of the medial femoral condyle. The contralateral knee served as a control with its defect either left empty or filled with collagen free gel. Upon analysis, relative to the control groups, the BM-MSC group produced reparative tissue more similar to hyaline cartilage, showing better integration by 4 weeks. However, by 24 weeks the quality of this tissue progressively declined as the thickness of the articular cartilage portion reduced below that of normal cartilage. The underlying subchondral bone however, was fully restored; histological grading scores indicated a markedly inferior repair throughout the assessment for the control group. Repair tissue from the cell treated group was stiffer than the control but less so than normal hyaline cartilage. PD-MSCs yielded results very similar to BM-MSCs but in addition exhibited a progressive increase in surface irregularity(Wakitani et al. 1994).

Hybrid designs for scaffolds have also been conceived. Shao et al. (2006) seeded BM-MSCs into a Polycaprolactone (PCL) scaffold for the cartilage part and a tricalcium phosphate-reinforced PCL scaffold for the bone portion. With fibrin glue, the seeded scaffolds were implanted into large osteochondral defects in the load bearing medial femoral condyle of rabbits. Controls received a cell free scaffold. After 6 months, repair tissue from the BM-MSC group was well integrated with host bone in all specimens. Most samples were hyaline like in nature with identifiable collagen type II and glycosaminoglycan, and an almost normal physiological stiffness. Conversely, unlike the control defects were incompletely filled with less stiff, predominantly fibrous repair tissue with little resemblance to cartilage or bone. Nevertheless, some repair tissues in the BM-MSC group experienced fissures and cracks at the integration site and a lack of typical zonal arrangement (Shao et al. 2006).

Similarly, repair of large osteochondral defects has been attempted using poly-lactic-glycolic acid (PLGA) scaffolds seeded with BM-MSCs (Uematsu et al. 2005). Bilateral, full thickness defects were made in the femoropatellar groove of rabbit knee joints. Control defects were treated with cell free PLGA scaffolds or left empty. The findings of this study were similar to the previous scaffold studies. Although in support of Wakitani et al, it did not, however, report the trend in thinning of the reparative cartilage at 12 weeks. Unlike Shao et al there were signs of zonal organisation of the newly formed cartilage. The PLGA scaffold also provided a way of preventing leaking of the cells from the defect as seen with injection procedures (Im et al. 2001). Additionally, the scaffold promoted cell differentiation, structure and orientation. However, there were unsuccessful cartilage repairs in the treatment group due to the detachment of the scaffold. Thus this procedure has scope for improvement. The repair of large osteochondral defects may be achievable when used in the presence of other growth factors. Wang et al (2010) showed that when the defect size was enlarged to 4 mm, it could not be effectively repaired by the TGF-β1 absent constructs but could be completely repaired by the TGF-β1 loaded constructs.

Contrary to current treatments, BM-MSCs have been implicated in repair of larger cartilage defects, in a reduction of invasiveness and the production of physiologically comparable reparative tissue. The quality of articular cartilage regeneration is varied where as successful subchondral bone regeneration is consistent across studies. The use of scaffolds should be an important consideration in any future therapy due to its synergistic role with BM-MSCs. However these proposed procedures still have profound flaws that must be overcome before any clinical treatment is developed.

Osteoarthritis

OA is both a consequence and causative factor of sport injuries (Buckwalter et al. 2004). Typical sport injuries such as isolated ACL ruptures affect the biomechanics of the medial side thus stressing the medial meniscus which ultimately leads to premature medial compartment OA (Sherman et al. 1988). Athletes involved in endurance, mixed and power sports are approximately 2.5 times more at risk of hospital admission due to OA (Kujala et al. 1994). There is currently no established regenerative treatment for OA, several studies have implicated BM-MSCs as potential therapy.

One such study (Murphy et al. 2003)practiced a scaffold-free approach using autologous, culture expanded BM-MSCs added to sodium hyaluronan. The suspension was injected intrarticularly. The ACL and medial meniscus were removed from goats to induce OA. The subjects were randomized into a treatment group receiving BM-MSC seeded sodium hyaluronan and a control group receiving just sodium hyaluronan. At 20 weeks the reparative tissue in the control was disorganised and attached to the proximal tibia. Substantial fibrillation, loss of ECM and osteophytic remodelling were apparent relative to the to contralateral joint. In comparison, the tissue in the treatment group was organised and detached from the femoral and tibial surfaces. The meniscal insertional ligaments were repaired with formation of functional entheses with the tibial bone. Gross and histological osteoarthritic changes were reduced compared to control groups suggesting BM-MSCs had a protective effect. Regardless of this reduction, significant OA lesions and absent repair of the severed ACLs were observed in both groups at 20 weeks.

Twenty four patients with medial unicompartmental OA, when undergoing high tibial osteotomy, received either BM-MSC seeded collagen gel, or collagen gel alone onto an articular cartilage defect on the medial femoral condyle. Clinical outcomes were measured using the Hospital for Special Surgery (HSS) knee rating scale. After a 16 month follow-up period after surgery, significant improvement was observed within each group, with no significant differences between groups. 42 weeks after surgery the repair tissue in the control group had an irregular surface, poor matrix production and areas of visible underlying bone. In the treatment group some areas of the tissue resembled hyaline cartilage with widely distributed matrix production. These observations were quantified using an arthroscopic and histologic grading scale: the treatment group scored 75% as opposed to the 50% achieved by the controls, this difference was significant.

No significant difference in clinical improvements was observed. Nevertheless histological analysis reported a significant improvement when BM-MSCs were used. However this conclusion is based on a small study sample with further omission of subjects at the analysis stage (Wakitani et al. 2002).

In a further study (Grigolo et al. 2009)rabbits were allocated to 3 groups: group 1 underwent a sham operation; group 2 had an ACL transection with no further treatment; group 3, in addition to an ACL transection, received BM-MSCs seeded onto a Hyaff-11 scaffold (BM-MSCs-HA) in the left femoral condyle and a hyaff-11 scaffold (HA) alone in the right. All animals experiencing ACL transection developed OA. The BM-MSC-HA group produced hyaline-like cartilage which featured collagen type II intra- and extracellularly; no collagen type I or MMP-1 was present. An inferior degree of tissue remodelling occurred in the HA group, with only mild amounts of collagen type II extracellularly. Additionally, uncharacteristic of normal cartilage, MMP-1 and type I collagen were present. In the BM-MSC-HA group mild surface irregularities and a mild loss of proteoglycans occurred. This took place to a greater extent in the HA group.

Osteoarthritis cannot be cured by BM-MSCs, they can merely hinder the progression of degeneration. This hindrance is consistently observed at a histological level, however it is not always translated clinically.

Conclusion

Several characteristics of BM-MSCs make them ideal candidates for treatment of sports injuries. Unlike other sources of stem cells, bone marrow is easy to obtain requiring minimal donor site morbidity, invasiveness and anaesthetic. For example, to obtain ACL fibroblasts an arthroscopy is required in an already injured knee (Van Eijk et al. 2004), whereas BM-MSCs can be aspirated from the iliac crest. BM-MSCs are relatively easy to isolate due to their superior ability to bind to tissue culture plastic relative to other bone marrow cells (Petite et al. 2000). Once isolated, BM-MSCs can be easily proliferated *in vitro* without losing their capacity for differentiation. Due to their multi-lineage potential, repair of complex injuries is possible. For example, when injected into a knee joint with injuries to the ACL, medial meniscus and cartilage of the femoral condyles, BM-MSCs mobilize to affected areas and contribute to regeneration(Agung et al. 2006). Their autologous nature eliminates the issue of immunoreactions and ethical problems.

In comparison with aminiotic fluid (AF-MSC) and embryonic umbilical cord MSCs (EUC-MSC), BM-MSCs undergo a higher degree of mineralisation when differentiating down an osteogenic lineage. They undergo a moderate chondrogenic differentiation as opposed to an almost non-existent differentiation by EUC-MSCs and an occasional differentiation by AF-MSCs (Lovati et al. 2011).

BM-MSC advantages are further enhanced by their insertion. In natural wound healing the activation of BM-MSCs is the rate-limiting step. Thus implanting already activated BM-MSCs overcomes this stage and increases the rate of healing (Kavalkovich et al. 2000).

The studies explored in this review highlight several considerations. A high density of BM-MSCs is needed to optimise the desired results. The majority of these studies used small animal models to demonstrate the effects of BM-MSCs. This reduces the applicability of the findings to a clinical setting due to the different gait patterns and biomechanics felt by the joint tissues. The injuries inflicted were not parallel with clinical injury. Further work in larger animal and ideally human models should be explored before any clinical relevance can be assessed.

Any successful future therapy is likely to involve the use of scaffolds, of which their efficacy has been illustrated by these studies. Scaffolds provide architectural support and prevent leakage of cells from the defect. However, the reparative effect of BM-MSCs when injected alone is also documented.

References

Agung, M., Ochi, M., Yanada, S., Adachi, N., Izuta, Y., Yamasaki, T., and Toda, K. 2006, "Mobilization of bone marrow-derived mesenchymal stem cells into the injures tissues after intraarticular injection and their contribution to tissue regeneration.", *Knee Surg Sports Traumatol Arthrosc*, vol. 14, pp. 1307-1314.

Angele, P., Johnstone, B., Kujat, R., Zellner, J., Nerlich, M., Goldberg, V., and Yoo, J. 2008, "Stem cell based tissue engineering for meniscus repair", *Journal of Biomedical Materials Research Part A*, vol. 85A, no. 2, pp. 445-455.

Angelidis, I.K., Thorfinn, J., Connolly, I.D., Lindsey, D., Pham, H.M., Chang, J. 2010 "Tissue Engineering of Flexor Tendons: The Effect of a Tissue Bioreactor on Adipoderived Stem Cell–Seeded and Fibroblast-Seeded Tendon Constructs.", *The Journal of Hand Surgery*, vol. 35, no. 9, pp. 1466-1472.

Aroen, A., Loken, S., Heir, S., Alvik, E., Ekeland, A., Granlund, O., and Engebretsen, L. 2004, "Articular cartilage lesions in 993 consecutive knee arthroscopies", *American journal of sports medicine*, vol. 32, pp. 211-215.

Awad, H., Butler, D., Boivin, G., Smith, F., Malaviya, P., Huibregtse, B., and Caplan, A. 1999, "Autologous mesenchymal stem cell-mediated repair of tendon.", *Tissue Engineering*, vol. 5, no. 3, pp. 267-277.

Ben-David, D., Kizhner, T.A., Kohler, T., Müller, R., Livne, E., Srouji, S. 2011, "Cell-scaffold transplant of hydrogel seeded with rat bone marrow progenitors for bone regeneration.", *Journal of Cranio-Maxillofacial Surgery*, vol. 39, no. 5, pp. 364-371.

Bennell, KL., Malcolm, SA., Thomas, SA., Wark, JD., and Brukner, PD. 1996, "The Incidence and Distribution of Stress Fractures in Competitive Track and Field Athletes", *The American Journal of Sports Medicine*, vol. 24, no. 2, pp. 211-217.

Bruder, SP., Kraus, KH., Goldberg, V., and Kadiyala, S. 1998a, "The Effect of Implants Loaded with Autologous Mesenchymal Stem Cells on the Healing of Canine Segmental Bone Defects", *Journal of Bone and Joint Surgery*, vol. 80, no. 7, pp. 985-996.

Bruder, SP., Kurth, AA., Shea, M., Hayes, WC., Jaiswal, N., and Kadiyala, S. 1998b, "Bone regeneration by implantation of purified, culture-expanded human mesenchymal stem cells", *Journal of Orthopaedic Research*, vol. 16, no. 2, pp. 155-162.

Buckwalter, JA. and Martin, JA. 2004, "Sports and osteoarthritis", *Current Opinion in Rheumatology*, vol. 16, no. 5.

Charbord, P., Livne, E., Gross, G., Häupl, T., Neves, N.M., Marie, P., Bianco, P., Jorgensen, C. 2010. "Human bone marrow mesenchymal stem cells: a systematic reappraisal via the genostem experience.", *Stem Cell Reviews,* vol. 7(1): pp. 32-42.

Chong, A., Ang, A., Goh, J., Hui, J., Lim, A., Lee, E., and Lim, B. 2007, "Bone marrow-derived mesenchymal stem cells influenced early tendon-healing in a rabbit Achiles tendon model.", *The Journal of Bone and Joint Surgery*, vol. 89, pp. 74-81.

de la Garza-Rodea, A.S., van der Velde-van Dijke, L., Boersma, H., Gonçalves, M.A., van Bekkum, D.W., de Vries, A.A., Knaän-Shanzer, S. 2011, "Myogenic properties of human mesenchymal cells derived from three different sources.", *Cell Transplantation.* (in press).

de Loes, M. 1990, "Medical treatment and costs of sports-related injuries in a total population", *Int. J. Sports Med.*, vol. 11, no. 1, pp. 66-72.

Ferrari, G., Cusella-De Angelis, G., Coletta, M., Paolucci, E., Stornaiuolo, A., Cossu, G., and Mavilio, F. 1998, "Muscle regeneration by bone marrow-derived myogenic progenitors", *Science*, vol. 279, pp. 1528-1530.

Fithian, DC., Kelly, M., and Mow, V. 1990, "Material Properties and Structure-Function Relationships in the Menisci", *Clinical Orthopaedics and Related Research*, vol. 252.

Frank, C. 2004, "Ligament structure, physiology and function", *J Musculoskel Neuron Interact*, vol. 4, no. 2, pp. 199-201.

Fukashiro, S., Komi, P., Jarvinen, M., and Miyashita, M. 1995, "In vivo achilles tendon loading' during jumping in humans", *European Journal of Applied Physiology and Occupational Physiology*, vol. 71, no. 5, pp. 453-458.

Gillquist, J. and Messner, K. 1999, "Anterior cruciate ligament reconstruction and the long-term incidence of gonarthrosis", *Sports Med.*, vol. 27, no. 3, pp. 143-156.

Gobbi, A., Bathan, L., and Boldrini, L. 2009, "Primary Repair Combined With Bone Marrow Stimulation in Acute Anterior Cruciate Ligament Lesions", *The American journal of sports medicine*, vol. 37, no. 3, pp. 571-578.

Granero-Molto, F., Weis, JA., Miga, M., Landis, B., Myers, T., O'Rear, L., Longobardi, L., Duco Jansen, E., Mortlock, D., and Spagnoli, A. 2009, "Regenerative effects of transplanted mesenchymal stem cells in fracture healing.", *Stem cells*, vol. 27, pp. 1887-1898.

Grigolo, B., Lisignoli, G., Desando, G., Cavallo, C., Marconi, E., Tschon, M., Giavaresi, G., Fini, M., Giardino, R., and Facchini, A. 2009, "Osteoarthritis treated with mesenchymal stem cells on hyaluronon-based scaffold in rabbit.", *Tissue Engineering*, vol. 15, no. 4, pp. 647-658.

Gulotta, L.V., Kovacevic, D., Montgomery, S., Ehteshami, J.R., Packer, J.D., Rodeo, S.A. 2010, "Stem cells genetically modified with the developmental gene MT1-MMP improve regenration of the supraspinatustendon-to-bone insertion site.", *American Journal of Sports Medicine,* vol. 38(7): pp. 1429-1437.

Hangody, L., Rathonyi, G., Duska, Z., Vasarhelyi, G., Fules, P., and Modis, L. 2003, "Autologous Osteochondral Mosaicplasty: Surgical technique", *Journal of Science and Medicine in Sport*, vol. 85a, no. 2, pp. 25-32.

Hunt, S., Jazrawi, L., and Sherman, O. 2002, "Arthroscopic management of osteoarthritis of the knee", *J Am Acad Orthop Surg*, vol. 10, pp. 356-363.

Im, G., Kim, D., Shin, J., Hyun, C., and Cho, W. 2001, "Repair of cartilage defect in the rabbit with cultured mesenchymal stem cells from bone marrow.", *Journal of Bone and Joint Surgery*, vol. 83b, pp. 289-294.

Izuta, Y., Ochi, M., Adachi, N., Deie, M., Yamasaki, T., and Shinomiya, R. 2001, "Meniscal repair using bone marrow-derived mesenchymal stem cells: experimental study using green fluorescent protein transgenic mice.", *The Knee*, vol. 12, pp. 217-223.

Jakob, R., Franz, T., Gautier, E., and Mainil-Varlet, P. 2002, "Autologous osteochondral grafting in the knee: indications, results, and reflections.", *Clin Orthop Relat Res*, vol. 401, pp. 170-184.

Kagami, H., Agata, H., Tojo, A. 2011, "Bone marrow stromal cells (bone marrow-derived multipotent mesenchymal stromal cells) for bone tissue engineering: Basic science to clinical translation" *The International Journal of Biochemistry and Cell Biology,* Volume 43, Issue 3, pp 286-289.

Kanaya, A., Deie, M., Adachi, N., Nishimori, M., Yanada, S., and Ochi, M. 2007, "Intra-articular injection of mesenchymal stromal cells in partially torn anterior cruciate ligaments in a rat model.", *Arthroscopy*, vol. 23, no. 6, pp. 610-617.

Kavalkovich, K., Murphy, J., and Barry, F. 2000, "Adhesion of mesenchymal stem cells to fibrilated osteoarthritic cartilage.", *Osteoarthritis and Cartilage*, vol. 8.

Koen, H. and Roeland, J. 2005, "Patellar tendinopathy in athletes: Current diagnostic and therapeutic recommendations", *Sports Medicine*, vol. 35, no. 1, pp. 71-87.

Kujala, U., Kaprio, J., and Sarno, S. 1994, "Osteoarthritis of weight bearing joints of lower limbs in former elite male athletes", *BMJ*, vol. 308, no. 6923, pp. 231-234.

Kujala, U., Sarna, S., and Kaprio, J. 2005, "Cumulative incidence of achilles tendon rupture and tendinopathy in male former elite athletes", *Clinical Journal of Sport Medicine*, vol. 15, no. 3, pp. 133-135.

Kvist, M. 1994, "Achilles tendon injuries in athletes", *Sports Med*, vol. 18, no. 3, pp. 173-201.

LaBarge, M.A., Blau, H.A. 2002, "Biological progression from adult bone marrow to mononucleate muscle stem cell to multinucleate muscle fiber in response to injury", *Cell*, vol. 111(4), pp. 589–601.

Lim, J., Hui, J., Li, L., Thambyah, A., Goh, J., and Lee, E. 2004, "Enhancement of tendon graft osteointegration using mesenchymal stem cells in a rabbit model of anterior cruciate ligament reconstruction.", *The Journal of Arthroscopic and Related Surgery.*, vol. 20, no. 9, pp. 899-910.

Lindqvist, K., Timpka, T., and Bjurulf, P. 1996, "Injuries during leisure physical activity in a Swedish municipality", Scand. J. Public Health, vol. 24, no. 4, pp. 282-292.

Lovati, A., Corradetti, B., Lange, C., Recordati, C., Bonacina, E., Bizzaro, D., and Cremonesi, F. 2011, "Comparison of equine bone marrow-, umbilical cord matrix and amniotic fluid-derived progenitor cells", *Veterinary Research Communications,* vol. 35, no. 2, pp. 103-121.

Murphy, J., Fink, D., Hunziker, E., and Barry, F. 2003, "Stem cell therapy in a caprine model of osteoarthritis.", *Arthritis and Rheumatism*, vol. 48, no. 12, pp. 3464-3474.

Nejadnik, H., Hui, J., Feng Choong, E., Tai, B., and Lee, E. 2010, "Autologous Bone Marrow-Derived Mesenchymal Stem Cells Versus Autologous Chondrocyte Implantation", *The American journal of sports medicine*, vol. 38, no. 6, pp. 1110-1116.

Nielsen, A. and Yde, J. 1991, "Epidemiology of acute knee injuries: a prospective hospital investigation", *J. Trauma*, vol. 31, no. 12, pp. 1644-1648.

Noyes, F., Basset, R., Grood, E., and Butler, D. 1980, "Arthroscopy in acute traumatic hemarthrosis of the knee. Incidence of anterior cruciate tears and other injuries", *The Journal of Bone and Joint Surgery*, vol. 62, pp. 687-695.

O'Donaghue, D. 1950, "Surgical treatment of fresh injuries to the major ligaments of the knee", *Journal of Bone and Joint Surgery*[Am], vol. 32, pp. 721-737.

Orchard, J., Wood, T., Seward, H., and Broad, A. 1998, "Comparison of Injuries in Elite Senior and Junior Australian Football", *Journal of Science and Medicine in Sport,* vol. 1, no. 2, pp. 83-88.

Ouyang, H. W., Goh, J. C., Thambyah, A., Teoh, S. H., and Lee, E. H. 2003, "Knitted poly-lactide-co-glycolide scaffold loaded with bone marrow stromal cells in repair and regeneration of rabbit Achilles tendon", Tissue Engineering, vol. 9, no. 3, pp. 431-439.

Ouyang, H. W., Goh, J., and Lee, E. 2004, "Use of bone marrow stromal cells for tendon graft-to-bone healing: histological and immunohistochemical studies in a rabbit model.", *The American journal of sports medicine*, vol. 32, pp. 321-327.

Petite, H., Viateau, V., Bensaid, W., Meunier, A., Pollack, C., Bourguignon, M., Oudina, K., Sedel, L., and Guillemin, G. 2000, "Tissue-engineered bone regeneration", *Nature Biotechnology,* vol. 18, pp. 959-963.

Pittenger, M., Mackay, A., Beck, S., Jaiswal, R., Douglas, R., Mosca, J., Moorman, M., Simonetti, D., Craig, S., and Marshak, D. 1999, "Multilineage Potential of Adult Human Mesenchymal Stem Cells", *Science*, vol. 284, pp. 143-147.

Port, J., Jackson, DW., Lee, TQ., and Simon, TM. 1996, "Meniscal Repair Supplemented With Exogenous Fibrin Clot and Autogenous Cultured Marrow Cells in the Goat Model", *The American journal of sports medicine*, vol. 24, no. 4, pp. 547-555.

Redman, S., Oldfield, S., and Archer, C. 2005, "Current strategies for articular cartilage repair", *European Cells and Materials,* vol. 9, pp. 23-32.

Roos, H., Ornell, M., Gardsell, P., Lohmander, L., and Lindstrand, A. 1995, "Soccer after anterior cruciate ligament injury- an incompatible combination? A national survey of incidence and risk factors and a 7-year follow up of 310 players.", *Acta Orthop Scand,* vol. 66, no. 2, pp. 107-112.

Shao, X., Goh, J., Hutmacher, D., Lee, E., and Zigang, G. 2006, "Repair of large osteochondral defects using hybrid scaffolds and bone marrow-derived mesenchymal stem cells in a rabbit model.", *Tissue Engineering*, vol. 12, no. 6, pp. 1539 1551.

Sherman, M., Warren, R., Marshall, J., and Savatsky, G. 1988, "A clinical and radiographical analysis of 127 anterior cruciate insufficient knees.", *Clinical Orthopaedics and Related Research*, vol. 227, pp. 229-237.

Uematsu, K., Hattori, K., Ishimoto, Y., Yamauchi, J., Habata, T., Takakura, Y., Ohgushi, H., Fukuchi, T., and Sato, M. 2005, "Cartilage regeneration using mesenchymal stem cells and a three-dimensional poly-lactic-glycolic acid (PLGA) scaffold", *Biomaterials*, vol. 26, pp. 4273-4279.

Van Eijk, F., Saris, D., Riesle, J., Willems, W., van Blitterswijk, C., Verbout, A., and Dhert, W. 2004, "Tissue Engineering of Ligaments: A Comparison of Bone Marrow Stromal Cells, Anterior Cruciate Ligament, and Skin Fibroblasts as Cell Source.", *Tissue Engineering*, vol. 10, no. 5-6, pp. 893-903.

Wakitani, S., Goto, T., Pineda, S., Young, R., Mansour, J., Kaplan, A., and Goldberg, V. 1994, "Mesenchymal cell-based repair of large, full-thickness defects of articular cartilage", *Journal of Bone and Joint Surgery*, vol. 76, pp. 579-592.

Wakitani, S., Imoto, K., Yamamoto, T., Saito, M., Murata, N., and Yoneda, M. 2002, "Human autologous culture expanded bone marrow mesenchymal cell transplantation for repair of cartilage defects in osteoarthritic knees.", *Osteoarthritis and Cartilage*, vol. 10, pp. 199-206.

Walsh, C., Goodman, D., Caplan, A., and Goldberg, V. 1999, "Meniscus Regeneration in a Rabbit Partial Meniscectomy Model", *Tissue Engineering*, vol. 5, no. 4, pp. 327-337.

Wang. W., Li, B., Yang, J., Xin, L., Li, Y., Yin ,H., Qi, Y., Jiang, Y., Ouyang, H., Gao, C.. 2010, "The restoration of full-thickness cartilage defects with BMSCs and TGF-beta 1 loaded PLGA/fibrin gel constructs" *Biomaterials,* vol. 31(34), pp. 8964-8973.

Williams, R., Peterson, L., and Cole, B. 2007, *Cartilage repair strategies.* Humana Press Inc.

Wiss, DA. and Stetson, WB. 1995, "Unstable Fractures of the Tibia Treated With a Reamed Intramedullary Interlocking Nail", *Clinical Orthopaedics and Related Research*, vol. 315.

Zellner, J., Mueller, M., Berner, A., Dienstknecht, T., Kujat, R., Nerlich, M., Hennemann, B., Koller, M., Prantl, L., Angele, M., Angele, P. 2010, "Role of mesenchymal stem cells in tissue engineering of meniscus", *Journal of Biomedical Material Research A,* vol. 94(4): pp.1150-61.

In: Stem Cells in Disease
Editor: Prasad S. Koka

ISBN: 978-1-62257-169-7
© 2012 Nova Science Publishers, Inc.

Chapter XVII

The Challenges of Cartilage Repair and the Potential of Stem Cell Applications

Matthew P. Newton Ede and Wasim S. Khan
University College London Institute of Orthopaedics and Musculoskeletal Sciences, Royal National Orthopaedic Hospital, Stanmore, Middlesex, UK

Abstract

Articular cartilage injuries pose a treatment challenge. These injuries are a direct cause of pain and loss of function and may precipitate osteoarthritis in the affected joint. Typically affecting a younger, more active population whose expectations of treatment and need for long term joint preservation are high. Articular cartilage poses a treatment challenge in that its capacity for satisfactory healing is limited. The common endpoint of conservative management and traditional surgical interventions is the generation of biomechanically inferior fibrocartilage. Regenerative techniques using human stem cells would appear to represent an exciting modality for the production of true hyaline cartilage with material and biological properties suited for lasting function. This review article summarises the current research regarding the use of human stem cells in the treatment of such injuries.

Keywords: (MeSH) Articular Cartilage; Hyaline Cartilage; Joints; Mesenchymal Stem Cells; Regeneration

Introduction

Hyaline articular cartilage injury represents a unique problem based on its privileged biological characteristics. Whilst bone beneath the calcified layer has rich vascular supply, above the calcified layer, the hyaline cartilage is completely avascular. Hyaline (glass-like) articular cartilage is composed of scant cellular components entombed in elegantly arranged extracellular matrix. The matrix component is primarily of Type II collagen and proteoglycans. The collagen are arranged in "loops", first described by Benninghoff in 1925, which describes a progression from vertical to horizontally aligned fibres moving from deep to superficial. These loops provide a firm structure within which the hydrophilic proteoglycans are arranged. This allows for limited water saturation of the articular cartilage, but the collagen loops, binding the proteoglycans and associated water, resist excessive saturation. This gives hyaline cartilage its unique shock absorbing and viscoelastic behaviour that allows dissipation of physiological forces throughout the joint.

Whilst the cells are locked in the matrix tomb (chondron), they are vital to maintenance of the anisotropic matrix. The avascular nature of hyaline cartilage makes for poor repair after injury. Insults above the tidemark initiate some chondrocyte proliferation, but no substantial matrix repair, the defect will remain. Injuries crossing the tidemark result in bleeding, inflammation and healing by scar. Scar is characterised by fibrocartilage (type I cartilage) with impaired material properties regarding shock absorbsion and resistance to shear.

The Consequence of Cartilage Injury

Chondral injuries are common injuries, being encountered in about 20% of arthroscopic procedures [1]. The natural history of chondral injury is the focus of debate and the reader is directed to the thorough review article on this subject by Dell'Accio and Vincent [2]. This is an injury that was noted even in the 18th century as being special with regard to regeneration: Hunter observed that "an ulcerated Cartilage is universally allowed to be a very troublesome disease and when destroyed, it is never recovered" [3]. Belber found the incidence of osteoarthritis in the knee was roughly doubled (13.9%) in those who had a knee injury compared to those who did not (6.0%) [4]. However Messener and Maletius found that of 28 athletes with severe chondral injuries 22 had excellent or good function at 14-year follow-up, suggesting a more benign natural history. There was not however a control group and the average age was young [5]. There may be a difference in the type of chondral injuries incurred experimentally with those occurring "naturally". Indeed, whilst in experimental models there is little evidence of cartilage healing, in clinical follow-up studies there appears to be some healing occurring, particularly amongst those partial-thickness injuries [5-7]. This contrasts with the conventional wisdom that partial injuries will not heal. Further, the accepted view of a tissue with little or no healing potential has been challenged by the discovery of stem cell markers (Notch-1 and Sto-1) in the superficial zone of hyaline cartilage. Whether these markers represent functioning stem cells with the potential for chondrogenic differentiation and whether they can be manipulated to differentiate and function as matrix producing chondrocytes remains to be explored. However it represents an interesting avenue of innate cartilage healing potential [8]. The end result of a chondral injury must be a complex relationship involving defect morphology, the existing mechanical environment and host factors (notably genetics, age, activity and obesity). Indeed, predicting which patients with chondral injuries are at risk of developing premature osteoarthritis and developing screening markers presents an avenue for further investigation to allow sensible rationing of resources.

Current Treatment Modalities

Existing treatment modalities include microfracture, autologous chondrocyte implantation (with or without matrix assistance), mosaicplasty and osteochondral allografting. Of these microfracture and ACI are stem cell therapies and will therefore be discussed in more detail.

Microfracture converts a superficial/partial thickness injury to a full thickness one. In essence it is the most basic stem cell mediated technique. By breaching the subchondral bone and allowing bleeding, so MSC's are recruited to the zone of injury. The resulting inflammatory response, with MSC's differentiating into fibroblasts, generates a fibrocartilage (Type I collagen) scar. Fibrocartilage has inferior material properties as a bearing surface and the repaired cartilage tends to be thinner. Addition of hyaluronic acid (an endogenous polymer found in human tissue) in a rabbit model improved the hyaline properties of the microfracture regenerate [9]. Microfracture augmented for 2 weeks with an indwelling pump administering fibroblast growth factor-2 (FGF-2) resulted in complete healing of large (5mm) full-thickness defects in rabbits [10]. These augmentations of microfracture may be an alternative to culture-expanded MSC techniques. They may be cheaper and have the advantage of requiring fewer operations.

Which Stem Cells?

Bone marrow derived MSC's are most commonly obtained from the iliac crest. This has the potential for donor-site morbidity and it seems preferable to obtain tissue from the site of primary pathology. The most commonly treated joint is the knee. This has lead to methodology to obtain MSC's from tissues within the knee. Bone marrow MSC's from under the defect can be obtained arthroscopically, however this usually would involve exposing subchondral bone which may generate an inflammatory reaction resulting in fibrocartilage scar as detailed above. Therefore there has been work looking at alternative sources of MSCs which require neither a second operative site, nor exposure of subchondral bone at the same site [11]. Within the knee, abundant tissue that is readily accessible to the surgeon is synovium from the inside of the joint capsule and adipose tissue from the infrapatellar fat pad. Both of these tissue sources can be harvested through the arthroscope at the time of initial arthroscopic assessment of the knee, with no additional morbidity. Both of the tissues contain stem cells and their ease of access has lead to these cell lines being explored for their suitability as a chondrogenic tissue.

Adult adipose tissue is a readily accessible source of stem cells that can be manipulated to differentiate into hyaline cartilage and bone in vivo [12]. Surface characteristics and differentiation characteristics are similar to bone marrow MSCs. Chondrogenic differentiation of Adipose Derived Stem Cells (ASLs) can be stimulated by low oxygen tension and Bone Morphogenic Protein-6 (BMP-6) [13]. English et al compared ASLs with MSCs and chondrocytes cultured from osteoarthritic tissue within knees. ASLs had good chondrogenic properties, were stable in their phenotype after serial expansion and maintained multipotency when compared to chondrocytes expanded from arthritic tissue. ASLs were comparable in surface expression and function to MSCs [14]. ASLs in an alginate gel produce hyaline cartilage in rabbits that is superior to no treatment or gel alone [15]. However Jakobsen et al. demonstrated in a hyaluronic acid scaffold that whilst ASLs were superior to autologous chondrocytes, they were inferior to MSCs when assessing Collagen II gene expression as a marker for chondrogenic properties [16].

Synovium is another potential site of stem cells [17,18]. It contains fibroblast-like stem cells which can be directed down chondrocyte differentiation pathways. Cells cultured even from elderly synovial tissue have the potential to differentiate into chondrogenic cells and thus the potential for stem cell and gene therapy for osteoarthritis is exciting [19]. Although synovium derived cells in a gel matrix can be induced to express chondrocyte genes when exposed to BMP-2, collagen I genes (fibrocartilage) continue to be expressed and is thus suboptimal as a source under these conditions [20]. There have been some direct comparisons of tissue sources. In a human source; compared with bone marrow, skeletal muscle, periosteum and fat; synovium was found to be superior regarding chondrogenic behaviour [17]. A rabbit model comparing similar sources to the above study, found synovial-MSCs to have the highest proliferation potential and highest cartilage production. These expansions were then implanted into chondral defects in vivo; again synovium and bone MSCs favoured best, this was maximised by implanting under a periosteal patch [21].

Given the apparent inferiority of adipose cells compared with synovium or bone, it seems unlikely that under existing expansion conditions, adipose cells will be appropriate in a clinical setting. Indeed the harvesting of bone marrow cells now involves only percutaneous aspiration from the iliac crest. This can be performed under anaesthetic and aseptic conditions simultaneously with the arthroscopic joint evaluatio. With this in mind, the complications and morbidity of bone marrow harvesting are minimal and we question whether there is a requirement for an alternative source.

Tracking MSC's is extremely useful for assessing success of therapies. As the transition occurs into human subjects, a useful non-invasive technique has been developed by Heymer et al. Commercially available Very Small Superparamagnetic iron oxide particles can be added to hMSCs seemingly without affecting their function. These can then visualised on Magnetic Resonance Imaging once in the human subject. This represents a non-invasive and relatively cheap cellular follow-up protocol [22].

Quality of MSCs appears to decline as we get older. Potential for chondrogenic behaviour reduces and senescence increases. Senescence represents the limitation of MSCs to undergo culture expansion whilst maintaining a undifferentiated phenotype. Thus when obtaining tissue from older people, the numbers of MSCs that can be implanted from a single source as well as the quality of the cells with regard to cartilage production declines [23,24].

Similarly osteoarthritic tissue has diminished properties similar to "older" articular tissue. The age of 40 is quoted as the point at which qualities diminish. Osteoarthritic tissue behaves like "healthy" tissue 20 years older [23].

Scaffolds and Matrix

Scaffold-cell-host relationships are complex. Essentially a scaffold must be mechanically stable and biocompatible with both recipient and seeded cells. The surface properties of the material must allow passage and interaction of extracellular matrix and cell signalling chemicals (integrins). Scaffolds can be biopolymers such as bone matrix, collagen, hyaluronan and alginate or they can be synthetic polymers. These synthetic compounds encompass polyglycolic acid (PGA) and polylactic acid (PLA) and co-polymers of them (PLGA). These polymers have a long history of safe use in vivo commonly used as a dissolvable suture material. They hydrolyse in the presence of water into the monomers glycolic acid and lactic acid which are natural metabolic products. This makes them attractive as scaffolds as they are already proven safe [25]. In the scaffold process, these polymers are arranged by a process of electrospinning to produce nanofibers (diameter of 500-100nm) in a porous three-dimensional scaffold. This arrangement appears to be well suited with regard to cellular ongrowth with rapid incorporation by seeded cells. Polycaprolactone (PCL) is also in extensive use already as a implanted biomaterial. It is used as a suture (Monocyl) which is long tried and accepted in clinical practice. PCL has been used to model some more complex material behaviours of native cartilage. This includes anisotropic and viscoelastic behaviours. Anisotropy is the asymmetrical material property based on orientation of load. This is a natural phenomenon found in most musculoskeletal tissues and is related to the orientation of fibres, resulting in different shear and compressive properties. Viscoelasticity is another material property in which deformation of the material is related to the rate of load. These are critical material properties of hyaline cartilage and have profound effects on joint lubrication and wear. Moutos and Guilak used PCL on a gel scaffold with ASLs. After 28 days they found that the experimental tissue displayed material properties very similar to natural cartilage regarding anisotropic compression, shear and friction coefficient [26]. Wise et al, again using a PCL nano-spun scaffold, found that by manipulating the orientation of the scaffold, the cellular orientation of the seeded and proliferating chondrocytes could be maintained [27]. This represents an exciting prospect of recreating the anisotropic qualities of hyaline cartilage. However the relative importance of scaffold orientation vs exogenous load was noted. Indeed whether it is necessary to manipulate cell orientation with a "bespoke" scaffold when physiological joint loading may indeed subsequently achieve the same result is undefined [28]. The complex interplay between loading, scaffold orientation and resultant material properties represents an interesting avenue for further work.

The MSCs need a template on which to deposit matrix, but also need to remain in contact with the defect. Simply injecting MSCs into a joint is unlikely to be successful. A radiolabeled MR follow-up study in rabbits showed no migration of autologous MSCs when injected into the knee [29]. Scaffolds also have a key role to play in maintaining chondrogenic behaviour. We know that physical properties can encourage or prevent chondroid production of MSCs. For example MSC pellet formation with MSCs being tightly packed seems to promote chondrogenesis via SOX-9 activation, whereas monolayers appear to be deficient through a similar mechanism [30,31]. Another environmental factor which appears relevant is pressure. Chondrogenic behaviour is optimised by cyclical loading mimicking the synovial joint [32]. Lower oxygen tension also promotes cartilage production and reduces senescence [33,34]. There is some evidence that a scaffold alone (ie without cultured MSCs or chondrocytes), when combined with microfracture is capable of resulting in hyaline cartilage repair and is superior to microfracture alone [35].

Where injuries involve underlying bone as well as cartilage, scaffolds are required to provide a support for the cartilage regenerate. Transplantation of cartilage with underlying bone from organ donors has been successful, but carries inherent risks of disease transmission. Where engineered hyaline cartilage is to be used, synthetic materials such bioglasses have shown superiority to autologous bone as a scaffold with regard to recipient-graft integration and production of hyaline cartilage [36].

Advantages of a natural scaffold are acceptance by licensing bodies and increased biocompatibility. Cheng investigated an entirely native cartilage derived porous scaffold. Additionally there was no use of exogenous growth factors. Good results were obtained with regard to chondrogenic markers and biomechanical properties of resultant tissue [37].

Silk has shown promise as a natural scaffold. When compared to collagen, MSCs seeded onto silk scaffold showed superior chondrogenesis regarding GAG and Collagen II expression. The structural strength of silk, high porosity and slow absorbsion compared with collagen were proposed as positive attributes [38]. Hyaluronate derived scaffolds have proven successful and again do not require licensing as it is a endogenous natural polymer [39]. In a rat model, human embryonic stem cells on a hyaluronate hydrogel showed regenerate tissue similar to non-injured rats [40].

Regulation and Controlling Differentiation

Controlling the local environment is key to maintaining differentiation into type II collagen producing chondrocyte-like cells. Whilst MSCs can survive in an environment without additional growth factors, early differentiation into chondrocytes is not maintained and Collagen I producing cells soon predominate [41]. Key to the differentiation and maintenance of MSCs into chondrogenic cell lines is the SOX-9 gene. Activation of this gene encourages chondrogenic differentiation and inhibition of it prevents cartilage production [42,43]. Controlling differentiation and preventing hypertrophy remains a challenge. Co-culture with mature chondrocytes in equine an equine model improves chondrogenic differentiation. TGF-β1 addition to the co-culture did not [44]. Co-culture in a human ex vivo study with embryonic derived MSCs with mature chondrocytes maintained better chondrogenic behaviour than MSCs alone, additionally there was reduced osteogenic (bone-forming) behaviour in co-culture [45]. [45]. BMP-4 in a rabbit model was found to be more potent in maintaining differentiation than BMP-7. In the same experiment, BMP-4 delivered in vivo to cartilage defects on a collagen bilayer scaffold showed good hyaline cartilage formation [46]. Glucosamine enhances in vitro chondrogenic behaviour by MSCs in terms of expression of Coll II and agrecan [47].

The location of differentiation may have a role. Fan et al contrasted 1. in vitro differentiation and expansion seeded onto a natural scaffold, compared with 2. The same scaffold seeded with undifferentiated MSC allowed to differentiate in vivo, both were impregnated with TGF-β1. Better early morphological and phenotypical properties were observed with cells allowed to differentiate in vivo although this difference disappeared at 6 weeks [48]. Contrasting this, Zscharnack et al found that in a sheep model, MSCs allowed to pre-differentiate for 14 days prior to implantation performed best regarding histological and morphological properties compared with those implanted as undifferentiated MSCs. However unlike Fan et al they did not augment their in vivo scaffold with regard to growth factors and thus one might expect a less controlled differentiation in vivo [49].

TGF-β3 impregnation into synthetic scaffolds improves macroscopic and histological appearance of cartilage regenerate and demonstrates mechanical properties similar to native hyaline cartilage in a rat model [50].

Gene Therapy

It is important to recognise that gene therapy modalities is where genes coding for desirable protein synthesis are transduced into MSCs as viral vectors and these are introduced into the diseased environment. Desirable genes may be those that produce useful proteins (such as Coll II or agrecan) or the genes may code for proteins that will maintain the chondrogenic differentiation (IGF, SOX-9) Similar growth factors are used extensively in co-culture as a way to encourage differentiation and maintenance of chondrocytes. These are however additions of actual proteins into the local environment and are not gene therapies. It is easy to confuse the two techniques when reading the literature, but they are quite different.

Pagnotto et al demonstrated that using adeno-associated virus (AAV) as a vector for gene transduction into MSCs. The transduction of Transforming Growth Factor Beta 1 (TGF β1) improved cartilage repair in a rat model [51]. Park et al found embedding MSCs in a hydrogel containing TGF-β3 enhanced chondrogenic behaviour in vivo [52]. Insulin-like Growth factor-1 when virally transduced into equine MSCs showed prolonged production of IGF-1 and hyaline cartilage [53]. Transduction with BMP-2 genes in mice produces bone which is useful where defects are osteochondral (ie they involve underlying bone in addition to cartilage) [12]. Kubo et al demonstrated that MSCs engineered with an inhibitor of Vascular Endothelial growth factor (VEGF) showed improved chondrogenic gene expression and within a rat model demonstrate superior clinical properties compared with MSCs without VEGF inhibition [54]. Transduction of anti-apoptotic genes (Bcl-xl) into MSC's reduces cell death. Hu et al demonstrated superior results morphologically and histologically compared with un-engineered controls [55].

The physical mechanism of gene application appears to alter histological outcome. Han et al found better expression of Coll II, improved mechanical and histological properties when TGF-β1 was delivered as a co-culture hybrid microsphere as compared to gelatine delivered TGF-β1 [56].

An interesting avenue arises in the delivery of gene vectors in vivo. Diao et al impregnated TGF-β1 gene-carrying plasmids into a chitosan/gelatine scaffold with MSCs seeded onto the scaffold. In a rabbit model it improved chondrogenic differentiation and hyaline cartilage regeneration. This technique has the interesting advantage of providing a prolonged delivery of gene engineered vectors [57]. Might it also be possible to impregnate gene vectors at different levels on the scaffold to vary the differentiation by level? For example, in the case of the osteochondral defect where bone is required at a deep level and cartilage at a superficial level.

Clinical Studies

Clinical studies in humans are currently limited [58]. There are Phase 1 clinical trials being conducted currently in Norway, Iran and Egypt. Completion of these will take a few years and Phase 1 trials are small studies to assess patient safety and efficacy. Successful completion is needed before proper randomised studies could be conducted. Considering the expense of MSC therapies the obvious control comparator would be microfracture (detailed above). We believe that benefit would have to be demonstrated against this established technique before in vitro culture expansion MSC therapies could be advocated.

Conclusion

Stem cells represent the human body's most profound tool for "scarless" repair. In the situation of cartilage injury, where scar formation results in impaired biomechanical properties, reduced function, pain and potential for premature arthritis, stem cell therapies must represent an exciting prospect for regeneration.

There remain important questions to be answered, not least the histological and clinical benefits of relatively expensive culture-expanded tissues from stem cell lines, vs. augmentation of the most basic in vivo stem cell technique of microfracture.

References

[1] Curl WW, Krome J, Gordon ES, Rushing J, Smith BP, Poehling GG. Cartilage injuries: a review of 31,516 knee arthroscopies. *Arthroscopy.* 1997 Aug;13(4):456-460.].

[2] Dell'accio F, Vincent TL. Joint surface defects: clinical course and cellular response in spontaneous and experimental lesions. *Eur. Cell Mater.* 2010;20:210-217.]

[3] On the structure and diseases of articular cartilage. 1743;42B:514-21.]

[4] Gelber AC, Hochberg MC, Mead LA, Wang NY, Wigley FM, Klag MJ. Joint injury in young adults and risk for subsequent knee and hip osteoarthritis. *Ann. Intern. Med.* 2000 Sep 5;133(5):321-328.]

[5] Messner K, Maletius W. The long-term prognosis for severe damage to weight-bearing cartilage in the knee: a 14-year clinical and radiographic follow-up in 28 young athletes. *Acta Orthop. Scand.* 1996 Apr;67(2):165-168.]

[6] Nakamura N, Horibe S, Toritsuka Y, Mitsuoka T, Natsu-ume T, Yoneda K, et al. The location-specific healing response of damaged articular cartilage after ACL reconstruction: short-term follow-up. *Knee Surg Sports Traumatol Arthrosc.* 2008 Sep;16(9):843-848.]

[7] Ding C, Cicuttini F, Scott F, Cooley H, Boon C, Jones G. Natural history of knee cartilage defects and factors affecting change. *Arch. Intern. Med.* 2006 Mar 27;166(6):651-658.]

[8] Karlsson C, Lindahl A. Articular cartilage stem cell signalling. *Arthritis Res. Ther.* 2009;11(4):121.]

[9] Kang S-W, Bada LP, Kang C-S, Lee J-S, Kim C-H, Park J-H, et al. Articular cartilage regeneration with microfracture and hyaluronic acid. *Biotechnol. Lett.* 2008 Mar;30(3):435-439.]

[10] Hiraki Y, Shukunami C, Iyama K, Mizuta H. Differentiation of chondrogenic precursor cells during the regeneration of articular cartilage. *Osteoarthr. Cartil.* 2001;9 Suppl A:S102-108.]

[11] Elvenes J, Knutsen G, Johansen O, Moe BT, Martinez I. Development of a new method to harvest chondroprogenitor cells from underneath cartilage defects in the knees. *J. Orthop. Sci.* 2009 Jul;14(4):410-417.]

[12] Dragoo JL, Samimi B, Zhu M, Hame SL, Thomas BJ, Lieberman JR, et al. Tissue-engineered cartilage and bone using stem cells from human infrapatellar fat pads. *J. Bone Joint Surg B*r. 2003 Jul;85(5):740-747.]

[13] Guilak F, Estes BT, Diekman BO, Moutos FT, Gimble JM. 2010 Nicolas Andry Award: Multipotent adult stem cells from adipose tissue for musculoskeletal tissue engineering. *Clin.. Orthop. Relat. Res.* 2010 Sep;468(9):2530-2540.]

[14] English A, Jones EA, Corscadden D, Henshaw K, Chapman T, Emery P, et al. A comparative assessment of cartilage and joint fat pad as a potential source of cells for autologous therapy development in knee osteoarthritis. *Rheumatology* (Oxford). 2007 Nov;46(11):1676-1683.]

[15] Zhang H-N, Li L, Leng P, Wang Y-Z, Lv C-Y. Uninduced adipose-derived stem cells repair the defect of full-thickness hyaline cartilage. Chin. *J. Traumatol.* 2009 Apr;12(2):92-97.]

[16] Jakobsen RB, Shahdadfar A, Reinholt FP, Brinchmann JE. Chondrogenesis in a hyaluronic acid scaffold: comparison between chondrocytes and MSC from bone marrow and adipose tissue. *Knee Surg Sports Traumatol Arthrosc.* 2010 Oct;18(10):1407-1416.]

[17] Sakaguchi Y, Sekiya I, Yagishita K, Muneta T. Comparison of human stem cells derived from various mesenchymal tissues: superiority of synovium as a cell source. *Arthritis Rheum.* 2005 Aug;52(8):2521-2529.]

[18] Teramura T, Fukuda K, Kurashimo S, Hosoi Y, Miki Y, Asada S, et al. Isolation and characterization of side population stem cells in articular synovial tissue. *BMC Musculoskelet Disord.* 2008;9:86.]

[19] Kurth T, Hedbom E, Shintani N, Sugimoto M, Chen FH, Haspl M, et al. Chondrogenic potential of human synovial mesenchymal stem cells in alginate. *Osteoarthr. Cartil.* 2007 Oct;15(10):1178-1189.]

[20] Park Y, Sugimoto M, Watrin A, Chiquet M, Hunziker EB. BMP-2 induces the expression of chondrocyte-specific genes in bovine synovium-derived progenitor cells cultured in three-dimensional alginate hydrogel. *Osteoarthr. Cartil.* 2005 Jun;13(6):527-536.]

[21] Koga H, Muneta T, Nagase T, Nimura A, Ju Y-J, Mochizuki T, et al. Comparison of mesenchymal tissues-derived stem cells for in vivo chondrogenesis: suitable conditions for cell therapy of cartilage defects in rabbit. *Cell Tissue Res.* 2008 Aug;333(2):207-215.]

[22] Heymer A, Haddad D, Weber M, Gbureck U, Jakob PM, Eulert J, et al. Iron oxide labelling of human mesenchymal stem cells in collagen hydrogels for articular cartilage repair. *Biomaterials.* 2008 Apr;29(10):1473-1483.]

[23] Freemont AJ, Hoyland JA. Morphology, mechanisms and pathology of musculoskeletal ageing. *J. Pathol.* 2007 Jan;211(2):252-259.]

[24] Barbero A, Grogan S, Schäfer D, Heberer M, Mainil-Varlet P, Martin I. Age related changes in human articular chondrocyte yield, proliferation and post-expansion chondrogenic capacity. *Osteoarthritis and Cartilage.* 2004 Jun;12(6):476-484.]

[25] Li W-J, Laurencin CT, Caterson EJ, Tuan RS, Ko FK. Electrospun nanofibrous structure: a novel scaffold for tissue engineering. *J. Biomed. Mater. Res.* 2002 Jun 15;60(4):613-621.]

[26] Moutos FT, Guilak F. Functional properties of cell-seeded three-dimensionally woven poly(epsilon-caprolactone) scaffolds for cartilage tissue engineering. *Tissue Eng Part A.* 2010 Apr;16(4):1291-1301.]

[27] Wise JK, Yarin AL, Megaridis CM, Cho M. Chondrogenic differentiation of human mesenchymal stem cells on oriented nanofibrous scaffolds: engineering the superficial zone of articular cartilage. *Tissue Eng Part A.* 2009 Apr;15(4):913-921.]

[28] Guilak F. The deformation behavior and viscoelastic properties of chondrocytes in articular cartilage. *Biorheology.* 2000;37(1-2):27-44.]

[29] Jing X-hong, Yang L, Duan X-jun, Xie B, Chen W, Li Z, et al. In vivo MR imaging tracking of magnetic iron oxide nanoparticle labeled, engineered, autologous bone marrow mesenchymal stem cells following intra-articular injection. *Joint Bone Spine.* 2008 Jul;75(4):432-438.]

[30] Kavalkovich KW, Boynton RE, Murphy JM, Barry F. Chondrogenic differentiation of human mesenchymal stem cells within an alginate layer culture system. *In Vitro Cell. Dev. Biol. Anim.* 2002 Sep;38(8):457-466.]

[31] Freemont AJ, Hoyland J. Lineage plasticity and cell biology of fibrocartilage and hyaline cartilage: its significance in cartilage repair and replacement. *Eur. J. Radiol.* 2006 Jan;57(1):32-36.]

[32] Angele P, Yoo JU, Smith C, Mansour J, Jepsen KJ, Nerlich M, et al. Cyclic hydrostatic pressure enhances the chondrogenic phenotype of human mesenchymal progenitor cells differentiated in vitro. *Journal of Orthopaedic Research.* 2003;21(3):451-457.]

[33] O'Driscoll SW, Fitzsimmons JS, Commisso CN. Role of oxygen tension during cartilage formation by periosteum. *J. Orthop. Res.* 1997 Sep;15(5):682-687.]

[34] Moussavi-Harami F, Duwayri Y, Martin JA, Moussavi-Harami F, Buckwalter JA. Oxygen effects on senescence in chondrocytes and mesenchymal stem cells: consequences for tissue engineering. *Iowa Orthop J.* 2004;24:15-20.]

[35] Erggelet C, Neumann K, Endres M, Haberstroh K, Sittinger M, Kaps C. Regeneration of ovine articular cartilage defects by cell-free polymer-based implants. *Biomaterials.* 2007 Dec;28(36):5570-5580.]

[36] Bal BS, Rahaman MN, Jayabalan P, Kuroki K, Cockrell MK, Yao JQ, et al. In vivo outcomes of tissue-engineered osteochondral grafts. *J. Biomed. Mater. Res. Part B Appl. Biomater.* 2010 Apr;93(1):164-174.]

[37] Cheng N-C, Estes BT, Awad HA, Guilak F. Chondrogenic differentiation of adipose-derived adult stem cells by a porous scaffold derived from native articular cartilage extracellular matrix. *Tissue Eng Part A.* 2009 Feb;15(2):231-241.]

[38] Meinel L, Hofmann S, Karageorgiou V, Zichner L, Langer R, Kaplan D, et al. Engineering cartilage-like tissue using human mesenchymal stem cells and silk protein scaffolds. *Biotechnol. Bioeng.* 2004 Nov 5;88(3):379-391.]

[39] Facchini A, Lisignoli G, Cristino S, Roseti L, De Franceschi L, Marconi E, et al. Human chondrocytes and mesenchymal stem cells grown onto engineered scaffold. *Biorheology*. 2006;43(3-4):471-480.]

[40] Toh WS, Lee EH, Guo X-M, Chan JKY, Yeow CH, Choo AB, et al. Cartilage repair using hyaluronan hydrogel-encapsulated human embryonic stem cell-derived chondrogenic cells. *Biomaterials*. 2010 Sep;31(27):6968-6980.]

[41] Tatebe M, Nakamura R, Kagami H, Okada K, Ueda M. Differentiation of transplanted mesenchymal stem cells in a large osteochondral defect in rabbit. *Cytotherapy*. 2005;7(6):520-530.]

[42] Tsuchiya H, Kitoh H, Sugiura F, Ishiguro N. Chondrogenesis enhanced by overexpression of sox9 gene in mouse bone marrow-derived mesenchymal stem cells. *Biochemical and Biophysical Research Communications*. 2003 Feb 7;301(2):338-343.]

[43] Bi W, Huang W, Whitworth DJ, Deng JM, Zhang Z, Behringer RR, et al. Haploinsufficiency of Sox9 results in defective cartilage primordia and premature skeletal mineralization. *Proceedings of the National Academy of Sciences*. 2001 Jun 5;98(12):6698 -6703.]

[44] Lettry V, Hosoya K, Takagi S, Okumura M. Coculture of equine mesenchymal stem cells and mature equine articular chondrocytes results in improved chondrogenic differentiation of the stem cells. *Jpn. J. Vet. Res.* 2010 May;58(1):5-15.]

[45] Bigdeli N, Karlsson C, Strehl R, Concaro S, Hyllner J, Lindahl A. Coculture of human embryonic stem cells and human articular chondrocytes results in significantly altered phenotype and improved chondrogenic differentiation. *Stem Cells*. 2009 Aug;27(8):1812-1821.]

[46] Jiang Y, Chen LK, Zhu DC, Zhang GR, Guo C, Qi YY, et al. The inductive effect of bone morphogenetic protein-4 on chondral-lineage differentiation and in situ cartilage repair. *Tissue Eng Part A*. 2010 May;16(5):1621-1632.]

[47] Derfoul A, Miyoshi AD, Freeman DE, Tuan RS. Glucosamine promotes chondrogenic phenotype in both chondrocytes and mesenchymal stem cells and inhibits MMP-13 expression and matrix degradation. *Osteoarthr. Cartil.* 2007 Jun;15(6):646-655.]

[48] Fan H, Liu H, Zhu R, Li X, Cui Y, Hu Y, et al. Comparison of chondral defects repair with in vitro and in vivo differentiated mesenchymal stem cells. *Cell Transplant.* 2007;16(8):823-832.]

[49] Zscharnack M, Hepp P, Richter R, Aigner T, Schulz R, Somerson J, et al. Repair of chronic osteochondral defects using predifferentiated mesenchymal stem cells in an ovine model. *Am. J. Sports Med.* 2010 Sep;38(9):1857-1869.]

[50] Han SH, Kim YH, Park MS, Kim IA, Shin JW, Yang WI, et al. Histological and biomechanical properties of regenerated articular cartilage using chondrogenic bone marrow stromal cells with a PLGA scaffold in vivo. *J. Biomed. Mater Res A*. 2008 Dec 15;87(4):850-861.]

[51] Pagnotto MR, Wang Z, Karpie JC, Ferretti M, Xiao X, Chu CR. Adeno-associated viral gene transfer of transforming growth factor-beta1 to human mesenchymal stem cells improves cartilage repair. *Gene Ther.* 2007 May;14(10):804-813.]

[52] Park JS, Woo DG, Yang HN, Lim HJ, Park KM, Na K, et al. Chondrogenesis of human mesenchymal stem cells encapsulated in a hydrogel construct: neocartilage formation in animal models as both mice and rabbits. *J. Biomed. Mater Res A*. 2010 Mar 1;92(3):988-996.]

[53] Nixon AJ, Brower-Toland BD, Bent SJ, Saxer RA, Wilke MJ, Robbins PD, et al. Insulinlike growth factor-I gene therapy applications for cartilage repair. *Clin. Orthop. Relat. Res*. 2000 Oct;(379 Suppl):S201-213.]

[54] Kubo S, Cooper GM, Matsumoto T, Phillippi JA, Corsi KA, Usas A, et al. Blocking vascular endothelial growth factor with soluble Flt-1 improves the chondrogenic potential of mouse skeletal muscle-derived stem cells. *Arthritis Rheum*. 2009 Jan;60(1):155-165.]

[55] Hu B, Ren J-L, Zhang J-R, Ma Q, Liu Y-P, Mao T-Q. Enhanced treatment of articular cartilage defect of the knee by intra-articular injection of Bcl-xL-engineered mesenchymal stem cells in rabbit model. *J. Tissue Eng Regen* Med. 2010 Feb;4(2):105-114.]

[56] Han Y, Wei Y, Wang S, Song Y. Cartilage regeneration using adipose-derived stem cells and the controlled-released hybrid microspheres. *Joint Bone Spine*. 2010 Jan;77(1):27-31.]

[57] Diao H, Wang J, Shen C, Xia S, Guo T, Dong L, et al. Improved cartilage regeneration utilizing mesenchymal stem cells in TGF-beta1 gene-activated scaffolds. *Tissue Eng Part A*. 2009 Sep;15(9):2687-2698.]

[58] Matsumoto T, Okabe T, Ikawa T, Iida T, Yasuda H, Nakamura H, et al. Articular cartilage repair with autologous bone marrow mesenchymal cells. *J. Cell. Physiol*. 2010 Nov;225(2):291-295.]

In: Stem Cells in Disease
Editor: Prasad S. Koka
ISBN: 978-1-62257-169-7
© 2012 Nova Science Publishers, Inc.

Chapter XVIII

Current Cell Based Strategies for Knee Cartilage Injuries

***P. K. Jaiswal*[1], *K. Wong*[2] *and Wasim S. Khan*[3]**
[1]University College London Institute of Orthopaedics and Musculoskeletal Sciences, Royal National Orthopaedic Hospital, Stanmore, Middlesex, UK
[2]Department of Trauma and Orthopaedics, Princess Alexandra Hospital NHS Trust, Harlow, Essex, UK
[3]University College London Institute of Orthopaedics and Musculoskeletal Sciences, Royal National Orthopaedic Hospital, Stanmore, Middlesex, UK

Abstract

Cartilage is frequently damaged and shows little or no capacity for repair. Injuries that extend to the subchondral level show some capacity for repair due to the release of bone marrow derived mesenchymal stem cells. This technique is employed in techniques like the microfracture but they are only appropriate for smaller cartilage defects. Autologous Chondrocyte Implantation (ACI) and Matrix-carried Autologous Chondrocyte Implantation (MACI) are currently used in clinical practice to treat larger full thickness chondral defects in the knee with similar results. MACI does however have a number of advantages including its amenability to be performed arthroscopically or through a more limited approach without requiring arthrotomy. More definitive studies showing the long-term effects of the two cell-based treatments and comparing them are however awaited. There are a small number of studies using mesenchymal stem cells and further in vitro and in vivo studies are needed before this treatment is optimised. This review discussed these treatment options and provides an evidence-based approach to current clinical treatments.

Keywords*:* ACI; MACI; mesenchymal stem cells; clinical studies

Introduction

A variety of surgical options exist for the treatment of osteochondral defects in the knee. A number of techniques endeavour to replace the defect with hyaline cartilage, including using osteochondral allografts, osteochondral autografts, or mosaicplasty. To date, none have been proven to provide a long term and reproducible improvement in pre-operative function, and concerns such as disease transmission and donor-site morbidity remain.

The challenge of recreating the special properties of hyaline articular cartilage is still ongoing, since it is so resilient and non-uniform. A cellular approach to the treatment of cartilage damage in the knee appears an attractive proposition, since it offers the best possibility of replacing damaged articular cartilage with hyaline-like cartilage. This review will discuss the origins of cell therapy for the treatment of osteochondral defects in the knee, namely in the form of autologous chondrocyte implantation and also look to the future and current literature regarding the use of mesenchymal stem cells.

History of Autologous Chondrocyte Implantation

The origins of Autologous Chondrocyte Implantation (ACI) can be tracked back to 1965, following the isolation of adult articular chondrocytes in suspension (Smith, 1965). Three years later, Chesterman and Smith (1968) demonstrated that isolated epiphyseal chondrocytes survived when implanted into experimentally-produced intra-articular humerus fractures in rabbits. Further advancement in chondrocyte implantation was made when Bentley and Greer (1971) repaired chondral defects in a rabbit model using autologous epiphyseal and articular chondrocytes. Chondrocytes were taken from immature rabbits as it was previously shown that these cells had the potential to divide, whereas chondrocytes from mature rabbits did not (Mankin, 1962a, 1962b, 1963).

The next logical progression in the development of ACI was to be able to expand the number of chondrocytes without losing their ability to produce type II collagen. Green described a technique of culturing chondrocytes after they had been isolated from the extracellular matrix by enzymatic digestion (Green, 1977). However, during expansion, the cells gradually de-differentiated and lost their ability to manufacture type II collagen. Chondrocytes regained this ability once they were exposed to agarose gels (Benya and Shaffer, 1982). Aston and Bentley showed that by growing the chondrocytes at high density, the phenotype was reserved and the cells produced type II collagen (Aston and Bentley, 1982, 1986). The ability to expand the numbers of adult chondrocytes in a monolayer culture proved a significant advancement in the treatment of osteochondral defects using autologous cells. Peterson et al. (2002) reported on the repair of defects in skeletally mature rabbits with autologous or homologous cultured chondrocytes. Cartilage plugs were removed from the mid-patellae and enzymatically-digested and grown in a monolayer culture for two weeks. Following this, the pellets of chondrocytes were implanted into artificially-created defects and covered with either a layer of fascia, synovium, blood clot, tendon or periosteum. Results were encouraging with a total reconstitution of full thickness 3mm defects with hyaline cartilage. Using autoradiography, Grande et al. (1989) proved that autologous chondrocytes grown in *vitro* were responsible for the repair tissue in artificially-created defects in rabbits.

Brittberg's (Brittberg et al., 1994) original technique for ACI involved covering the chondral defect with periosteum harvested from the proximal tibia during the second stage procedure. Once the defect is covered and the periosteum sutured, the chondrocytes injected, and the repair process is completed by sealing the periosteum with fibrin glue to ensure there is a watertight seal. Minas and Nehrer (1997) speculated that growth factors secreted by the periosteum stimulated cultured chondrocytes to divide. Another possible mechanism speculated was that the periosteum and cultured chondrocytes stimulated adjacent cartilage, in the subchondral bone or in the periosteum itself to enter the defect and repair it. The later can probably be disregarded since the results of treatment of chondral defects in both animal models and human subjects have been poor with the use of a periosteal patch alone (Brittberg et al., 1996 and Angermann, 1998). Evidence for the dual action of periosteum with cultured chondrocytes was confirmed when dead periosteum was sutured to the rim of the chondral defect in rabbits and chondrocyte suspension was injected into sealed defects (Brittberg et al. 1996). Only 1 out of 8 rabbits developed good repair tissue, thus suggesting that periosteum and chondrocytes work together to repair the defect.

The first use of ACI in humans originated in Sweden in 1994 (Brittberg et al., 1994). In the original cohort of 23 patients, none of the defects extended beyond the subchondral bone. The mean age of the patients was 27, and the mean defect size was 3.1cm^2. In the original post-operative protocol, the patients were placed in a small elastic bandage and active movement without weight bearing was initiated at 2-3 days following surgery. Weight bearing was introduced gradually with exercises to strengthen the quadriceps mechanism over the 8 week period post-surgery. Of the 16 patients that had defects in the femoral condyle, 14 reported good or excellent results and the biopsy results revealed hyaline cartilage formation in 11 out of the 15 patients. The treatment of patella defects was not so encouraging. Only 2 out of 7 patients reported a good or excellent result. The suggestion for such poor outcomes in the patella was the co-existence of additional pathology such as abnormal patella-femoral joint mechanics that were not corrected at the time of the procedure.

In 2002, Peterson and Brittberg reported on the long term results of ACI. They evaluated 61 patients who had been treated for isolated chondral defects over the femoral condyle or patella, with a mean follow-up of 7.4 years. Defects ranged from 1.3 to 12cm^2. After 2 years, 50 out of 61 patients had good or excellent results. A subsequent report on the same cohort of patients revealed good or excellent results in 51 out of 61 patients (Peterson et al., 2002). These results suggest that long-term relief of symptomatic chondral defects in the knee can be achieved with ACI. In general, other techniques for the treatment of symptomatic chondral defects have been shown to be not as durable. Hubbard reported 80% success at 1 year following debridement, but this reduced to 59% at 5 years (Hubbard, 1996). Similarly, defects repaired by fibrocartilage as a result of arthroscopic abrasion arthroplasty tended not to last beyond 4 years (Bert, 1993).

Several concerns were raised with the use of the periosteal flap technique (ACI-P). This so-called first generation technique required a second surgical procedure at the proximal tibia, causing additional pain and risks to the patient. In addition, the periosteal flap had to be fixed by sutures 3mm apart, hereby damaging healthy cartilage. Further disadvantages are low mechanical stability as well as the unequal distribution of the cultured chondrocytes (especially due to gravity). Furthermore, hypertrophy, delamination and even graft failure may occur (Wood et al., 2006).

Second generation techniques involved using a synthetic type I/III collagen porcine membrane (ACI-C). This avoided the removal of the periosteum from the tibia. Though the synthetic membrane still requires suturing to adjacent cartilage, it has been shown that ACI-C has significantly lower rates of graft hypertrophy requiring secondary surgery than ACI-P (Gooding et al. 2006, and Wood et al., 2006). A prospective study of 63 patients treated with ACI-C found significant improvements to International Cartilage Repair Society and Modified Cincinnati Scores that were maintained at 3 years with no incidence of graft hypertrophy (Steinwachs and Kreuz, 2007). Robertson et al. (2007) also found a positive correlation between Knee Injury and Osteoarthritis Outcome Score (KOOS) and MRI outcome scores in a prospective study of 31 patients followed-up to 24 months. The favourable results with ACI-C suggest that the implanted chondrocytes repopulate the defect and synthesize a new cartilage matrix. The periosteal patch acts simply as a seal, ensuring the cells stay within the defect.

Matrix-Carried Autologous Chondrocyte Implantation

Concerns regarding the unequal distribution of cells, suturing of membrane to adjacent healthy cartilage, and also the possibility of cell leakage beyond the periosteal flap or collage membrane led to the development of Matrix-Carried Autologous Chondrocye Implantation (MACI; Verigen, Leverkusen, Germany). MACI has a similar porcine-derived type I/III collagen membrane. One surface has a roughened appearance because of widely-spaced collagen fibres, between which the chondrocytes are seeded. The other side has a smooth surface due to the high density of collagen fibres (Zheng et al., 2007). The MACI membrane can be secured to the defect directly with fibrin glue and therefore does not require additional cover. There is no need for additional sutures or harvesting of periosteum. The procedure can be performed faster and with less extensive exposure (Bartlett et al., 2005).

A concern regarding the MACI technique is the number of chondrocytes present in the collagen bilayer. It is estimated that there are 1 million chondrocytes per mm^3. In the ACI-C technique, there are approximately 5 million cells/ml suspension. Le Baron and Athanasiou performed a study seeding a manufactured scaffold with chondrocytes. They reported that scaffolds with less than 10 million cells/ml resulted in poor cartilage formation (LeBaron and Athanasiou, 2000). Puelacher et al. noted that scaffolds seeded with 20-100 million cells/ml resulted in cartilage formation when implanted subcutaneously into nude mice (Puelacher et al, 1994). Normal articular cartilage however contains only 10,000 cells/mm^2. Possible reasons for the need for such high concentrations of implanted chondrocytes may be because a proportion of implanted cells undergo apoptosis once they are implanted onto the defect or perhaps it is the physical crowding of cells that is needed for them to redifferentiate into type II secreting chondrocytes. In their recent review, the Swedish group have advocated using 30 million cells/ml in the clinical setting. Despite these reservations, several studies have shown that MACI is as efficacious as the first and second generation techniques (Bartlett et al., 2005 and Zeifang et al., 2010).

Outcome Following ACI / MACI

There are few randomised trials comparing two different techniques of cartilage transplant. Gooding et al. (2006) compared ACI using a periosteal flap (33 patients) with ACI using synthetic collagen membrane (ACI-C) such as the one used in this study (35 patients). The clinical results were similar in the two groups, though a significant number of patients in the ACI-P required a re-operation for graft hypertrophy. This difference in the re-operation rates resulted in the trial being stopped prematurely.

A randomised controlled trial compared outcome in patients treated with ACI or MACI for symptomatic osteochondral defects in the knee. One year following surgery, the mean Modified Cincinnati Score in the ACI-C group (n=44) was 59 (mean increase 17.5 points) and in the MACI group (n=47) was 64.1 (mean increase 19.4 points). However, this difference was not statistically significant. Analysed another way, 72.3% of patients reported a good or excellent outcome in the MACI group compared with 59.1% in the ACI-C group.

More recently, 21 patients were randomised to have either ACI-P or MACI using a resorbable scaffold of polyglactin 910 or poly-p-dioxanon (Zeifang et al., 2010). Knee function was assessed according to the International Knee Documentation Committee (IKDC) score at 24 months. Secondary outcome parameters used were the SF-36, Lysholm and Gillquist and Tegner Activity scores. The mean IKDC score changed from 51.1 to 72 in the ACI-P group and from 52 to 76.6 in the MACI group at 12 months, and this improvement was maintained at 2 years. There was no significant difference in the IKDC with respect to the treatment received. The only scoring system that demonstrated significant difference between the two treatment groups was the Lysholm and Gillquist scores, which favoured the ACI-P group. MRI scoring to evaluate cartilage repair had shown that there was a significant difference in favour of MACI at 6 months but not at 12 and 24 months. This was confirmed by another study which showed complete attachment of MACI grafts in 14 out of 16 patients at a mean of 34.7 days (range 22 to 47 days) (Marlovits et al., 2004).

For a randomised study, it was interesting to read that the ACI-P group comprised 10 males and the MACI group consisted of 6 men and 5 women. The number of patients in this study is questionable even though they had performed sample size calculations and stated that their study had 80% power. In their discussion, they have admitted that the standard deviation of 3.5 for IKDC scores used to calculate the sample size required was grossly underestimated and hence their sample size calculations were incorrect. There are two other weaknesses of the study; firstly, there were no women in the MACI group and secondly, there were no lateral femoral condyle lesions in the ACI-P group. As this is a randomised study with few patients, these discrepancies are likely to have occurred by chance, but results from this study have to be interpreted with caution.

In a prospective cohort study, 20 patients received two different types of MACI; 10 patients had a MACI graft with a synthetic collagen membrane (similar to the one used in this study) and 10 patients had a MACI graft based on hyaluronic acid (Welsch et al., 2010). They reported that the collagen MACI had higher quality superficial repair tissue according to a magnetic resonance imaging scoring system, though this did not translate clinically as there were equal proportions of good or excellent outcome (80%) in both treatment groups according to the Brittberg Score. Once again, due to the use of different scoring systems, a comparison between this study and ours is difficult. Ferruzzi et al. (2008) had demonstrated superior results with the use of MACI on a hyaluronic acid scaffold implanted arthroscopically (50 patients) compared with ACI-P (48 patients) implanted in the traditional manner (open arthrotomy). In both groups, there was statistically-significant increase in IKDC scores at 6, 12, 24, 36, 48 and 60 months following surgery. Between the two groups, the arthroscopic MACI group had significantly better scores that ACI-P until 18 months. At 24 months, the scores were slightly higher in the arthroscopy group but were not statistically-significant. However, complications and re-operation rates were significantly lower in the arthroscopy group (9 complications in the open series versus 2 in the arthroscopy group, p=0.008). The authors' speculated that the use of hyaluronic acid as a scaffold and its adhesive properties could explain no graft delamination or loose body formation. The design of this study has a fundamental flaw. It can not conclude that arthroscopic implantation is better than the open technique since here are two different types of ACI used. It would have been more appropriate to have used MACI in the open series.

MACI was shown to be efficacious in two other studies assessing traditional versus accelerated approaches to post-operative rehabilitation. 16 patients were randomised to have an accelerated weight-bearing whereas 15 patients underwent delayed weight-bearing following surgery (Wondrasch et al., 2009). Clinical assessment was performed using the IKDC, the Knee Osteoarthritis and Outcome Score (KOOS) and the Tegner Score. Compared to the pre-operative status, all clinical scores showed an improvement in both treatment groups with no statistically-significant differences. These were supported by a larger randomised controlled trial of 62 patients randomised to have traditional versus accelerated weight-bearing following MACI (Ebert et al., 2008). In their study, it was shown that accelerated weight-bearing resulted in significantly lower knee pain according to the KOOS.

The ultimate goal of ACI is to restore function in the relatively young, fit and active patient population. The secondary, more long-term goal is to avoid the development of secondary degenerative changes in the affected knee that may require a more radical surgical procedure such as tibial osteotomy or partial/total joint arthroplasty. Zaslav et al. (2009) deomonstrated 75% survivorship of ACI grafts at 48 months (though they used different end points). The 10-year survivorship in 72 patients was 83.3% with the end point being any operation to remove the implanted ACI graft (Moseley et al., 2010).

The Use of Mesenchymal Stem Cells

An open biopsy of articular cartilage is necessary in order to obtain the chondrocytes necessary for expansion and re-implantation. This exposes the patient to the morbidity of two surgical procedures. Stem cells are ideal alternative to chondrocytes since they are easily accessible, expandable in culture and mutlipotent and can be inserted in a single stage. Mesenchymal stem cells (MSCs) have been isolated from many tissues including bone marrow (Pittenger et al., 1999), synovial membrane (De Bari et al., 2004), periosteum (De Bari et al., 2006) and articular cartilage (Dowthawaite et al., 2004).

There are two important studies concerning the use of MSCs to engineer cartilage. Caplan's group developed an *in vitro* method of inducing both animal (Johnstone et al., 1998) and human (Yoo et al., 1998) into the chondrogenic pathway. The second important study was by Wakitani et al. (1994) in which rabbit MSCs were placed in full thickness OCDs in the medial condyle of young mature rabbits. Since then, considerable work has been performed on larger animal models (Liu et al., 2006, Wilkes et al., 2007, Bonfield et al., 2009) but to date there are few studies in humans.

Wakitini's group advanced their studies by transplanting autologous culture-expanded bone marrow mesenchymal cells into nine full-thickness articular cartilage defects of the patello-femoral joints (including two kissing lesions) in the knees of three patients. Three weeks before transplantation, bone marrow blood was aspirated from the iliac crest. Adherent cells were cultured with media containing autologous serum. Six months after transplantation, the patients' clinical symptoms had improved and the improvements have been maintained over the follow-up periods (17-27 months). Histology of the first patient 12 months after the transplantation revealed that the defect had been repaired with the fibrocartilaginous tissue. Magnetic resonance imaging of the second patient 1 year after transplantation revealed complete coverage of the defect, but they were unable to determine whether or not the material that covered the defects was hyaline cartilage.

Haleem et al. used platelet-rich fibrin glue as a scaffold to deliver autologous culture-expanded bone marrow MSCs for cartilage repair. All five patients had statistically-improved clinical scores 1 year following surgery. Only two of the five patients had agreed to an arthroscopic assessment of their grafts one year following surgery and they had improved arthroscopic (ICRS) scores from 8/12 to 11/12 (Haleem et al., 2010).

The source of stem cells is an important issue when considering cartilage repair. MSCs from bone marrow appear to have high propensity to cartilage hypertrophy and bone formation (Peltari et al., 2006) and hence may not be the ideal chondroprogenitors. MSCs from synovial membrane appear to have a greater propensity to form cartilage *in vitro* than MSCs from bone marrow and periosteum (Sakaguchi et al., 2005).

Recent work by Bosetti et al. (2011) have identified several growth factors such as bone morphogenic proteins that can induce the differentiatiation of human bone marrow MSCs into mature chondrocytes, with the additional effect of increased expression of collagen type II and Sox9, the markers for chondrogenesis. However, the more recent discovery of its immunomodulation capacity is just as exciting. Several publications indicate that MSCs and their secretions affect dendritic cells, T-cells, B-cells and Natural Killer cells (Iyer et al., 2008). Therefore the possibility exists of using MSCs to eliminate chronic inflammation from joints.

Discussion

The recent literature indicates that both ACI and MACI are equally effective in treating full thickness chondral defects in the knee and seem to be better than other techniques such as microfracture for larger defects (Bentley et al, 2003, Visna et al, 2004, Saris et al, 2008, Saris et al, 2009). High rates of graft hypertrophy in the ACI technique with periosteum suggest that we should be using a synthetic scaffold. (Gooding et al, 2006). Good to excellent long term outcomes on the use of ACI have been reported by Peterson (2010), but no other studies have reproduced similar results. There is no difference in short term results between ACI versus MACI (Bartlett et al 2005). There is currently ongoing work by Bentley, Briggs and colleagues in Stanmore, UK, on a prospective cohort randomised to ACI versus MACI, with data for both techniques being collected since 2003. However, the undisputable advantage of MACI is its amenability to be performed via arthroscopic or a more limited approach, without requiring arthrotomy. The positive results seen with an accelerated weight-bearing rehabilitation programme are also encouraging because it reduces the functional deficit in the patient who tends to be young and fit. It is also currently believed that MACI may provide a superior rate of clinical improvement compared to ACI (Gikas et al., 2008).

The further emergence of data is expected, encouraged by NICE recommendations to enrol all patients receiving ACI into new or ongoing clinical studies (NICE, 2005). There are currently no long term reports confirming that cell-based treatment of osteochondral defects limits progression to symptomatic primary, or as the case may be, secondary osteoarthritis.

As the work on MSCs is still in early stages, there is no consensus regarding the optimum source of harvesting of stem cells. The elucidation of the factors influencing chondrogenetic differentiation of MSCs is a step further into this technology. However, there is currently no evidence to suggest that the repair produced by MSCs is of histological quality comparable to ACI/MACI. In practice, the use of MSCs itself depends on not only the propensity for those cells to differentiate into hyaline as opposed to fibro-cartilage, but also the surgical technique in implantation, clinical effectiveness and donor site morbidity.

The role of these cell-based strategies for treating osteochondral defects in the knee will be clearer as new data emerges from follow-up studies and head-to-head trials, opening the door for patients to receive these increasingly-established treatments.

Key Points

- Only cartilage injuries that extend to the subchondral level show some capacity for repair due to the release of bone marrow derived mesenchymal stem cells.
- Autologous Chondrocyte Implantation (ACI) and Matrix-carried Autologous Chondrocyte Implantation (MACI) are currently used in clinical practice to treat larger full thickness chondral defects in the knee.
- There are a small number of studies using mesenchymal stem cells MSCs) and further in vitro and in vivo studies are needed before this treatment is optimised.

References

Angermann, P., Riegels-Nielson, P., Pederson, H., (1998) Osteochondritis dissecans of he femoral condyle treated with periosteal transplantation. Poor outcome in 14 patients followed for 6-9 years. *Acta Orthop. Scand* 69(6) 595-7.

Aston, J.E., Bentley, G. (1982) Culture of articular cartilage as a method of storage: assessment of maintenance of phenotype. *J. Bone Joint Surg.* 64 B, 384.

Aston, J.E., Bentley, G., (1986) Repair of articular surfaces by allografts of articular and growth-plate cartilage. *J. Bone Jt Surg.* 68B, 29-35.

Bartlett, W., Gooding, C.R., Carrington, R.W., Skinner, J.A., Briggs, T.W., Bentley, G., (2005) Autologous chondrocyte implantation at the knee using a bilayer collagen membrane with bone graft. A preliminary report. *J. Bone Joint Surg. Br.* 87(3) 330-2.

Bentley, G., Greer, R.B., (1971) Homotransplantation of isolated epiphyseal and articular cartilage chondrocytes into joint surfaces of rabbits. *Nature* 230, 385-388.

Bentley, G., Biant, L.C., Carrington, R.W., Akmal, M., Goldberg, A., Williams, A.M., Skinner, J.A., Pringle, J., (2003) A prospective, randomised comparison of autologous chondrocyte implantation versus mosaicplasty for osteochondral defects in the kee. *J. Bone Joint Surg. Br.* 85(2) 223-30.

Benya, P.D., Shaffer J.D. (1982) Dedifferentiated chondrocytes reexpress the differentiated collagen phenotype when cultured in agarose gels. *Cell* 30, 215-224.

Bert, J.M., (1993) Role of abrasion arthroplasty and debridement in the management of osteoarthritis of the knee. *Rheum. Dis. Clin. North Am.* 19(3) 725-39.

Bosetti, M., Boccafoschi, F., Leigheb, M., Bianchi A.E., Cannas, M., (2011 Feb 28) Chondrogenic induction of human mesenchymal stem cells using combined growth factors for cartilage tissue engineering. *J. Tissue Eng. Regen. Med.* (Epub ahead of print).

Brittberg, M., Lindahl, A., Nilsson, A., Ohlsson, C., Isaksson, O., Peterson, L., (1994) Treatment of deep cartilage defecs in the knee with autologous chondrocyte implantation. *N. Engl. J. Med.* 6;331(14) 889-95.

Brittberg, M., Nilsson, A., Lindahl, A., Ohlsson, C., Peterson, L., (1996) Rabbit articular cartilage defects treated with autologous cultured chondrocytes. *Clin. Orthop. Relat. Res.* (326) 270-83.

Chesterman, P.J., Smith, A.U., (1968) Homotransplantation of articular cartilage and isolated chondrocytes – an experimental study in rabbits. *J. Bone Joint Surg.* 50 B 1 184-197.

De Bari, C., Dell'Accio, F., Luyten, F.P., (2004) Failure of in vitro-differentiated mesenchymal stem cells from the synovial membrane to form ectopic stable cartilage in vivo. *Arthritis Rheum.* 50(1) 142-50.

De Bari, C., Dell'Accio, F., Vanlauwe, J., Eyckmans, J., Khan, I.M., Archer, C.W., Jones, E.A., McGonagle, D.,, Mitsiadis, T.A., Pitalis, C., Luyten, F.P., (2006) Mesenchymal multipotency of adult human periosteal cells demonstrated by single cell lineage analysis. *Arthritis Rheum.* 54(4) 1209-21.

Douthwaite, G.P., Bishop, J.C., Redman, S.N., Khan, I.M., Rooney, P., Evans, D.J.R., Haughton, L., Bayram, Z., Boyer, S., Thomson, B., Wolfe, M.S., Archer, C.W., (2004) The surface of articular cartilage contains a progenitor cell population. *J. Cell Sci.* (117) 889-897.

Ebert, J.R., Robertson, W.B., Lloyd, D.G., Zheng, M.H., Wood, D.J., Ackalnd, T., (2008) Traditional vs accelerated approaches to post-operative rehabilitation following matrix-induced autologous chondrocyte implantation (MACI): comparison of clinical, biomechanical and radiographic outcomes. *Osteoarthritis cartilage* 16(10) 1131-40.

Ferruzzi, A., Buda, R., Faldini, C., Vannini, F., Di Caprio, F., Luciani, D., Giannini, S., (2008) Autologous chondrocyte implantation in the knee joint: open compared with arthroscopic technique. Comparison at a minimum follow-up of five years. *J. Bone Joint Surg. Br.* 90(4) 90-101.

Gikas, P.D., Aston, W.J.S., Briggs, T.W.R., (2008) Autologous chondrocyte implantation: where do we stand now? *J. Orthop Sci.* (13) 283-292.

Gooding, C.R., Bartlett, W., Bentley, G., Skinner, J.A., Carrington, R., Flanagan, A. (2006) A prospective, randomised study comparing two techniques of autologous chondrocyte implantation for osteochondral defects in the knee: periosteum covered versus type I/III collagen covered. *Knee* 13(3) 203-10.

Grande, D.A., Pitman, M.I., Peterson, L., Menche, D., Klein, M., (1989) The repair of experimentally produced defects in rabbit articular cartilage by autologous chondrocyte transplantation. *J. Orthop. Res.* 7 208-18.

Green, W.T., (1971) Behavior of articular chondrocytes in cell culture. *Clin. Orthop. Rel. Res.* 75, 248-260.

Haleem, A.M., Singergy, A.A., Sabry, D., Atta,, H.M., Rashed, L.A., Chu, C.R., El Shewy, M.T., Azzam, A., Abdel Aziz, M.T., (2010) The clinical use of human culture-expanded autologous bone marrow mesenchymal stem cells transplanted on platelet-rich fibrin glue in the treatment of articular cartilage defects: a pilot study and preliminary results. *Cartilage* 1(4) 253-261.

Hubbard, M.J., (1996) Articular debridement versus washout for degeneration of the medial femoral condyle. A five-year study. *J. Bone Joint Surg. Br.* 78 (2) 217-9.

Iyer, S.S., Rojas, M., (2008) Anti-inflammatory effects of mesenchymal stem cells: novel concept for future therapies. *Expert Opin. Biol Ther.* (8) 569-81.

Johnstone, B., Hering, T.M., Caplan, A.I., Goldberg, V.M., Yoo, J.U., (1998) In vitro chondrogenesis of bone marrow-derived mesenchymal progenitor cells. *Exp. Cell Res.* 238(1) 265-72.

LeBaron, R.G., Athanasiou, K.A., (2000) Ex vivo synthesis of articular cartilage. *Biomaterials* 21(24) 2575-87.

Lindahl, A., Brittberg, M., Peterson, L., (2003) Cartilage repair with chondrocytes: clinical and cellular aspects. *Novartis Found Symp.* 249 175-86.

Liu, H., Kemeny, D.M., Heng, B.C., Ouyang, H.W., Melendez, A.J., Cao, T., (2006) The immunogenicity and immunomodulatory function of osteogenic cells differentiated from mesenchymal stem cells. *J. Immunol.* 176(5) 2864-71.

Mankin, H.J. (1962a) Localization of tritiated thymidine in articular cartilage of rabbits. I. Growth in immature cartilage of rabbits. *J. Bone Jt Surg.,* 44A 682.

Mankin, H.J. (1962b) Localization of tritiated thymidine in articular cartilage of rabbits. II. Repair in immature cartilage. *J. Bone Jt Surg.,* 44A 688.

Mankin, H.J. (1963) Localization of tritiated thymidine in articular cartilage of rabbits. III. Mature articular cartilage. *J. Bone Jt Surg*., 45A 529.

Marlovits, S., Striessnig, G., Kutsha-Lissberg, F., Resinger, C., Aldrian, S.M., Vécsei, V., Trattnig, S., (2005) *Knee Surg. Sports Traumatol. Arthrosc.* 13(6) 451-7.

Minas, T., Nehrer, S., (1997) Current concepts in the treatment of articular cartilage defects. *Orthopaedics* 2(6) 525-38.

Moseley, J.B. Jr., Anderson, A.F., Browne, J.E., Mandelbaum, B.R., Micheli, L.J., Fu, F., Erggelet, C., (2010) Long-term durability of autologous chondrocyte implantation: a multicenter, observational study in US patients. *Am. J. Sports Med.* 38(2) 238-46.

National Institute of Clinical Excellence Technology (NICE) (2005) Appraisal 89 The use of autologous chondrocyte implantation for the treatment of cartilage defects in knee joints.

Pelttari, K., Winter, A., Steck, E., Gotzke, K., Hennig, T., Ochs, B.G., Aigner, T., Richter, W., (2006) Premature induction of hypertrophy during in vitro chondrogenesis of human mesenchymal stem cells correlates with calcification and vascular invasion after ectopic transplantation in SCID mice. *Arthrit Rheum.* (54) 3254-326.

Peterson, L., Brittberg, M., Kiviranta, I., Akerlund, E.L., Lindahl, A., (2002) Autologous chondrocyte transplantation. *Biomechanics and long-term durability* 30(1) 2-12.

Peterson, L., Vasiliadis, H.S., Brittberg, M., Lindahl, A., (2010) Autologous chondrocyte implantation: a long term follow-up. *Am. J. Spors Med.* 38(6) 1117-24

Pittenger, M.F., Mackay, A.M., Beck, S.C., Jaiswal, R.K., Douglas, R., Mosca, J.D., Moorman, M.A., Simonette, D.W., Craig, S., Marshak, D.R., (1999) Multilineage potential of adult human mesenchymal stem cells. *Science* 284(5411) 143-7.

Puelacher, W.C., Kim, S.W., Vacanti, J.P., Schloo, B., Mooney, D., Vacanti, C.A., (1994) Tissue-engineered growth of cartilage: the effect of varying the concentration of chondrocytes seeded onto synthetic polymer matrices. *Int. J. Oral Maxillofac. Surg.* (23)49-53.

Robertson, W.B., Fick, D., Wood, D.J., Linklater, J.M., Zheng, M.H., Ackland, T.R., MRI and clinical evaluation of collagen-covered autologous chondrocyte implantation (CACI) at two years. *Knee* 14(2) 117-27.

Sakaguchi, Y., Sekiya, I., Yagishita, K., Muneta, T., (2005) Comparison of human stem cells derived fro various mesenchymal tissues: superiority of synovium as a cell source. *Arthrit. Rheum.* (52) 2521-2529.

Saris, D.B., Vanlauwe, J., Victor, J., Haspl, M., Bohnsack, M., Fortems, Y., Vanderkerckhove, B., Almqvist, K.F., Claes, T., Handelberg, F., Lagae, K., van der Bauwhede, J., Vandenneucker, H., Yang, K.G., Jelic, M., Verdonk, R., Veulemans, N., Bellemans, J., Luyten, F.P., (2008) Characterized chondrocyte implantation results in better structural repair when treating symptomatic cartilage defects of the knee in a randomized controlled trial versus microfracture. *Am. J. Sports Med.* 36 (2) 235-46.

Saris, D.B., Vanlauwe, J., Victor, J., Almqvist, K.F., Verdonk, R., Bellemans, J., Luyten, F.P., TIG/ACT/01/2000andEXT Study Group (2009) Treatment of symptomatic cartilage defects of the knee: characterized chondrocyte implantation results in better clinical outcome at 36 months in a randomized trial compared to microfracture. *Am. J. Sports Med.* 37 Suppl1 10S-19S.

Smith, A.U., (1965) Survival of frozen chondrocytes isolated from cartilage of adult mammals. *Nature* 205,782.

Steinwachs, M., Kreuz, P.C., (2007) Autologous chondrocyte implantation in chondral defects of the knee with a type I/III collagen membrane: a prospective study with a 3-year follow-up. *Arthroscopy* 23(4) 381-7.

Visna, P., Pasa, L., Cizmár I., Hart, R., Hoch, J., (2004) Treatment of deep cartilage defects of the knee using autogous chondrograft transplantation and by abrasive techniques—a randomized controlled study. *Acta Chir Belg* 104(6) 709-14.

Wakitani, S., Goto, T., Pineda, S.J., Young, R.G., Mansour, J.M., Goldberg, V.M., (1994) Mesenchymal cell-based repair of large, full-thickness defects of articular cartilage. *J. Bone Joint Surg. Am.* 76(4) 579-92.

Welsch, G.H., Mamisch, T.C., Zak, L., Blanke, M., Olk, A., Marlovits, S., Trattnig, S., (2010) Evaluation of cartilage repair tissue after matrix-associated autologous chondrocyte transplantation using a hyaluronic-based or a collagen based scaffold with morphological MOCART scoring and biochemical T2 mapping: preliminary results. *Am. J. Sports Med.* 38(5) 934-42.

Wilke, M.M., Nydam, D., Nixon, A.J., (2007) Enhanced early chondrogenesis in articular defecs following arthroscopic mesenchymal stem cell implantation in an equine model. *J. Orthop. Res.* 25(7) 913-925.

Wondrasch, B., Zak, L., Welsch, G.H., Marlovits, S., (2009) Effect of accelerated weightbearing after matrix-associated autologous chondrocyte implantation on the femoral condyle on radiographic and clinical outcome after 2 years: a prospective, randomised controlled pilot study. *Am. J. Sports Med.* 37 (1) 88S-96S.

Wood, J.J., Malek, M.A., Frassica, F.J., Polder, J.A., Mohan, A.K., Bloom, E.T., Braun, M.M., Coté, T.R., (2006) Autologous cultured chondrocytes: adverse events reported to the United States Food and Drug Administration. *J. Bone Joint Surg. Am.* 88(3) 503-7.

Yoo, J.U., Barthel, T.S., Nishimura, K., Solchaga, L., Caplan, A.I., Goldberg, V.M., Johnstone, B., (1998) The chondrogenic potential of human bone-marrow-derived mesenchymal progenitor cells. *J. Bone Joint Surg. Am.* 80(12) 1745-57.

Zaslav, K., Cole, B., Brewster, R., DeBerardino, T., Farr, J., Fowler, P., Nissen, C., STAR Study Principal Investigators. (2009) A prospective study of autologous chondrocyte implantation in patients with failed prior treatment for articular cartilage defecs of the knee: results of the Study of the Treatment of Articular Repair (STAR) clinical trial. *Am. J. Sports Med.* 37(1) 42-55.

Zeifang, F., Oberle,, D., Nierhoff, C., Richter, W., Moradi, B., Schmitt, H., (2010) Autologous chondrocyte implantation using the original periosteum-cover technique versus matrix-associated autologous chondrocyte implantation: a randomised clinical trial. *Am. J. Sports Med.* 38(5) 924-33.

Zheng, M.H., Willers, C., kirilak, K., Yates, P., Xu, J., Wood, D., Shimmin, A., (2007) Matrix-induced autologous chondrocyte implantation (MACI): biological and histological assessment. *Tissue Eng.* 13(4) 737-46.

In: Stem Cells in Disease
Editor: Prasad S. Koka
ISBN: 978-1-62257-169-7
© 2012 Nova Science Publishers, Inc.

Chapter XIX

Stem Cells for Tendon and Ligament Tissue Engineering and Regeneration

***N. A. Siddiqui*[1],**
***J. M. L. Wong*[1],**
***Wasim S. Khan*[2*] *and A. Hazlerigg*[3]**

[1]Department of Trauma and Orthopaedics, Royal Free Hampstead NHS Trust, London, UK
[2]University College London Institute of Orthopaedics and Musculoskeletal Sciences, Royal National Orthopaedic Hospital, Stanmore, Middlesex, UK
[3]Kingston Hospital NHS Trust, Kingston, London, UK

Abstract

Tendons and ligaments are frequently injured. Due to their relatively avascular nature, repair is slow and often incomplete. Stem cells offer a new approach to augment healing of native tissues, as well as providing materials to surgically replace injured structures that are beyond repair. Here we discuss the various roles of stem cells in natural repair processes compared to engineered tissues to assist healing or replace tissues.

Keywords: Healing; materials; scaffolds; stem cells

* Corresponding Author: Mr Wasim S Khan, Clinical Lecturer, University College London Institute of Orthopaedics and Musculoskeletal Science, Royal National Orthopaedic Hospital, Stanmore, Middlesex, London, HA7 4LP, UK. Telephone number: +44 (0) 7791 025554. Fax number: +44 (0) 20 8570 3864. E-mail address: wasimkhan@doctors.org.uk.

Introduction

Tendon and ligament injuries occur frequently. They are a significant cause of patient morbidity, with reduced quality of life and increased financial burden. Over 200,000 Anterior Cruciate Ligament (ACL) reconstructions per year are carried out in the US (Shelton 2011), and 40,000 in-patient procedures were performed in the USA for rotator cuff repair in 2002 (Oh *et al* 2007). In 2007, Achilles tendon injuries had an incidence of 11.3/100,000 per year in the UK (Clayton and Court-Brown 2008).

Healing of tendons and ligaments results in a poorer quality tissue with a high risk of re-injury. Laboute *et al* (2010) found a re-rupture rate of 12.7% for ACL reconstructions performed with hamstring tendon autografts.

The clinical challenge is in improving functional outcomes for patients following these injuries, attempting to match their pre-morbid state. This is the driving force behind the concept of "tissue engineering". Langer and Vacanti (1993) described tissue engineering as applying "the principles of engineering and the life sciences toward the development of biological substitutes that restore, maintain, or improve tissue function". The three main components of this concept are (1) cells/cell substitutes, (2) tissue inducing chemicals, and (3) scaffolds to contain the cells.

Stem cells are naturally occurring cells that have the ability to both self-replicate as well as differentiate into another cell type. Therefore, they have an important role to play as the basic building block of any tissue that needs to be engineered.

Normal Structure

Human ligaments and tendons share some structural and microscopic properties but are still very different tissues. They are highly resistant to stretching, and have a molecular structure which is specialised to fulfil this property.

They both consist of cells and an extracellular matrix. The cells constitute approximately 20% of the tissue, and are specialised fibroblasts. The remaining 80% is extracellular matrix, which consists of 70% water and 30% collagen, ground substance, and elastin. The collagen present in ligaments and tendons is predominantly type I. There is also a small amount (less than 10%) of type III collagen, but this is more often found in healing tissues, before most of it is converted to type I collagen. There is also a very small amount of type IV collagen present. Type I collagen contains two alpha-1 and one alpha-2 polypeptide chains, formed within the fibroblast as separate molecules before aggregation into a triple-helix structure and further processing to form collagen molecules. Stable cross-links create well aligned bundles.

In tendons these collagen bundles are usually arranges into fascicles, enveloped by layers of connective tissue: endotenon and then epitenon. Ground substance stabilises the collagen microfibrils, and consists of a variety of molecules including proteoglycans, glycoproteins, and plasma proteins. It has the ability to bind water, resulting in a gel-like substance with increased strength. A small amount of elastin is also produced by fibroblasts. It is highly cross-linked and organised multi-directionally, and can stretch and recoil back to its original shape.

The insertion of ligaments and tendons into bone is of great importance, and is fairly constant. There are four zones:

1. Collagen fibres lying parallel
2. Unmineralized fibrocartilage interwoven with the collagen
3. Fibrocartilage becomes increasingly mineralised as it approaches the surface of the bone (Sharpey's fibres)
4. Cortical bone interwoven with the mineralized fibrocartilage before being full transition into cortical bone

There is also some contribution to the strength of ligaments by direct incorporation of the collagen fibres with the periosteum.

A tendon links muscle to bone, allowing specific advantages over muscle directly attaching to bone. Tendons must often pass over angled surfaces just as joints, and therefore must be able to resist forces when angled, and allow the muscle to exert its force at a different angle to its contraction.

A ligament is a structure that attaches one bone to another bone. It requires its strength to be maximal in several different directions, so the collagen is organised in a slightly less aligned direction to that of tendons, which are only required to exert a force in the direction of pull of a muscle, which is less variable. The collagen fibres are both less parallel, as well as being arranged in layers of differing directions and having a crimped, or wavy, pattern to allow for better energy absorption. But this multi-directional arrangement also means that ligaments are generally weaker than tendons.

Reasons for Poor Naturally Healed Tissues

The blood supply to both tendons and ligaments is relatively poor. They have, therefore, adapted to have a very low metabolic rate. They have slightly different methods of vascular supply. Tendons are covered, either entirely or at least in part, by a paratenon, which is a form of loose areolar connective tissue. Ligaments also have a similar structure enveloping them. It contains a large number of cells and is also responsible for the majority of the vascular supply to these structures. The blood supply of a ligament is via a uniform supply from its insertion site, whereas blood supply to tendons is via small arterioles which run along with the paratenon, giving off segmental branches.

Tendons have some variability of this surrounding tissue, in some cases having a synovial sheath, but in many cases having a layer of epitenon just below the paratenon to facilitate gliding of the tendon over high friction areas such as around the wrist and hand. Tendons without a paratenon, i.e. those with a synovial sheath, receive their blood supply via segmentally arranged vinculae which carry a vessel to supply only a segment of tendon, adjacent areas being dependent on diffusion. For this reason, tendons with a paratenon have an advantageous blood supply.

The musculo-tendinous junction is an area of particular weakness. However, there is an abundant blood supply to assist with healing. To provide additional strength, the muscle is infolded in order to provide a greater surface area for interdigitation with the basement membrane and the tendon.

When considering the strength of a tendon or ligament, the load-to-failure force is an indicator of its likelihood to rupture when compared to peak *in vivo* forces. The Ultimate Tensile Strength of the human Achilles tendon is 1,189N (Louis-Ugbo *et al* 2004). As peak *in vivo* forces are usually higher than the load-to-failure force of healed tendons and ligaments, there is, inevitably, a risk of re-rupture due to inadequacies in the quality of a tissue once it has healed.

The specialised structure of tendons and ligaments thus make them ideally suited to their function, but these hypocellular, relatively avascular structures also result in a relatively poor ability to regenerate and heal. Whether after healing naturally or via surgical repair, the resultant tissue is of relatively poor quality, is prone to re-rupture and requires protection before resuming normal activities with physiological loads.

Various techniques have been employed to try to improve the poor healing of tendons and ligaments. Options for current therapy using grafts may be autologous, cadaveric, or artificial. Problems include donor site morbidity, immunological and infection risks, foreign body reactions to artificial grafts. ACL reconstruction can be performed using various grafts, and the technique performed is dependant on the surgeon. Allografts are popular as they avoid morbidity from the donor site, yet it is recognised that there is an inherent risk of immunological reactions and infection. Greenberg *et al* (2010) studied 861 patients undergoing primary ACL reconstruction either with an autograft or allograft and found no significant difference in the incidence of infection between the two groups. However, Romanini *et al* (2010) found that allografts were associated with a higher rate of failure.

Stem Cells

Stem cells are currently an item of great interest in both scientific research as well as the popular media. Stem cells are naturally occurring cells that must have two fundamental abilities:

1. Replicate to produce exactly the same cell type, i.e. 'self-renewal'
2. Differentiate into another cell type given various stimuli

There are a number of different cells which may be classed as stem cells. These may be broken down into different types, with varying capacities for differentiation:

Totipotent – only the early embryo (zygote) may be truly called totipotent, it has the ability to form any cell, i.e. the foetus as well as the placenta. It is up to approximately the 4-day stage when the zygote has a totipotent ability.

Pluripotent – Embryonic Stem Cells (ESCs), derived from the Inner Cell Mass (ICM) are able to differentiate into any of the foetal tissues, i.e. into ectoderm, mesoderm, and endoderm, as well as germ cells

Multipotent – able to differentiate into a large but limited number of cell types

Oligopotent – able to differentiate only into a few types of cell

These differ from the Unipotent cell type, which has the ability only to differentiate into a single cell type, e.g. skin or hepatocytes. These have the property of self-renewal, as opposed to terminally differentiated cells, but cannot differentiate into any other cell type and so cannot be regarded as a true stem cell. Oligopotent stem cells have limited use as they have only a limited ability to differentiate, e.g. vascular stem cells may differentiate into smooth muscle or endothelial cells.

When cultured *in vitro* Totipotent and Pluripotent stem cells have similarities in their gene expression to that of tumour cells (Knoepfler 2009), and have been associated with a greater risk of uncontrolled growth, and therefore risk of tumorigenic change. For this reason, their use is limited at present. They must be harvested from the embryo or foetus, and therefore pose significant ethical and moral issues.

The greatest promise lies with Multipotent stem cells. Examples are haematopoietic stem cells present in bone marrow, which can produce almost any type of blood cell, and mesenchymal stem cells (MSCs), which can produce a wide variety of connective tissues such as osteocytes, chondrocytes, tenocytes, and myocytes (Pittenger *et al* 2002). Human umbilical cord blood has the advantage of being an accessible source of MSCs (Arien-Zakay, 2010). Ohnishi et al (2011) found that the limitations in MSCs of proliferation/differentiation could be overcome by producing Induced Pluripotent Stem Cells from frozen stocked bone marrow and MSCs. Lee and Hui (2006) have suggested characteristics for successful use of stem cells in therapy, which include:

- Adequate numbers of correct cell phenotypes
- Animal-free culture
- Better characterisation of cells
- Better differentiation of cells
- Better expansion of cells
- Appropriate three-dimensional structure
- Produce extra-cellular matrix
- Structurally and biomechanically compatible with the demands placed on it
- Fully integrate with host tissue
- Immunologically compatible

When stem cells are cultured with various stimuli they have the ability to change into a particular cell type. Stimuli that induce such change include:

- Terminally differentiated cells included in culture medium
- Type of culture medium
- Genetic modification of stem cells
- Scaffold containing the stem cell
- Molecular stimulants such as Growth Factors, hormones, signalling proteins such as Smads, and matrix metalloproteinases
- Mechanical stimulation.

MSCs are a form of adult stem cell and can be harvested without resorting to foetal/embryonic sources. They may be found in non-haematopoietic bone marrow stroma, as well as periosteum, fat, and skin. They have been used to create tendon and ligament-like structures *in vitro* using scaffolds, and have been used as local injections of the cells into areas requiring regeneration.

Tissue Engineering Approach to Tendon and Ligament Augmentation and Replacement

Strategies to improve the repair of ligaments and tendons include:

1. Replace the tendon with a graft (autologous, allogenic, or tissue engineered)
2. Deliver cells locally to induce a better quality repair
3. Deliver chemicals locally to induce a better repair

The United States National Committee on Biomechanics (USNCB) has suggested six principles of tissue engineering, as reported by Butler *et al* (2000):

1. Measurement of normal tissue stress and strain patterns *in vivo*
2. Measurement of normal tissue failure properties
3. Identify a subset of the properties to focus research on
4. Establish a minimum standard that these properties much achieve
5. Investigate which stimuli cells react to *in vivo*
6. Investigate the role of physical factors on cell stimulation in bioreactors during the production of such engineered tissues

Factors that may play a significant role in producing tissues that are effective substitutes for normal healthy tissues include proteins present in normal extracellular matrix, as well as those with a role in intracellular signalling. Growth factors are also known to generate improved properties (Hertel *et al* 2005, Schwitzer *et al* 2010). Hou *et al* (2009) investigated the effects of transforming growth factor (TGFβ-1) on Achilles tendon healing in rabbits. They showed that by transfecting the bone marrowed-derived MSCs, the tendons showed higher concentrations of collagen and rapid matrix remodelling.

Wei *et al* (2011) showed local administration of TGFβ-1/VEGF165 gene-transduced bone MSCs in Achilles allograft replacement of the ACL in rabbits improved vascularisation and promoted mechanical strength on biomechanical testing.

Juncosa *et al* (2003) implanted force transducers into the patellar ligament of rabbits in order to establish normal values for standing and activities to assess what the resting and peak forces would be *in vivo*. This would establish the benchmark with which any engineered tissues could be compared. There is a continuous pursuit to increase the quality of structures that are engineered to replace injured tissues. This is illustrated by the work of Butler *et al* (2000), who showed how, through a systematic approach to changing the production of a ligament substitute, material properties can be improved to try to match the strength and behaviour of normal tissue. Early tissue engineering involved growth of cells *in vitro* in a gel-like culture medium with a tensioned suture in order to help orientate the cells correctly, provide an anchor for cellular attachment, and assist with contraction. A decade later, Butler *et al* (2010) described the patella tendon as a reproducible model for studying healing, by using collagen-based scaffolds for tissue-engineered repair of tendons.

Awad *et al* (2003) cultured MSCs in this way and implanted the resulting tissue into rabbit patellar ligament defects, after labelling the MSCs with a fluorescent dye. A defect was made in the contralateral side as a control at the same time. After sacrifice at 12 and 26 weeks they found that the strength of the construct was greater than that of naturally healing tissue in the contralateral side. Compared to healthy tissue, the cultured MSCs had 23-27% strength, whereas the healed tissue managed only 15-19% strength. Original MSCs were still present, as evidenced by the fluorescent stained cells. However, they found ectopic bone formation on the cultured side, a result of poorly constrained cellular differentiation. Inducing *in vitro* differentiation of the MSCs into tendon-forming cells prior to introduction is thought to reduce the incidence of ectopic bone formation and tumour formation (Lui *et al* 2011).

Juncosa-Melvin *et al* (2005) altered the ratio of cells to collagen in the culture medium and found that, by reducing the cell: collagen ratio from up to 2.67×10^6 cells/mg collagen to a minimum 0.04×10^6 cells/mg collagen, as well as changing the sutures to anchor posts to maintain an axial strain on the gel, all ectopic bone was eliminated. In addition, there was an improvement in maximum stress to 30% and modulus of elasticity to 20%. The failure forces were greater than peak *in vivo* forces, thereby making the substance strong enough to withstand normal mobility forces. Surgical management of repair of tendon bone interfaces is challenging. Using viral modification, Shahab-Osterloh *et al* (2010) showed how the tenogenic, osteo-/chondrogenic properties of MSCs could be manipulated to form stem cell dependant tendon-bone interfaces, entheses. In order to improve the stiffness, and to match the 'Tangent Stiffness' of normal tissue, i.e. to match the normal stress-strain curve, they then experimented with different collagen sponges instead of a gel. This resulted in tissues that were very similar in their behaviour to normal tissue, as well as being strong enough to withstand peak forces, and, therefore, suitable for normal activities. Awad *et al* (2003) were able to further improve tissue properties by intermittent stimulation by applying increased strain for one second every five minutes for eight hours a day for twelve days. This reinforced theories that tissue properties may be improved by stimulating the tissue while still in the bioreactor by not only providing chemical stimuli such as growth factors, but also by providing mechanical stimulation.

Similarly, Ju (2008) used MSCs derived from synovium to accelerate healing of an Achilles tendon graft in murine models. When the Achilles tendon was grafted into a bone tunnel filled with MSCs, integration of tendon to bone was accelerated. Okamoto N (2010) compared the mechanical impact, collagen immunohistochemistry and histological changes that MSCs produced to that of whole Bone Marrow Cells (BMCs) in rat models. Whole BMCs possess multipotentiality, and by treating Achilles tendon ruptures with injections of these cells, they showed that the BMC group withstood more loading, stronger type-III collagen staining after a week, and stronger type-I collagen staining at 28 days, suggesting that this treatment may be a better alternative for Achilles tendon rupture.

Chong *et al* (2007) have also used MSCs successfully to promote tendon healing in an animal model. Rabbit Achilles tendon was sectioned and then immediately repaired and treated with bone marrow derived MSCs. This study showed improved tendon healing and structure in the first few weeks after surgery and receiving MSCs, although there no long term benefits were observed when compared to control groups.

Conclusion

Injuries to tendons and ligaments are a challenge to treat effectively and provide a result which has adequate strength, able to withstand peak forces applied during a variety of activities, ranging from standing to sporting activities. The treatment must be acceptable to the patient and care provider. It must be safe, effective, simple enough for the patient to comply with, and have minimal associated morbidity.

Current treatments do not fulfil all these criteria, and this has led to a search for the optimal way of managing these injuries. Autografts carry a significant risk of morbidity from donor sites. For example, Anterior Cruciate Ligament grafts for reconstruction harvested from patellar ligaments results in pain and numbness to surrounding skin, amongst others (Hertel et al 2005, Shelton et al 2011).

Artificial substitutes for the ACL have been tried, including carbon fibre, polypropylene, Dacron and polyester but have been unsuccessful for a variety of reasons, including immunological reactions and debris generation causing synovitis (Legnani *et al* 2010).

Cadaveric grafts have grown in popularity but do have a small risk of transmission of disease. Díaz-de-Rada *et al* took cultures from cadaveric ACL allografts at the time of implantation and found 24 of 181 allografts to have positive cultures, even though they had initially been screened and found to be negative for bacterial and viral infections. All positively cultured patients received antibiotic treatment and none resulted in deep infection.

Other than structural properties, the property of proprioception has not been addressed (Hoffman and Gross, 2007) when tendon and ligament tissues have been engineered. The incorporation of mechanoreceptors may be the focus of further tissue engineering projects.

Tissue engineering offers a promising answer to this difficult problem. We are learning more and more about the methods in which tissues can be produced to emulate natural tissues, with properties that match natural healthy tissues in terms of peak strength, as well as other behavioural properties such as modulus of elasticity and *in vivo* displacement under stress.

With research aimed initially at obtaining information about healthy tissues, naturally healed damaged tissues, and the resistance to forces required by engineered tissues, we are able to create treatment modalities which are able to deliver to areas of damaged tissues a variety of options: chemical stimulation of the patient's own tissues; stem cells implanted locally to the site of injury; or completely engineered tissues for grafting.

Although there are some concerns about the potential for uncontrolled growth by Pluripotent Stem Cells, which ultimately have the potential for indefinite self-renewal, the role of MSCs is being explored and has not been found to have the same problem. The problem of ectopic bone formation at the site of MSC treatment is due to differentiation of these cells into another phenotype, the very reason why they are of such great use, but this problem has been avoided by alterations in the method of production of the engineered tissue (Juncosa-Melvin *et al* 2005).

One important factor to consider is that the vast majority of studies in this field have been performed using animal models. We still do not know how the data obtained from animal models may be translated into information we may use in human trials, and there are no large trials, as yet, looking at the application of stem cells and engineered tissues for ligaments and tendons in humans. At present there is still controversy over which animal would be best to use in these studies. Most authors would agree that the animal should vary according to what aspect of the tendon is being studied. Tapper *et al* (2008) describes the similarity in biomechanical stresses of a knee of a sheep to that of a human, yet porcine knees seem to share more characteristics with its human counterpart for the healing process (Murray *et al* 2010).

Although in its relative infancy, tissue engineering and the use of stem cells is very likely to hold the answer to the problem of how to improve the healing of tendons and ligaments, or to replace damaged tissues. As these are relatively simple structures, compared to tissues such as liver or neural tissue, there remains a greater possibility of a successful treatment which can be used to restore full function following such common and debilitating injuries.

References

Awad HA, Boivin GP, Dressler MR, et al (2003) Repair of patellar tendon injuries using a cell-collagen composite. *Journal of Orthopaedic Research* 21: 420-431.

Arien-Zakay H, Lazarovici P, Nagler A (2010). Tissue regeneration potential in human umbilical cord blood. *Best Practice Research in Clinical Haematology* 23(2): 291-303.

Butler DL, Goldstein SA, Guilak F (2000) Functional tissue engineering: the role of biomechanics. *Journal of Biomechanical Engineering* 122: 570–575.

Butler DL, Gooch C, Kinneberg KR, Boivin GP, Galloway MT, Nirmalanandhan VS, et al (2010) The use of mesenchymal stem cells in collagen-based scaffolds for tissue-engineered repair of tendons. *Nature Protocols* 5(5): 849-863.

Chong AKS, Ang AD, Goh JCH, Hui JHP, Lim AYT, Lee EH, Lim BH (2007). Bone Marrow-Derived Mesenchymal Stem Cells Influence Early Tendon-Healing in a Rabbit Achilles Tendon Model. *Journal of Bone and Joint Surgery (Am)* 89: 74-81.

Clayton RA, Court-Brown CM. (2008) The epidemiology of musculoskeletal tendinous and ligamentous injuries. *Injury* 39(12):1338-1344.

Díaz-de-Rada P, Barriga A, Barroso JL, García-Barrecheguren E, Alfonso M, Valentí JR (2003) Positive culture in allograft ACL-reconstruction: what to do? *Knee Surgery, Sports Traumatology and Arthroscopy*. 11(4): 219-222.

Greenberg DD, Robertson M, Vallurupalli S, White RA, Allen WC (2010). Allograft compared with autograft infection rates in primary anterior cruciate ligament reconstruction. *Journal of Bone and Joint Surgery (Am)* 92(14): 2402-2408.

Hertel P, Behrend H, Cierpinski T, Musahl V, Widjaja G (2005) ACL reconstruction using bone-patellar tendon-bone press-fit fixation: 10-year clinical results. *Knee Surgery, Sports Traumatology and Arthroscopy* 13(4): 248-255.

Hoffman A, Gross G (2007) Tendon and ligament engineering in the adult organism: mesenchymal stem cells and gene-therapeutic approaches. *International Orthopaedics* 31:791-797.

Hou Y, Mao Z, Wei X, Lin L, Chen L, Wang H, Fu X, Zhang J, Yu C (2009) The roles of TGF-beta1 gene transfer on collagen formation during Achilles tendon healing. *Biochemical and Biophysical Research Communications* 383(2): 235-239.

Ju Y-J, Muneta T, Yoshimura H, Koga H, Sekiya I. (2008). Synovial mesenchymal stem cells accelerate early remodelling of tendon-bone healing. *Cell and Tissue Research*. 332: 469–478.

Juncosa N, West JR, Galloway MT, Boivin GP, Butler DL (2003) In vivo forces used to develop design parameters for tissue engineered implants for rabbit patellar tendon repair. *Journal of Biomechanics* 36:483–488.

Juncosa-Melvin N, Boivin GP, Galloway MT, Gooch C, West JR, Butler DL (2005) Effects of cell to collagen ratio in mesenchymal stem cell-seeded implants on tendon repair biomechanics and histology. *Tissue Engineering* 11: 448–457.

Knoepfler PS (2009) Deconstructing Stem Cell Tumorigenicity: A Roadmap to Safe Regenerative Medicine. *Stem Cells* 27, 1050-1056.

Laboute E, Savalli L, Puig P, Trouve P, Sabot G, Monnier G, et al (2010) Analysis of return to competition and repeat rupture for 298 anterior cruciate ligament reconstructions with patellar or hamstring tendon autograft in sportspeople. *Annals of Physical and Rehabilitation Medicine* 53(10): 598-614.

Langer R, Vacanti JP (1993) Tissue engineering. *Science*, 260 (5110): 920-926.

Lee EH, Hui JHP (2006) The potential of stem cells in orthopaedic surgery. *Journal of Bone and Joint Surgery* (Br) 88-B: 841-851.

Legnani C, Ventura A, Terzaghi C, Borgo E, Albisetti W (2010) Anterior cruciate ligament reconstruction with synthetic grafts. A review of literature. *International Orthopaedics.* 34(4):465-471.

Louis-Ugbo J, Leeson B, Hutton WC (2004) Tensile properties of fresh human calcaneal (Achilles) tendons. *Clinical Anatomy* 17, 30-35.

Lui PP, Rui YF, Ni M, Chan KM (2011) Tenogenic differentiation of stem cells for tendon repair-what is the current evidence? *Journal of Tissue Engineering and Regenerative Medicine.* (in press).

Murray MM, Margarian E, Zurakowski D, Fleming BC (2010) Bone-to-Bone fixation enhances functional healing of the porcine anterior cruciate ligament using a collagen-platelet composite. *Arthroscopy-Journal of Arthroscopic and Related Surgery 26* (Suppl.1): S49-57.

Oh LS, Wolf BR, Hall MP, Levy BA, Marx RG (2007) Indications for rotator cuff repair: a systematic review. *Clinical Orthopaedics and Related Research* 455: 52-63.

Ohnishi H, Oda Y, Aoki T, Tadokoro M, Katsube Y, Ohgushi H, et al (2011) A comparative study of induced pluripotent stem cells generated from frozen, stocked bone marrow-and adipose tissue-derived mesenchymal stem cells. *Journal of Tissue Engineering and Regenerative Medicine.* (in press)

Okamoto N, Kushida T, Oe K, Umeda M, Ikehara S, Lida H (2010) Treating Achilles tendon rupture in rats with bone-marrow-cell transplantation therapy. *Journal of Bone and Joint Surgery.* 92(17): 2776-2784.

Pittenger MF, Flake AM, Deans RJ (2002) Stem cell culture: mesenchymal stem cells from bone marrow. In: *Methods of Tissue Engineering*. Eds Atala A, Lanza RP. San Diego: Academic Press 461-469.

Romanini E, D'Angelo F, De Masi S, Adriani E, Magaletti M, Lacorte E, Laricchuiuta P, Sagliocca L, Morciano C, Mele A (2010) Graft selection in arthroscopic anterior cruciate ligament reconstruction. *Journal of Orthopaedics and Traumatology* 11(4): 211-219.

Schwietzer R, Zelzer E, Volk T (2010) Connecting muscles to tendons: tendons and musculoskeletal development in flies and vertebrates. *Development* 137(17): 2807-2817.

Shahab-Osterloh S, Witte F, Hoffmann A, Winkel A, Laggies S, Neumann B, et al (2010) Mesenchymal stem cell-dependant formation of heterotopic tendon –bone insertions(osteotendinous junctions). *Stem Cells* 28(9): 1590-1601.

Shelton WR, Fagan BC (2011) Autografts commonly used in anterior cruciate ligament reconstruction. *Journal of the American Academy of Orthopaedic Surgeons* 19(5): 259-264.

Tapper JE, Fukushima S, Azuma H, Sutherland C, Marchuk L, Thornton GM, et al (2008) Dynamic in vivo three dimensional (3D) kinematics of the anterior cruciate ligament/medial collateral ligament transected ovine stifle joint. *Journal of Orthopaedic Research* 26(5): 660-672.

Wei X, Mao Z, Hou Y, Lin L, Xue T, Chen L, Wang H, Yu C (2011) Local administration of TGFβ-1/VEGF165 gene-transduced bone mesenchymal stem cells for Achilles allograft replacement of the anterior cruciate ligament in rabbits. *Biochemical and Biophysical Research Communications* 406(2): 204-210.

In: Stem Cells in Disease
Editor: Prasad S. Koka

ISBN: 978-1-62257-169-7
© 2012 Nova Science Publishers, Inc.

Chapter XX

Functional Tissue Engineering for Rotator Cuff Tendons

J. Donaldson[1], Wasim S. Khan[2*] and A. Hazlerigg[3]
[1]Royal Free Hospital NHS Trust, Hampstead, London, United Kingdom
[2]University College London Institute of Orthopaedics and Musculoskeletal Sciences, Royal National Orthopaedic Hospital, Stanmore, UK
[3]Kingston Hospital NHS Trust, Kingston, London, UK

Abstract

Rotator cuff disease is becoming more prevalent and is a significant source of pain and disability. Current methods of treating rotator cuff dysfunction have inconsistent results and there is a high rate of recurrent tear and failure. This has prompted the search for novel solutions and the use of tissue engineered strategies and approaches. This article looks at the current state of tissue engineering methods for rotator cuff regeneration.

Keywords: Rotator cuff, tissue engineering, rotator cuff augmentation, cell therapy

The rotator cuff is a group of muscles and associated tendons that contribute to shoulder movements and stability. The tendons of supraspinatus, infraspinatus, subscapularis and teres minor muscles merge with the shoulder joint capsule to form the rotator cuff. These muscles arise from the scapula and insert onto the head of the humerus (subscapularis to the lesser tuberosity and supraspinatus, infraspinatus and teres minor to the greater tuberosity), and, in addition to the deltoid and teres major muscles, make up the six scapulohumeral muscles.

Rotator cuff disease can vary from impingement syndrome and tendinitis to partial- and full thickness tears, which may also vary in size. The larger the tear, the less potential for

* Corresponding Author: Mr Wasim S Khan, Clinical Lecturer, University College London Institute of Orthopaedics and Musculoskeletal Science, Royal National Orthopaedic Hospital, Stanmore, Middlesex, London, HA7 4LP, UK Telephone number: +44 (0) 7791 025554. Fax number: +44 (0) 20 8570 3864. E-mail address: wasimkhan@doctors.org.uk

repair exists. Rotator cuff dysfunction can be associated with significant functional impairment and chronic disabling pain and is the commonest cause of upper limb disability. Partial and full thickness rotator cuff tears are known to occur more frequently with increasing age and from overhead traumatic injuries. In a recent study of 1,366 patients in Japan, rotator cuff tears were demonstrated in over 20%. Risk factors identified included dominant arm, trauma and age (Yamamoto et al, 2010). Between 30,000 and 75,000 rotator cuff repairs are performed annually in the United States (American Academy of Orthopaedic Surgery, 2005).

Aetiological factors for rotator cuff disease can be divided into either intrinsic or extrinsic factors. Intrinsic factors include age-related degeneration, intra-tendinous lesions and poor vascularity. Extrinsic factors include subacromial impingement, shoulder instability, internal impingement, acute trauma, and repetitive microtrauma (Matava et al, 2005).

Most tears can be surgically repaired with good results. The aim of surgery is to restore the anatomical footprint without tension using sutures, tendon-to-bone fixation, and tendon mobilising and sliding techniques (Nho et al, 2010). However failure rates in all patients remain high, despite improvements in the understanding of the disease process and in surgical techniques. The re-rupture rate is estimated at anywhere between 20% and 65% (Galatz et al, 2001; Harryman et al, 1991; Gerber et al, 2000; Gazielly et al, 1994) depending on patient age, tear size, muscle atrophy and degeneration, tendon quality, repair technique and post-operative rehabilitation (Bartolozzi et al, 1994; Iannotti, 1994). A five-year follow up of arthroscopic surgical repair showed that radiological defects are more prevalent with increased tear size, age of patient, or multiple tendon involvement. (Gulotta et al, 2011). In addition, the success rate for revision rotator cuff repair is low (Packer et al, 1986; Bigliani et al, 1992).

The most common mechanism of failure of rotator cuff repair is thought to be due to suture cutting through tendon due to excessive tension at the repair. Although this can be improved newer technologies and surgical techniques, the still high failure rate and inconsistent results has led to the evolution and application of tissue engineering principles in rotator cuff repair. In a systematic review looking at re-tear rates and surgical technique, Duquin et al (2010) found that re-tear rates were significantly reduced when using double row repair for tears greater that 1cm, compared to transosseus or single row suture anchor techniques.

Tendons seem to be the least complex of connective tissues with respect to their composition and architecture, and this leads to the expectation that they would be more amenable to tissue engineered approaches. The commonest approaches have been with the use of scaffolds, growth factors, cell therapy and seeding, or a combination of each.

Normal Tendons and Healing

Tendons are dense connective tissue structures that connect muscle to bone. They are composed of highly specialised mesenchyme-derived cells (tenocytes) embedded in an extracellular matrix, consisting predominantly of type 1 collagen - primarily responsible for the tendon's stiffness and strength. Tendons have poor spontaneous regenerative capabilities, as they are relatively hypocellular and hypovascular (Bray et al, 1996) and following an injury, regeneration is never fully achieved despite extensive remodelling. The alignment of the collagen fibrils is also noted to be disrupted in healing tendons. Using collagen V siRNA engineered tenocytes in scaffold free tissue, Lu et al (2011) showed improved tendon tissue healing.

The types and characteristics of the collagen fibres in reparative scar tissue are different from those of a normal tendon. There is reduced interdigitation of the collagen fibres with the presence of a large quantity (20-30%) of type 3 collagen (normally <1%). Type 3 collagen has inferior strength and biomechanical properties compared to type 1 collagen fibres. With maturation of the scar tissue better interdigitation of the collagen fibres, an increase in the type 1 to type 3 collagen ratio, and an enlargement of fibrillar diameter does improve the tendon, but the mechanical properties still remain suboptimal due to the disorganised structure and poor matrix formation. Subsequently, a larger amount of fibrous tissue is needed to compensate for this mechanical inefficiency, which results in a thickened but less elastic tendon.

Tissue Engineering Strategies

1. Growth Factors

Growth factors present in platelets and fibroblasts can stimulate collagen deposition and tendon regeneration (Mishra and Pavelko, 2006). Growth factors such as platelet derived growth factor-BB (PDGF-BB), insulin-like growth factor-1 (IGF-1) and basic fibroblast growth factor (bFGF) have been used previously to promote tendon healing and tendon cell proliferation (Costa et al, 2006). Dose dependent increases have been demonstrated in cell populations of synovial sheath, epitenon, and endotenon by PDGF-BB. In addition, the combination of two or more of these growth factors showed a synergistic dose-dependent rise in all three cell populations.

Studies have looked into modulating the local repair environment with the addition of growth factors in an effort to improve healing in rotator cuff dysfunction. Kim et al (2011) introduced isoforms of TGFβ into transected supraspinatus tendons in rats. TGF-β1 isoform delivered via an osmotic pump showed increased type III collagen production, indicative of a scar mediated response. In a sheep infraspinatus tear model, growth factors from bovine cortical bone extract (BMP-2 to BMP-7, TGF-ß1 to TGF-ß3, and FGF) were implanted into healing rotator cuff with a type 1 collagen sponge (Rodeo et al, 2007). The augmented group showed numerous advantages with increased bone and soft tissue volume and improved failure loads compared to the non-augmented group. They did note however that when the loads were normalised for tissue volume, there were no differences between the augmented and the control group, suggesting the growth factors may accelerate tendon healing but do not actually improve the quality of tendon healing. Similar results using BMP-12 were observed in another sheep rotator cuff repair model (Seeherman et al, 2008). Comparing BMP-2 and BMP-7 *in vitro*, Pauly et al (2011) found an increased tenocyte cell activity and collagen type 1 production and expression with BMP-7.

It is probable that the cascade of growth factors work synergistically and much interest has therefore been shown in platelet rich plasma (PRP) injections, with an inherent high number of growth factors, including TGF-β1, PDGF, VEGF and IGF-1. Their use has been proposed since the early 1980s and has gained popularity over the last decade for a number of tendon disorders. The proposed mechanism is that the growth factors encourage tenocyte migration and differentiation at the site of tendon injury, and thus enhance repair. A recent prospective double blinded randomized controlled trial by Randelli et al (2011), applied autologous PRP intraoperatively to arthroscopic rotator cuff repairs. In the two year follow up they found that in the treated group, there was less pain in the immediate post operative period and, in grade 1 and 2 tears, PRP application positively affected cuff healing. Similarly, Geng et al (2011) found that PRP applied to transected Achilles tendons in rabbits improved the healing quality. They found expression of TGFβ-1 on immunohistochemistry staining was upregulated in the immediate post operative period for up to two weeks. This correlated to significant differences in fibroblast counts and a higher collagen content in the parenchyma compared to that of the control. To date, however, PRP has yet to prove itself in rotator cuff regeneration, or indeed in many other tendon disorders (Maffulli et al, 2010), although it has been shown to be safe, without any adverse side effects (Randelli et al, 2008).

Uggen et al (2005) isolated cells from rat rotator cuff tendons and transduced the cells with the genes of either platelet-derived growth factor-beta (PDGF-ß) or insulin-like growth factor-1 (IGF-I) by retroviral vectors. An *in vitro* model demonstrated an increase in collagen and DNA synthesis forming highly cellular tissue constructs by attaching to a polyglycolic acid scaffold. In addition when the cells were implanted into an experimental group of torn and then sutured rotator cuffs, excellent results were shown with almost complete repair.

Dines et al (2007) similarly used the same growth factors transduced in rat rotator cuff tendon fibroblasts in an effort to improve healing. The repaired tendons were harvested and histologically examined 6 weeks after surgery. The repaired tendons with the added growth factors were cellular with well organised collagen bundles; in contrast to the repair controls, which were relatively acellular, with little in the way of repair. In addition, the repaired tendons with the added growth factors were tougher and tolerated more load before failure (statistically significant in the IGF-1 group and a trend in the PDGF-ß group) than the control repaired tendons.

These results suggest that tendon fibroblasts can be tissue engineered to deliver therapeutic growth factors locally with positive effects on the repair response.

2. Cell Therapy

Recent advances in cell therapy have directed attention towards the use of multipotential progenitor cells (such as embryonic stem cells, periosteal cells, and mesenchymal stem cells) in repairing injured tendons. It is technically possible to harvest tissue cells, culture them to expand the cell population, and allow them to differentiate, under exogenous and endogenous factors control, into the appropriate cell type required for tendon repair.

Mesenchymal stem cells (MSCs) are cells that have the ability to proliferate and differentiate into progenitors of different mesenchymal tissues. They actively home to damaged tissues (Porada et al, 2010) and have the advantage of being hypoimmunogenic, as they lack major histocompatibility complex-II molecular expression and are widely found in many tissues.

Pelinkovic et al (2003) used genetically engineered highly purified muscle derived cells (MDCs) and injected them into the tendinous part of surgically torn supraspinatus tendons in nude rats. The MDCs were transfected with a plasmid carrying the ß-galactosidase marker gene, which was used to distinguish cultivated cells from normal surrounding cells in the tendons. The injected cells were monitored for three weeks and then checked histologically and immunohistochemically with fluorescence in-situ hybridization.

From day seven the cell nuclei became spindle shaped, cells were integrated into the tendon collagen bundles, and the cells showed differentiation into vimentin-expressing fibroblastic cells (normal supraspinatus cells stain positive for vimentin; clonal MDCs do not).

Their results suggest that the rotator cuff tendon matrix and its original cellular components modulate the injected MDCs towards a fibroblastic phenotype. They conclude that the compatibility and ability of MDCs to differentiate into other cell lineages, such as fibroblasts, might therefore have potential in tissue engineering applications, and in *ex-vivo* gene therapy for the treatment of rotator cuff lesions.

3. Scaffolds and Augmentation Grafts

Scaffolds and tendon augmentation grafts for rotator cuff repair are not new. Autografts, allografts, xenografts and tendon prostheses have all been used in the past with limited success.

Scaffolds and augmentation grafts are used on the premise that they may help to 'off-load the repair at the time of surgery and in the immediate post operative period, and to improve the rate and quality of biological healing.

In an analytical model for rotator cuff repairs, it was found that an estimated 70-80% of the load will be distributed to the repaired tendon, while the remaining 20-30% is distributed to the augmentation graft. (Aurora et al, 2010) The ideal scaffold should induce host-tissue in-growth and tendon regeneration during the process of degradation, which varies considerably depending on the properties of the scaffold.

In recent decades new tissue engineered scaffolds have been introduced. These scaffolds are either biological or synthetic. Biological scaffolds are protein based extracellular matrices (ECMs) that are usually derived from human or animal connective tissue (Chen et al, 2009). Synthetic scaffolds are manufactured from chemical compounds. Both have their advantages and disadvantages (see table 1).

Scaffold devices derived from ECM (biological), polyurethaneurea (synthetic) and polylactic acid (synthetic) are commercially available at this time and are US Food and Drug Administration (FDA) approved for rotator cuff repair augmentation.

Valentin et al (2006) compared several biological ECM scaffolds, differing in their species and tissue of origin, methods of processing, and methods of terminal sterilisation, in a rodent abdominal wall model. All ECM scaffolds were associated with an early, intense cellular response. However, each device elicited a distinct morphologic response over time with respect to cellularity, vascularity, the presence of multinucleate giant cells, and organisation of the remodelled tissue.

Rapidly degraded devices like Restore (DePuy Orthopaedics) and autologous tissue showed the greatest amount of cellular infiltration.

Table 1. Advantages and Disadvantages of Biological or Synthetic Scaffolds

Biological		Synthetic	
Advantages	Disadvantages	Advantages	Disadvantages
Well defined three-dimensional microstructure allowing host cell integration	Poor mechanical properties which may result in surgical failure	Permit better control of the chemical and physical properties	Poor biocompatibility as cannot be absorbed and integrated
Natural porosity allowing larger space for host cell attachment, proliferation and migration	Variation in biocompatibility which can cause an inflammatory response and even rejection	Stronger and more consistent in quality	High incidences of post-operative infection and chronic immune responses
Assists gas and metabolite diffusion	Undefined degradation rate Non-specific induction ability		
Quickly interact and induce new tissue formation	Potential risk of disease transmission		

Devices that degraded slowly like CuffPatch (Organogenesis), TissueMend (Stryker) and Permacol (Covidien) were associated with giant cells, chronic inflammation and/or the accumulation of dense poorly organised fibrous tissue.

Sandor et al (2009) showed similar findings when comparing chemically cross-linked porcine dermis versus non-cross linked porcine small intestinal submucosa (SIS). The non-cross linked SIS material had a more robust cellular infiltrate and an associated increase in strength over time. Cross-linking of ECM (and devices that degrade slowly) seems therefore to be associated with an unfavourable response and outcome. There is, of course, a trade off with loss of the mechanical properties of the scaffold as it degrades and this is likely to be a crucial step in clinical success.

Animal Studies

Schlegel et al (2006) performed infraspinatus repairs in sheep using a patch of small intestinal submucosa (SIS) over the repaired tissue and compared it to repaired tissue without the SIS scaffold. The authors commented that both repairs had evidence of gap formation. Similarly, Nicholson et al (2007) reported no benefit in ultimate load in partial supraspinatus tears in a sheep model between augmented and non-augmented repairs at 9 and 24 weeks of healing.

Several other studies have showed more promising results. Gumina et al (2009) used a porcine SIS to regenerate a 4mm full thickness supraspinatus tear in rats. The construct was then harvested for histological and biomechanical testing at both six and sixteen weeks. The SIS-regenerated group showed better behaviour in ultimate load to failure, toughness, stiffness, and yield strength than the defect group (Zalavras et al, 2006). Dejardin et al (2006) similarly looked at an SIS scaffold in infraspinatus tears in dogs. At both 3 and 6 months, the SIS-regenerated tendons histologically mimicked normal tendon. Biomechanically the SIS tendons were weaker than normal tendon, although similar to repaired tendon without SIS at 3 and 6 months. Perry et al (2007) examined full thickness supraspinatus tears and the effectiveness of SIS augmentation in both acute and chronic rat models. In the acute group with SIS augmentation the creation of a material similar to natural healing tendon was demonstrated; in the chronically injured group SIS augmentation demonstrated better mechanical behaviour than native tendon repair. Of note, Edelstein et al (2011) looked at 30 different species and determined that only the rat had a supraspinatus tendon that passes under an enclosed arch, similar to that of a human. This may suggest that the rat may be a superior model for animal studies.

Hee et al (2011) used recombinant human PDGF-BB (rhPDGF-BB) combined with a type 1 collagen bovine matrix in rotator cuff tears in a sheep model. They found that the anatomical appearance and biomechanical strength at 12 weeks were significantly improved compared to the control. A dose dependant response was also observed with increased tendon-to-bone interdigitation observed in the 75μg and 150μg compared to the 500μg rhPDGF-BB group.

Funakoshi et al (2006) used chitin fabric as a matrix for rotator cuff regeneration. The chitin fabric was used to cover tears in infraspinatus tendons in rabbits. Chitin is biocompatible and therefore has a lower immunogenicity than extracellular matrix. It also has the advantage that the pore size and thickness can be altered with relative ease. However, the authors noted the quality of collagen produced was inferior (type III collagen) to normal tendon collagen (type I) and the biomechanical properties of the chitin scaffold were poor. Synthetic ECMs are less likely to cause an inflammatory response than allograft or xenograft biological material. One study investigated a polyglycolic acid (PGA) sheet to augment rotator cuff repairs in white rabbits (Yokoya et al, 2008). Histologic improvement in tendon healing was demonstrated but this only correlated to a small improvement in tensile strength when compared to controls with another slowly absorbing synthetic material.

A further study by MacGillivray et al (2006) used another synthetic scaffold, polylactic acid patches, in goats. No difference was noted between the treated and the controls. Derwin et al (2009) performed a similar experiment using a woven poly-L-lactide device in bilateral dog infraspinatus tears. In one shoulder, the synthetic scaffold was used; in the contralateral shoulder the repair was left unaugmented and used as the control. The augmented repair showed improved biomechanical properties compared to the contralateral repaired side, with fewer tendon retractions, greater strength and increased stiffness. Repairs of a chronic tendon tear in a sheep model using polyurethane synthetic scaffold mesh compared to control have been shown in biomechanical analysis to provide greater mechanical strength (Santoni et al, 2010).

Scaffolds and Cell or Growth Factor Seeding

Funakoshi et al (2005) looked at the combination of fibroblast seeding and a chitosan-based hyaluronan hybrid scaffold. Fibroblasts from rabbit patella tendon were used on the scaffold for infraspinatus tears. Non-cell seeded scaffold was also used and a control group where the defect was not repaired. The fibroblast seeded group demonstrated best performance with improved tensile strength and type I collagen production four weeks post-operatively. The non-seeded group showed predominantly type III collagen with inferior biomechanical properties.

Autologous cell infiltration into either biological or synthetic scaffolds was examined by Chen et al (2007), who harvested purified tenocytes from patella ligaments and then implanted them onto xenogenic and synthetic ECMs after five days of cell harvesting. Infraspinatus tears were then repaired using either the cell infiltrated ECM, ECM alone or autologous tendon. The engineered autologous tendon resulted in increased type I and type III collagen deposition, decreased immunologic response, and improved absorption into the host tendon when compared to the ECM augmentation alone.

Autogenic cell constructs also have the advantage of being able to be manipulated using gene therapy. Dines et al (2007) used interposed genetically engineered autologous tendon in rat rotator cuff repairs. Tenocytes were isolated from the rotator cuff and transduced with the genes for PDGF-ß or IGF-1, both factors known to promote fibroblast proliferation and minimise inflammation. Successfully transduced cells were isolated and seeded onto PGA, and used to augment the rotator cuff repair. The tendons transduced with PDGF-ß showed no improvement over controls augmented with PGA alone or simple repair. However, the fibroblastic cells transduced to express IGF-1 demonstrated an improvement in both strength and maximum load.

Normal tendon collagen is a highly organised structure, and this in part adds to its mechanical properties. It has therefore been hypothesised that the nanofibre organisation of a tissue engineered scaffold would positively regulate cellular response and scaffold properties. Moffat et al (2009) looked into this by aligning fibroblasts on a nanofibre based polylactide-co-glycolide (PLGA) scaffold. They demonstrated that fibroblasts cultured on aligned scaffolds along the nanofibre axis showed improved mechanical properties compared to fibroblasts on an unaligned scaffold, which were polygonal and randomly orientated. Quantitative analysis showed cell alignment, distribution, and matrix deposition conformed to the aligned scaffold and these differences were maintained over time. They conclude scaffold design and cell orientation is therefore a critical parameter in scaffold design.

Clinical Studies

Few studies are available assessing the commercially available ECM grafts, and the ones that do exist have small numbers and no control subjects, offering level III-IV evidence at best.

Restore is a non-cross linked porcine SIS graft made by DePuy. Metcalf et al (2002) conducted a two year follow-up of twelve patients who underwent arthroscopic repair of massive chronic rotator cuff tears with Restore as an augment. Follow-up Magnetic Resonance Imaging (MRI) scans showed incorporation and functional improvement in eleven of the twelve patients. In the twelfth patient clinical failure was observed within twelve weeks. Conversely, more recent studies using Restore have showed better results in the non-augmented group with respect to healing and function (Iannotti et al, 2006; Sclamberg et al, 2004).

GraftJacket, a non-cross linked human dermis ECM (Wright Medical Technology) was retrospectively followed up in sixteen patients by Dopirak et al (2007). The ECM scaffold was used as an interposition graft to span the tendon edge and bone defect being repaired. All patients had improved post-operative function. Radiographically three failures were demonstrated on MRI scans, two failed within the first three months and the third failed following a fall at four months. Bond et al (2008) also used GraftJacket as an interpositional device with improved clinical outcome score. At one year three grafts of the thirteen performed had failed when a follow-up MRI scan was performed. Burkhead et al (2007) demonstrated similar results using GraftJacket to augment massive rotator cuff repairs, although they did note their three re-tears (out of twelve) were smaller and some connection between the repair and bone still remained.

Using Acellular Human Dermal Matrix (AHDM) as an augment in five cases, Rotini et al (2011) followed these patients up using Constant Murley scoring system and a control MRI performed at a year. There were no inflammatory or septic complications, and radiological assessment showed that three cases progressed to complete healing. One patient suffered from a re-tear secondary to trauma and one patient had a complete recurrence. The authors described ten ideal scaffold properties:

1. Biological activity
2. Biocompatible
3. Reabsorbable
4. No risk of infectious disease transmission
5. Mechanical strength
6. High suture retention quality
7. Available in different sizes and thicknesses
8. Easy to handle in open and arthroscopic surgery
9. Fit for augmentation and bridging
10. Easy to store in operating room

Badhe et al (2008) looked at Zimmer collagen repair, a cross linked porcine dermis ECM, used as an augmentation device and again showed improved clinical outcomes, despite two graft disruptions out of ten with follow up imaging. In contrast to this a further study following up Zimmer collagen repair reported early complications with the grafts failing in all four patients between three and six months post-operatively (Soler et al, 2007).

Conclusion

Rotator cuff degeneration and tears are becoming increasingly common. Symptoms include pain and restricted function. Those that fail to improve with conservative therapy may elect to undergo rotator cuff repair. Failure to heal and re-tearing after surgery are not uncommon, especially in an already degenerate and histologically abnormal tendon. Functional tissue engineering strategies have therefore been investigated in both animals and humans in an effort to improve rotator cuff healing and strength.

Many growth factors and cellular processes are involved in normal tendon healing. It is probably not possible to clearly define the function of each in the complex inflammation and healing cascades. The addition of growth factors and/or reparative cells, either directly or via genetic engineering, has shown promising results for tendon regeneration in animal models.

Much research has been directed towards scaffold devices designed to augment and enhance tendon healing. These devices used alone or in combination with genetically engineered tenocytes or growth factors, have shown encouraging results in animal models. The limited numbers of human studies using commercially available scaffolds have however shown mixed results, and further studies are required to investigate the clinical results and applications.

References

American Academy of Orthopaedic Surgery (2005). Number of patients, number of procedures, average patient stay – *National Hospital Discharge Survey* 1998-2005.

Aurora A, Gatica JE, van den Bogert AJ, McCarron JA, Derwin KA (2010). An analytical model for rotator cuff repairs. *Clin. Biomech.* 25: 751-758.

Badhe SP, Lawrence TM, Smith FD, Lunn PG (2008). An assessment of porcine dermal xenograft as an augmentation graft in the treatment of extensive rotator cuff repairs. *J. Shoulder Elbow Surg* 17: 35S-39S

Bartolozzi A, Andreychik D, Ahmad S (1994). Determinants of outcome in the treatment of rotator cuff disease. *Clin. Orthop. Relat Res:* 90-97.

Bigliani LU, Cordasco FA, McIlveen SJ, Musso ES (1992). Operative treatment of failed repairs of the rotator cuff. *J. Bone Joint Surg* (Am) 74: 1505.

Bond JL, Dopirak ML, Higgins J, Burns J, Snyder SJ (2008). Arthroscopic replacement of massive, irreparable rotator cuff tears using a GraftJacket allograft; technique and preliminary results. *Arthroscopy* 24: 403-4-9.

Bray RC, Rangayyan RM, Frank CB (1996). Normal and healing ligament vascularity: a quantitative histological assessment in the adult rabbit medial collateral ligament. *J. Anatomy* 188(1): 87-95

Burkhead WZ, Schiffern SC, Krishnan SG (2007). Use of GraftJacket as an augmentation for massive rotator cuff tears. *Semin Arthroplasty* 1: 11-18.

Chen J, Xu J, Wang A, Zheng M (2009). Scaffolds for tendon and ligament repair: review of the efficacy of commercial products. *Expert Rev. Med. Devices* 6: 61-73.

Chen JM, Willers C, Xu JK, Wang A, Zheng MH (2007). Autologous tenocyte therapy using porcine-derived bioscaffolds for massive rotator cuff defect in rabbits. *Tissue Eng* 13: 1479-1491

Costa MA, Wu C, Pham BV, Chong AK, Pham HM, Chang J (2006). Tissue engineering of flexor tendons: Optimisation of tenocyte proliferation using growth factor supplementation. *Tissue Eng* 12(7): 1937-1943.

Dejardin LM, Arnoczky SP, Ewers B et al (2006). Tissue engineered rotator cuff tendon using porcine small intestine submucosa. Histologic and mechanical evaluation in dogs. *Am. J. Sports* Med 29: 175-184.

Derwin KA, Codsi MJ, Milks RA, Baker AR, McCarron JA, Iannotti JP (2009). Rotator cuff repair augmentation in a canine model with use of a woven poly-L-lactide device. *J. Bone Joint Surg.* (Am) 91: 1159-1171.

Dines JS, Grande DA, Dines DM (2007). Tissue engineering and rotator cuff tendon healing. *J. Shoulder Elbow Surg* 16(5 suppl): S204-S207.

Dines JS, Grande DA, Dines DM (2007). Tissue engineering and rotator cuff tendon healing. J *Shoulder Elbow Surg* 16(5 suppl): S204-S207.

Dopirak R, Bond JL, Snyder SJ (2007). Arthroscopic total rotator cuff replacement with an acellular human dermal allograft matrix. *Int. J. Shoulder Surg* 1: 7-15.

Duquin TR, Buyea C, Bisson LJ (2010). Which method of rotator cuff repair leads to the highest rate of structural healing? A systematic review. *Am. J. Sports Med.* 38: 835-841.

Edelstein L, Thomas L, Soslowsky J (2011). Rotator Cuff Tears: What have we learned from animal models? *J. Musculoskelet Neuronal. Interact.* 11: 150-162.

Funakoshi T, Majima T, Suenaga N, Iwassaki N, Yamane S, Minami A (2006). Rotator cuff regeneration using chitin fabric as an acellular matrix. *J. Shoulder Elbow Surg* 15(1): 112-118.

Funakoshi T, Majima T, Iwassaki N, et al (2005). Application of tissue engineering techniques for rotator cuff regeneration using a chitosan-based hyaluronan hybrid fiber scaffold. *Am. J. Sports* Med 33(8): 1193-1201.

Galatz LM, Griggs S, Cameron BD, Iannotti JP (2001). Prospective longitudinal analysis of postoperative shoulder function: a ten-year follow-up study of full-thickness rotator cuff tears. *J. Bone Joint Surg. Am.* 83:1052-6.

Gazielly DF, Gleyze P, Montagnon C (1994). Functional and anatomical results after rotator cuff repair. *Clin. Orthop.* 304:43-53.

Gerber C, Fuchs B, Hodler J (2000). The results of repair of massive tears of the rotator cuff. *J. Bone Joint Surg Am* 82:505-15.

Geng Z, Wang C, Zhou H (2011). Effect of platelet–rich plasma on tendon healing. *Zhongguo Xiu Fu Chong Jian Wai Ke Za Zhi.* 25: 344-348.

Gulotta LV, Nho SJ, Dodson CC, Adler RS, Altchek DW, Macgillivray JD (2011). Prospective evaluation of arthroscopic rotator cuff repairs at 5 years;Part II-prognostic factors for clinical and radiographic outcomes. *J. Shoulder Elbow Surg.* (in press).

Gumina S, Patti AM, Vulcano A, Della Rocca C, Postacchini F (2009). Culture of human rotator cuff cells on orthobiologic support (porcine small intestinal submucosa) *Chir Organi Mov.* 93 Suppl 1: S65-S70.

Harryman DT 2nd, Mack LA, Wang KY, Jackins SE, Richardson ML, Matsen FA 3rd (1991). Repairs of the rotator cuff. Correlation of functional results with integrity of the cuff. *J. Bone Joint Surg. Am* .73:982-9.

Hee CK, Dines JS, Dines DM, et al (2011). Augmentation of a rotator cuff suture repair using rhPDGF-BB and a Type 1 Bovine Collagen Matrix in an Ovine Model. *Am. J. Sports Med.* (in press).

Iannotti JP (1994). Full thickness rotator cuff tears: factors affecting surgical outcome. *J. Am. Acad Orthop. Surg.* 2: 87-95.

Iannotti JP, Codsi MJ, Kwon YW, Derwin K, Ciccone J, Brems JJ (2006). Porcine small intestine submucosa augmentation of surgical repair of chronic two tendon rotator cuff tears. A randomised, controlled trial. *J. Bone Joint Surg* (Am). 88: 1238-1244.

Kim HM, Galatz LM, Das R, Havlioglu N, Rothermich SY, Thomopoulos S (2011). The role of transforming growth factor beta isoforms in tendon-to-bone healing. *Connect Tissue Res.* 52(2): 87-98.

Lu P, Zhang GR, Song XH, Zou XH, Wang LL, Ouyang HW (2011). Col V siRNA Engineered Tenocytes for Tendon Tissue Engineering. *PLoS One.* 6(6): e21154.

MacGillivray JD, Fealy S, Terry MA, Koh JL, Nixon AJ, Warren RF (2006). Biomechanical evaluation of a rotator cuff defect model augmented with a bioresorbable scaffold in goats. *J. Shoulder* Elbow *Surg.* 15: 63-64.

Maffulli N, Longo UG, Denaro V (2010). Novel approaches for the management of tendinopathy. *J. Bone Joint Surg. Am.* 92: 2604-2613.

Matava MJ, Purcell DB, Rudzki JR (2005). Partial thickness rotator cuff tears. *Am. J. Sports Med.* 33(9): 1405-1417.

Metcalf MH, Savoie FH III, Kellum B (2002). Surgical technique for xenograft augmentation of rotator cuff repair. *Oper. Tech Orthop.* 12: 204-208.

Mishra A, Pavelko T (2006). Treatment of chronic elbow tendinosis with buffered platelet rich plasma. *Am. J. Sports Med.* 34:1774-1778.

Moffat KL, Kwei AS, Spalazzi JP, Doty SB, Levine WN, Lu HH (2009). Novel nanofiber scaffold for rotator cuff repair and augmentation. *Tissue Eng Part A.* 15: 115-126.

Nho SJ, Delos D, Yadav H, Pensak M, Romeo AA, Warren RF, MacGillivray JD (2010). Biomechanical and biologic augmentation for the treatment of massive rotator cuff tears. *Am. J. Sports Med.* 38(3):619-629.

Nicholson GP, Breur GJ, Van SD, Yao JQ, Kim J, Blanchard CR (2007). Evaluation of a cross linked acellular porcine dermal patch for rotator cuff repair augmentation in an ovine model. *J. Shoulder Elbow Surg.* 16 (Suppl); S184-S190.

Packer NP, Calvert PT, Bayley JL, Kessel L (1986). Arthrography of the shoulder after operative repair of the torn rotator cuff. *J. Bone Joint Surg.* (Br). 68: 147.

Pauly S, Klatte F, Strobel C, Schmidmaier G, Greiner S, Scheibel M, Wildemann B (2011). BMP-2 and BMP-7 affect human rotator cuff tendon cells in vitro. *J. Shoulder Elbow Surg.* (in press).

Pelinkovic D, Lee JY, Engelhart M, Rodosky M, *Cummins J.,* Fu F, Huard.

J (2003). Muscle cell mediated gene delivery to the rotator cuff. *Tissue Eng.* 9(1): 143-151.

Perry SM, Gupta RR, Van Kleunen J, Ramsey ML, Soslowsky LJ, Glaser DL (2007). Use of small intestine submucosa in a rat model of acute and chronic rotator cuff tear. *J. Shoulder Elbow Surg.* 16: S179-S183.

Porada CD, Almeida-Porada G (2010). Mesenchymal stem cells as therapeutics and vehicles for gene and drug delivery. *Adv. Drug Deliv. Rev.* 62 (12): 1156-1166.

Randelli PS, Arrigoni P, Cabitza P, Volpi P, Maffuli N (2008). Autologous platelet rich plasma for arthroscopic rotator cuff repair: a pilot study. *Disabil Rehabil* 30: 1584-1589.

Randelli P, Arrigoni P, Ragone V, Aliprandi A, Cabitza P (2011). Platelet rich plasma in arthroscopic rotator cuff repair: a prospective RCT study, 2-year follow-up. *J. Shoulder Elbow Surg.* 20 (4): 518-528.

Rodeo SA, Potter HG, Kawamura S, Turner AS, Kim HJ, Atkinson BL (2007). Biologic augmentation of rotator cuff tendon healing with use of a mixture of osteoinductive growth factors. *J. Bone Joint Surg* (Am). 89: 2485-2497.

Rotini R, Marinelli A, Guerra E, Bettelli G, Castagna A, Fini M, Bondioli E, Busacca M (2011). Human dermal matrix scaffold augmentation for large and massive rotator cuff repairs: preliminary clinical and MRI results at 1 year follow-up. *Musculoskelt Surg.* (in press)

Sandor M, Xu H, Connor J, Lombardi J, Harper JR, Silverman RP, et al (2009). Host response to implanted porcine-derived biologic materials in a primate model of abdominal wall repair. *Tissue Eng Part A.* 14: 2021-2031.

Santoni BG, McGilvary KC, Lyons AS, Bansal M, Turner AS, Macgillivray JD, Coleman SH, Puttlitz CM (2010). Biomechanical analysis of an ovine rotator cuff repair via porous patch augmentation in a chronic rupture model. *Am. J. Sports Med.* 38 (4): 679-686.

Schlegel TF, Hawkins RJ, Lewis CW, Motta T, Turner AS (2006). The effects of augmentation with Swine small intestine submucosa on tendon healing under tension: histologic and mechanical evaluation in sheep. *Am. J. Sports Med.* 34: 275-280.

Sclamberg SG, Tibone JE, Itamura JM, Kasraeian S (2004). Six month magnetic resonance imaging follow up of large and massive rotator cuff repairs reinforced with porcine small intestinal submucosa. *J. Shoulder Elbow Surg.* 13: 538-541.

Seeherman HJ, Archambault JM, Rodeo SA, Turner AS, D'Augusta D, Li XJ, Smith E, Wozney JM (2008). rhBMP-12 accelerates healing of rotator cuff repairs in a sheep model. *J. Bone Joint Surg* (Am). 90: 2206-2219.

Soler JA, Gidwani S, Curtis MJ (2007). Early complications from the use of porcine dermal collagen implants (Permacol) as bridging constructs in the repair of massive rotator cuff tears. A report of 4 cases. *Acta Orthop. Belg.* 73: 432-436.

Uggen JC, Dines J, Uggen CW et al (2005). Tendon gene therapy modulates the local repair environment in the shoulder. *J. Am. Osteopath Assoc.* 105: 20-21.

Valentin JE, Badylak JS, McCabe GP, Badylak SF (2006). Extracellular matrix bioscaffolds for orthopaedic applications. A comparative histologic study. *J. Bone Joint Surg. (Am).* 88: 2673-2686.

Yamamoto A, Takagishi K, Oswara T (2010). Prevalence and risk factors of a rotator cuff tear in the general population. *J. Shoulder Elbow Surg.* 19:116-20.

Yokoya S, Mochizuki Y, Nagata Y, Deie M, Ochi M (2008). Tendon-bone insertion repair and regeneration using polyglycolic acid sheet in the rabbit rotator cuff injury model. *Am. J. Sports* Med. 36: 1298-1309.

Zalavras CG, Gardocki R, Huang E, Stevanovic M, Hedman T, Tibone J (2006). Reconstruction of large rotator cuff tendon defects with porcine small intestinal submucosa in an animal model. *J. Shoulder Elbow Surg.* 15(2): 224-231.

Index

B

C

D

E

F

G

H

I

M

N

O

P

Q

R

S

T

U

V

W

X

Y

Z